Nurses' Guide to Clinical Procedures

FOURTH EDITION

Jean Smith-Temple, MSN, RN
Clinical Assistant Professor
Adult Health Nursing
College of Nursing
The University of South Alabama
Mobile, Alabama

Joyce Young Johnson, PhD, RN, CCRN
Curriculum Consultant and Faculty
Department of Nursing
Georgia Perimeter College
Atlanta, Georgia
President
Johnson's Consulting Firm
Atlanta, Georgia

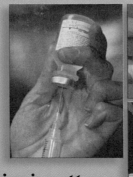

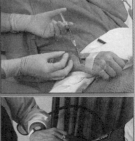

Lippincott
Philadelphia · New York · Baltimore

Acquisitions Editor: Ilze Rader
Managing Editor/Development: Hilarie Surrena
Senior Production Manager: Helen Ewan
Managing Editor/Production: Barbara Ryalls
Design Coordinator: Doug Smock
Manufacturing Manager: William Alberti
Indexer: Nancy Newman
Compositor: Peirce Graphic Services
Printer: Vicks Lithograph Printing Corp.

Edition 4

9   8   7   6   5

Library of Congress Cataloging-in Publication Data

Smith-Temple, Jean.
    Nurses' guide to clinical procedures / Jean Smith-Temple, Joyce Young Johnson.— 4th ed.
        p. ; cm.
    Includes bibliographical references and index.
    ISBN 0-7817-3228-X (alk. paper)
    1. Nursing—Handbooks, manuals, etc. I. Johnson, Joyce Young. II. Title.
    [DNLM: 1. Nursing Process—Handbooks. 2. Home Care Services—Handbooks. 3. Patient Care Planning—Handbooks. WY 49 S662n 2002]
RT51 .S655 2002
610.73—dc21

                                            2001044786

To my husband, Richard . . . for your encouragement, support, sacrifice, and love.

To my son, Benjamin, for his sacrifice and love.

Jean

To my husband, Larry, and my children, Virginia and Larry, Jr., for your hugs, love, and patience.

To my parents, Dorothy and Riley Young Sr., who taught me perserverance, and encourage me in everything I do.

Joyce

To our students and colleagues for contributing to our professional growth and development.

To our Lord and Savior, through whom we can do all things.

Jean and Joyce

Fourth Edition

LCDR Edward S. Bates, MSN, RN, CS, ACNP
Nurse Corps, United States Navy
U. S. Naval Hospital
Okinawa, Japan

Robin Bingham, RN, MSN, CWOCN
Clinical Specialist Wound Management
University of South Alabama Medical Center
Regional Burn and Wound Center
Mobile, Alabama

Ola Fox, RN, C, MSN, DSN
Clinical Assistant Professor, Adult Health
College of Nursing
University of South Alabama
Mobile, Alabama

Phyllis Prather Hicks, RN, BSN
Instructor
Harrisburg Area Community College
Harrisburg, Pennsylvania

Third Edition

Alfreda Bivins, RN, MS
Director, Medical-Surgical Services
Parkway Medical Center
Lithia Springs, Georgia

Rosie Calvin, RN, DNS
Associate Professor
University of Mississippi Medical Center
School of Nursing
Jackson, Mississippi

Frankie R. Dunmore, RN, MSN
Assistant Professor
Alcorn State University School of Nursing
Natchez, Mississippi

Ola Fox, RN, C, MSN
Clinical Assistant Professor
University of South Alabama
Mobile, Alabama

Phyllis Prather Hicks, RN, BSN
Instructor
Harrisburg Area Community College
Harrisburg, Pennsylvania

Lorelei Papke, RN, MSN, CRNI
Manager, Clinical Nursing, IV Therapy Services
University of Michigan Medical Center
Ann Arbor, Michigan

Daryl S. Todd, RN, MS
Clinical Nurse Specialist/Advance Practice Nurse
Department of Medical-Surgical Nursing
Grady Health Systems
Atlanta, Georgia

Contributors to Previous Editions

Second Edition

Rosie Calvin, RN, MSN
Clinical Specialist
University of Mississippi Medical Center
Jackson, Mississippi

Phyllis Prather Hicks, RN, BSN
Instructor
Harrisburg Area Community College
Harrisburg, Pennsylvania

Richard Temple, Jr., LPTA, BS
Licensed Physical Therapist Assistant
Mobile Infirmary Medical Center
Mobile, Alabama

First Edition

Louise Gore Grose, RN, PhD
Nurse Consultant
Board of Nurse Examiners for the State of Texas
Staff Nurse
Home Health Care Department
Holy Cross Hospital
Austin, Texas

LaDonna Powell, RN, MSN
Pediatric Clinical Nurse Specialist
University Medical Center
Children's Hospital
Jackson, Mississippi

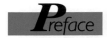
Preface

Nurses' Guide to Clinical Procedures, 4E is a quick-reference clinical-support tool designed to serve students in all types of educational programs and practicing nurses in any clinical setting. The book explains the key steps necessary to perform nursing skills and provides cues to the critical thinking needed for client care.

This guide contains information on nearly 200 skills and now includes more home health procedures. A detailed Table of Contents and Index are provided for easy reference to procedures. The procedures within the 12 chapters of *Nurses' Guide to Clinical Procedures* are organized in a nursing process format, with procedures listed at the beginning of each chapter for convenience. Chapter overviews review basic principles and concepts, including general delegation guidelines. A list of potential nursing diagnoses accompanies each procedure. Nursing procedures are organized as follows:

Equipment
Purpose(s)
Assessment
Nursing Diagnoses
Outcome Identification and Planning
   - Examples of desired outcomes
   - Highlighted special considerations
     General
     Pediatric
     Geriatric
     Home health
     Transcultural aspects
     Cost-cutting tips
     Delegation guidelines, when appropriate
Implementation (actions with rationales)
Evaluation
Documentation (includes examples of charting)

Actions are presented concisely, with clear illustrations to assist the user. Standard precautions are considered whenever applicable. A pictogram next to the procedure title indicates that gloves should be worn.

Nursing procedures have been organized to facilitate safe, expedient performance. *Nurses' Guide to Clinical Procedures* should be used as a clinical reference; it is not intended for initial in-

struction of nursing procedures. The user should review principles in the chapter overview before proceeding to the nursing
procedures. Procedures should be read in their entirety to ensure
that all relevant health-care matters are considered during performance. Narrative documentation format will be used for charting examples, although many other forms of documentation may
be used in the clinical setting. Illustrations, tables, and appendices
provide further support. Users should refer to these aids as well
as to related nursing procedures, as needed.

Jean Smith-Temple, RN, MSN
Joyce Young Johnson, RN, PHD, CCRN

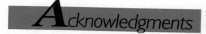
Acknowledgments

We would like to thank our contributors for their contributions of excellence.

We would like to thank Ilze Rader for her insight and support.

We would also like to thank Hilarie Surrena, Barbara Ryalls, and Nicole Walz for their guidance and patience.

We would also like to thank Patricia Knott Chapman, CEO-Owner, File-a-Claim Services, for her clerical input and organizational skills, and Clemmie Riggins for her excellent clerical skills.

We would also like to thank the many nurse colleagues and colleagues from other disciplines who provided us direction in the preparation of this guidebook.

*C*ontents

5 *Nutrition: Fluid and Nutrient Balance*   172

Overview
Procedure

12 Special Procedures 685

Overview
Procedure

Appendices 702

Bibliography 749

Index 751

*C*hapter *1*

Verbal Communication Skills

OVERVIEW

▶ Verbal communication involves a sender, a receiver, a message, and the environment in which the interaction takes place.

▶ Communication includes the attitude projected—gestures, voice tone, rhythm, volume, and pitch—in addition to words spoken (nonverbal and verbal aspects).

▶ Effective communication is:
- *Simple*—briefly and comprehensively relates data using commonly known and understood terms
- *Clear*—states exactly what is meant, covering the who, what, when, where, why, and how of the matter
- *Pertinent*—contains data that are important to the current situation and ties data to an apparent need to show significance
- *Sensitive*—considers readiness of the receiver and adapts depth and breadth of data to meet receiver's needs
- *Accurate*—includes factual information related with confidence and credibility

▶ Building effective communication skills requires a constant awareness of oneself as a sender and a receiver of messages.

► Communication approaches should be modified to meet the individual needs of the client (cultural, age-related, religious orientation, etc.).

► In general, some factors that should be considered in the communication process are knowledge level; personal perceptions, values, and beliefs; language; environmental setting; roles in the family and interpersonal relationships; space; and the general status of one's health.

► The home setting may provide unique challenges to verbal communication. Efforts should be made to minimize distractions and to include all family members in communication, as appropriate.

► Confidentiality is a major concern in all communication related to a client. All conversations about the client, including those with the client, family, or significant others, should take place in a private setting away from uninvolved parties and should be kept confidential. If a tape or other recording of client information is made, the recording should remain on the nursing unit or at the care service agency.

► All communication should take place over a secure, private channel when possible. Minimal personal client information should be provided over cellular phones or other open channels when unavoidable.

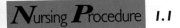

Interdisciplinary Information Exchange (Report)

 EQUIPMENT

- Client Kardex or plan of care/clinical pathway
- Client summary notes (kept throughout shift or visit)
- Tape recorder, if warranted by facility protocol
- Form to document verbal communication
- Provider or payor phone and fax numbers or e-mail address as indicated

Purpose

Facilitates continuity of client care through accurate and comprehensive communication of relevant client data among nurses and various care providers (may occur in the form of shift-to-shift updates, interdisciplinary consultation, and client-care conferences)

Assessment

Assessment should focus on the following:

Current status of client (comfort, medications/fluid infusions, etc.) and treatments pending
Identity and availability of care providers and payor sources involved in the client's care
Information needed by various care providers and payor sources
Desired method of communication (ie, phone, fax, or e-mail). Determine that method is secure and private.

Outcome Identification and Planning

Desired Outcomes (sample)

Appropriate treatments, medications, and other care measures and support consistent with plan of care are received as scheduled or needed.
All applicable care providers and payor sources will have accurate information concerning the client and any changes in client condition.

3

Special Considerations

When "walking rounds" are employed, visual verification of the client's condition should supplement reported data.

When reporting to caregivers with little previous exposure to the client, more background may be needed or desired. Caregivers with extensive previous exposure to the client may require only a brief update of pertinent changes. Take a few minutes to determine exactly what information is needed (eg, a medical supply company about to make a delivery will need a correct address, whereas a payor source will need to know client condition, care being received, and expected duration of care).

Remember to report data or occurrences from previous shifts, days, or visits, when pertinent.

Include concerns of the client, family members, or significant others.

Establish with the agency a method for routing information received from the physician's office. In some agencies, the field nurse is called directly by pager or by cellular phone, whereas, in others, the supervisor is the go-between. All parties involved in the communication must have the same information.

Home Health

The assessment and report of a homebound client should include the client's status at the time of the last home health visit, the client's response to interventions, any restrictions present in the environment (such as no running water or no electricity), and any adaptations that have been made in client-care procedures (such as irrigating a wound while in the bathtub).

The visit report should also include the client's address (with directions if it is difficult to locate), any special supplies or equipment to be taken on the next visit, and client-teaching needs.

It is rare that the home health nurse will speak directly with the physician during physician office hours. Establish a contact at the office who will reliably transfer information to the physician. Check with the office to determine the best time and method (ie, fax, voicemail, e-mail) to leave nonemergency messages for the physician.

 Transcultural

Pertinent data about the client's sociocultural background should be included if the data are significant to some aspect of the client's care.

 Cost-cutting Tip

Tape recording of report may be less time-consuming and, therefore, more cost-effective.

Delegation Issues

Direct communication ensures the greatest accuracy of information exchange. However, if information must be relayed to the doctor, another member of the health care team, a payor, or the client through a third party, the nurse should follow up as soon as possible to validate that the correct information was relayed.

IMPLEMENTATION

Action	Rationale

Inpatient Report

Action	Rationale
1. Gather information and equipment.	*Facilitates organizing report*
2. Report client identification data: - Name, room number, age - Medical diagnosis (primary and secondary) - Doctor's name	*Ensures association of reported data with correct client*
3. Record special circumstances of client. - Sight or hearing deficits - Language or cultural barriers - Safety needs (eg, client at high risk for falls) - Support needs - Family concerns - Religious concerns	*Promotes client safety and psychosocial well-being* *Recognizes ethical and legal concerns*
4. Summarize client's status using nursing diagnoses or outcomes to indicate active emotional or physical problems (see Display 1.1). BEGIN WITH DIAGNOSES OR OUTCOMES OF HIGHEST PRIORITY AND PROCEED TO THOSE OF LEAST PRIORITY.	*Validates established nursing diagnoses and outcomes and need for continued intervention* *Establishes priority of client's needs*
5. For each diagnosis or outcome, addressed, record the following: - Nursing diagnosis or outcome - Assessment data (complaints, wound/	*Summarizes current status of treatments*

DISPLAY 1.1	Report Format—Summary

Client identification data
Special circumstances
Client status—physical/emotional
   Priority nursing diagnoses
   Assessment data
   Interventions (treatments, teaching, monitoring needs)
   Evaluation (client response to interventions)
Recent diagnostic test results
New orders medical/nursing
Environmental concerns
   Tubes
   Infusions (fluid count)
   Drains
Immediately pending treatments
Family's or significant others' concerns or considerations

IMPLEMENTATION

Action	Rationale
dressing status, IVs, drains, O$_2$, etc.) - Interventions used (medications, IV, treatments, monitoring, teaching) - Evaluation (intake and output, client response to treatments, teaching, etc.)	
6. Report recent results of diagnostic procedures and lab tests.	*Provides status update*
7. Report new medical/ nursing orders (diagnostic tests, medications, treatments, surgery, dietary or activity restrictions, or discharge planning).	*Provides update on planned medical and nursing interventions*
8. Summarize general environmental concerns (tubes, drains, infusions with fluid counts, and mechanical supports [include settings]).	*Facilitates maintenance of support equipment*

Action	Rationale
9. Summarize treatments, fluid replacements, medication needs, tests, etc. required during first hour of oncoming shift.	*Facilitates punctuality and continuity in execution of treatment regimen*

Outpatient/Home Setting

Action	Rationale
1. Determine what information is needed before initiating a phone communication.	*Having needed information readily available increases the clarity and focus of the communication.*
2. Have all related information with you at the time of the call, and make the call in as quiet an environment as possible.	*Allows the nurse to answer questions and to hear and understand the other party*
3. Clearly state who you are, the agency you represent, and what the call is about.	*Allows party receiving the call to route you to the proper person*
4. Obtain the name of the person with whom you are speaking.	*Permits the nurse to followup with the same person, if needed*
5. Give all information in a clear and concise manner. If giving a condition report, know current vital signs, symptoms, medications, and doses, etc.	*Reduces the need for additional calls by having all needed information*
6. If receiving a phone order from a physician, repeat it back to the physician for verification, spell medications for clarity, and put it in writing immediately, to be sent out for physician signature.	*Reduces the chance of acting on a misunderstood order.*
7. Document all verbal and phone communication concerning any client.	*Provides a clear picture in the client record and reduces the reliance on any individual's memory.*

Evaluation

Were desired outcomes achieved?

DOCUMENTATION

Document all physician orders on the form specified by the agency. Document all client communication on the form designated for that function by the agency. All documentation must be dated.

SAMPLE DOCUMENTATION

DATE	TIME	
5/07/02	0530	**Physician order:** "Continue current daily wound irrigation and wound care × 7 days." Phone order Dr. Jones/N. Smith RN
		Phone conference with insurance co. case manager: Spoke with Tom Bridges, case manager re: John James. Reported increased drainage from wound, need for continued skilled nursing visits daily × 1 week to observe healing, perform sterile irrigation, packing, and wound dressing as ordered by Dr. Jones. Approval received from Tom Bridges. N. Smith RN

SAMPLE DOCUMENTATION

Sample Shift Report

Mr. Homes, Room 102, is a 75-year-old client of Dr. Smith admitted with diverticulitis; he has a history of hypertension and diabetes.

He is slightly hard-of-hearing in his left ear.

Priority nursing diagnosis: Altered comfort related to abdominal cramps. Mr. Homes complained of pain at 9:00 AM and 2:00 PM, was medicated with 4 mg morphine sulfate IV each time), and experienced relief within 30 minutes.

His potassium level was 3.7 this AM, and the last fingerstick glucose level was 140.

(continued)

(continued)

He is scheduled for a barium enema this PM at 5:00 and has received enemas till clear. Food and fluids are restricted (NPO).

He has dextrose 5% in water (D_5W) infusing at 50 ml/hr, with 400 ml left to count.

He is scheduled for a fingerstick glucose level test at 4:00 PM.

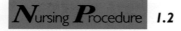
Client Education

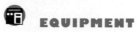 **EQUIPMENT**

Selected teaching tools (booklets, pamphlets, audiovisual materials, games, etc.)

Purpose

Assists client in learning information necessary for participation in self-care

Reduces anxiety

Assessment

Assessment should focus on the following:

Presence of those persons participating in client's care

Client's or significant others' readiness to learn and ability to comprehend

Age and education level of learner(s)

Amount and accuracy of client's and significant others' prior knowledge about content

Community resources for referral

Presence of any communication barriers such as visual, hearing, or speech problems

Presence of any physical or emotional barriers (conditions or medications that alter mental state or cause pain or stress)

Environmental distractions (TV, radio, noise, visitors not involved in client care or education session)

Nursing Diagnoses

The nursing diagnoses may include the following:

Knowledge deficit related to unfamiliarity with new illness
Anxiety related to knowledge deficit

Outcome Identification and Planning

Desired Outcomes (sample)

Client states purpose of procedure before beginning procedure.
Client demonstrates procedure correctly with 100% accuracy by
time of discharge from facility or agency service.
Client states solutions to potential complications of procedure by
time of discharge.

Special Considerations

Individuals with similar problems are frequently helpful in facilitating client learning.
A list of support or referral groups may be available through an
agency or a nursing association web site (see Appendix K).

Geriatric

Because of delayed reaction times that occur with normal aging,
elderly clients may require more response time during actual
teaching and evaluation. Consider response time when planning
time frame.

Pediatric

Visual aids and demonstrations are often effective when teaching
children.
Always include parents or other family members (for reinforcement), if available.
Same-age-group teaching can be used.

 Cost-cutting Tips

Group education is a cost-effective way to teach general principles to a large number of clients.
Video/DVD materials may be purchased to teach frequently
taught patient information; this may reduce staff teaching time
and will allow the client to review material repeatedly, as
needed or desired.

Home Health

Incorporate adaptations or modifications of procedures that are
likely to occur in the home setting.

 Transcultural

▪ Examples used for clarification or explanation of information
may, in some instances, be understood more easily if they relate
to some aspect of the client's culture. Pictures may be useful if a
different language is spoken. Many facilities have access to in-
terpreters of various languages, if needed.

. It is important to find out how the client views health. Many clients of various cultures view illness as a curse or bad luck. This may affect the nurse's ability to engage the client successfully in active learning.

IMPLEMENTATION

Action	Rationale
1. Establish verbal contract with client regarding teaching plans.	*Provides mutual goals for client and nurse*
2. Eliminate environmental distractions such as excess noise, poor lighting, uncomfortable room temperature, clutter in room, excess visitor and staff traffic, and clinical treatments and procedures.	*Creates environment for communication and learning*
3. Secure private environment.	*Maintains confidentiality and promotes free exchange of information*
4. During assessment and along with client, determine exactly what information client needs and is able to retain.	*Provides teaching focus* *Involves client* *Teaching is most effective when it occurs in response to specific needs expressed by the learner.*
5. Determine nursing diagnoses based on assessment findings.	*Provides focus for goal-setting*
6. Set realistic, measurable goals with client and significant others.	*Promotes client participation* *Provides focus for implementing teaching*
7. Develop teaching plan (Display 1.2) that specifically addresses:	
- Objectives to be met by the end of the teaching session	*Facilitates optimal learning*
- Content to be taught	
- Methods of teaching	
- Methods of evaluation	*Provides questions to guide teaching plan preparation*
8. Obtain all necessary equipment.	
9. Implement teaching plan.	
10. Evaluate plan and implementation.	

DISPLAY 1.2	Preparation Guide for Development of a Teaching Plan

Objectives to be met by end of session
Content
    What content will be taught to meet objectives?
    Will complex content need to be taught in divided stages?
Teaching methods
    What reading materials are needed?
    What audiovisual aids are needed?
    Will games or role-playing be used?
    Will support groups or group sessions be used?
    What equipment/supplies are needed?
    Will tours or visits to related agencies be helpful?
    How much time is needed to cover each section of material?
    Will practice time be needed?
    How much time is realistic for this client?
Evaluation methods
    How much time will be needed to evaluate learning?
    Will evaluation be:
        verbal?
        written?
        return demonstration?

Evaluation

Were desired outcomes achieved?

Documentation

The following should be noted on the client's chart:

- Extent to which each objective was met (fully, partially, not met)
- Nature of material taught
- Persons other than client included in session
- Client's response to teaching
- Client concerns expressed during teaching
- Need for additional teaching or alternate method of teaching
- Need for revision of plans with client input

SAMPLE DOCUMENTATION

DATE	TIME	
6/11/02	0900	Client teaching done regarding importance of low-sodium diet in relation to managing hypertension. Client demonstrated selection of low-sodium foods with 80% accuracy from list. Participated actively in learning. Denies concerns in relation to topic at this time.

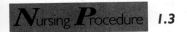

Therapeutic Communication

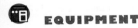 **EQUIPMENT**

- Calendars
- Clocks
- Picture or word boards
- Any items needed to add clarity to message

Purpose

Facilitates client's sense of well-being and control
Promotes beneficial nurse–client/family interaction

Assessment

Assessment should focus on the following:

Client's age, developmental level, cultural or ethnic background,
    educational level
Physical and mental barriers to communication, such as poor
    sight or hearing, speech impediment, pain, etc.
Client's use of nonverbal gesturing
Client's perceptions of people and situations
Sources of stress for client
Client's use of defense and coping mechanisms
Immediate environment (eg, noise, lighting, visitors)
Support systems (family, friends, community agencies)
(See Nursing Procedure 3.4—Support System Assessment.)

Nursing Diagnoses

The nursing diagnoses may include the following:

Anxiety related to inability to communicate needs
Noncompliance related to feeling of lack of control
Individual ineffective coping related to multiple stressors

Outcome Identification and Planning

Desired Outcomes (sample)

Client shows no signs of anxiety and communicates needs effectively.

Client complies with dietary, activity, or home health regimen.

Client discusses current major stressors in life.

Special Considerations

Anticipate questions and concerns when explaining factual information.

Plan interaction times to ensure privacy and avoid interruptions.

When planning interactions, consider the phase of the nurse–client relationship:

- *Orientation phase:* Initial meeting of client and nurse; verbal contract is made
- *Working phase:* Basic nurse–client trust established and relationship solidified through meeting of objectives
- *Termination phase:* Preparation for discharge and ending of relationship

When interacting with clients, consider their stage of coping or possible grief: denial, anger, bargaining, depression, and acceptance (Display 1.3).

Avoid statements or behaviors that might result in barriers to communication (Display 1.4).

Geriatric

Elderly clients may have one or more communication barriers that may readily be removed once discovered; necessary dentures, hearing aids, and glasses should be acquired, if possible.

With increasing age, a client's speech and comprehension may be slowed, requiring more time for communication.

Pediatric

A child may perceive sudden body movements by an adult as threatening; approach slowly after informing the child of your intentions.

When communicating with a child, consider developmental stage.

Home Health

Encourage the client and family to prepare a list of questions or concerns during the time between the nurse's visits. Use of a diary or journal may promote communication of content as well as context of client's concerns.

DISPLAY 1.3	Considerations for Interactions with Special Clients/Families

When interacting with an anxious client, recognize client's decreased ability to focus on and respond to multiple stimuli:
- maintain quiet, calm environment
- keep messages simple, concrete, and brief
- repeat messages often
- minimize need for extensive decision making
- monitor anxiety level, using verbal and nonverbal cues

When interacting with an angry client:
- use careful, unhurried, deliberate body movements
- provide an open, nonthreatening environment
- clear area of anger-provoking stimuli (persons, objects, etc.)
- maintain a nonthreatening demeanor, using open body language, soft voice tones, etc.

When interacting with a depressed client:
- allow additional time for interactions
- emphasize use of physical attending
- avoid giving client time-limited tasks due to slowed reflexes
- monitor closely for cues of self-destructive tendencies
- keep messages simple, concrete, and brief
- minimize need for extensive decision making

When interacting with a client exhibiting denial:
- use direct questions to determine the situation triggering use of coping mechanism
- do not avoid the reality of the situation, but allow client to maintain denial defense; it often serves a protective function
- recognize that denial may be the first of a series of crisis phases, to be followed by phases of increased tension, disorganization, attempts to reorganize, attempts to escape the problem, local reorganization, general reorganization, and possibly resolution
- be alert for cues that the phase is ending (ie, questions from client regarding the disturbing situation)

 Transcultural

- Use of an interpreter for clients whose native language is not English may reduce chances of miscommunication by client and nurse.
- Clients from some cultures may view direct eye contact as offensive and intrusive. It is best to follow the cues of the client in developing rapport.
- Sociocultural differences should be considered when interpret-

DISPLAY 1.4	Blocks to Therapeutic Communication

Giving advice
Using responses that imply approval or disapproval
Agreeing or disagreeing
Not listening attentively
Appearing distracted
Imposing judgment
Stereotyping
Providing false reassurance
Using clichés
Excessive probing
Questioning without bias
Responding defensively

ing a client's nonverbal behavior (eg, lack of eye contact may signify respect, not insecurity, and a shuffling gait may signify "cool" use of body language, not physical debilitation).

IMPLEMENTATION

Action	Rationale
1. Approach the client in a purposeful but unhurried manner.	*Facilitates controlled but nonthreatening interaction*
2. Identify self and relationship to client.	*Initiates orientation phase of nurse–client relationship*
3. Arrange environment so it is conducive to type of interaction needed (ask client or family permission and assistance if in the home setting).	*Eliminates environmental distractions*
4. Use physical attending skills throughout the interaction process: - Face directly and lean toward client. - Maintain eye contact and an open posture (do not cross legs or arms).	*Exhibits nonverbal body language consistent with verbalizations* *Conveys interest, attentiveness, sincerity, and nondefensiveness*
5. Begin interaction using therapeutic techniques	*Facilitates purposeful and mutually beneficial interaction*

IMPLEMENTATION

Action	Rationale
when eliciting or sharing information or responses:	*for nurse and client*
- Use open-ended statements and questions.	*Allows ventilation of those feelings and concerns most important to client at the time*
- Restate or paraphrase client statements when indicated.	*Confirms significance of client's comments*
- Clarify unclear comments	*Ensures intended message*
- Focus the statement when client tends to ramble or is vague.	*Promotes concreteness of message*
- Explore further when additional information is needed.	*Promotes more complete information gathering*
- Provide rationale why more information is needed, when appropriate.	*Maintains professional integrity of interaction*
- Use touch and silence, when appropriate.	*Conveys compassion and allows time for client to gain composure*
6. Use active listening techniques:	
- Do not interrupt client in the middle of comments.	*Prevents distraction*
- Use verbal indicators of acceptance and understanding ("um-hmm," "yes").	*Expresses interest*
- Focus on verbal and nonverbal messages.	*Facilitates receipt of complete message*
7. When client communicates, note use of gestures as well as facial expression and elements of speech (eg, tone, pitch, emphasis of words, etc.).	*Facilitates receipt of complete message*
8. Note client's nonverbal gestures as you are speaking (eg, facial grimacing, smiling, crossing arms or legs).	*Facilitates detection of cues indicating acceptance or nonacceptance of message*
9. Toward end of the interaction summarize important aspects of the conversation.	*Avoids abrupt and incomplete closure*

Evaluation

Were desired outcomes achieved?

Documentation

The following should be noted on the client's chart:

- Date, time, and place of interaction
- Nature and significant highlights of the discussion
- Communication barriers (if any) and interventions used
- Significant nonverbal gestures

SAMPLE DOCUMENTATION

DATE	TIME	
2/29/02	1400	Client in bed and tearful; upset because husband has not visited in 3 days. States concern about husband's feelings regarding loss of her breast. Reach to Recovery support group discussed. Nurse will contact husband this PM.

Chapter 2

Written Communication Skills

2.1 Nursing Process/Plan of
   Care Preparation
2.2 Nurses' Progress Notes

OVERVIEW

▶ Written communication is often the major and occasionally
  the only medium for data exchange between health care team
  members.
▶ Communication that is client oriented and reflects the
  nursing process will be more focused and organized than
  disjointed, task-oriented communication.
▶ Written communication often provides proof of practice or
  malpractice. **Legally speaking, if it wasn't documented, it
  wasn't done.** Focus charting or charting by exception may be
  used to minimize lengthy narrative charting through the use
  of checklists. Clear documentation is best proof that
  responsible, well-planned nursing care was given.
▶ Written communication should follow the guidelines of good
  communication and should be simple, clear, pertinent,
  sensitive, and, above all, accurate.
▶ Nurses' notes and plans of care often will be the only proof in
  future years that clients were monitored and cared for.
▶ Well-written plans of care, completed flow sheets, and notes
  lay a strong foundation for continuity of client care.
▶ Standardized plans of care may be used in some settings;

however, some individualization of the plan of care should be possible, and basic knowledge of plan of care preparation remains beneficial.

▶ The terms *goals, outcomes,* and *objectives* are often used interchangeably; however, distinctions are made between the terms in some settings. Nurses should be familiar with the use of the terms in the setting in which they work.

▶ Patient-outcome or critical-path time line plans may guide patient care. Documentation of patient outcomes remains important for evaluation.

▶ Although nursing diagnoses accepted by the North American Nursing Diagnosis Association (NANDA) are available as a reference, additional clinically useful diagnoses such as collaborative problems (Carpenito, 2000) may be used, if institutionally acceptable.

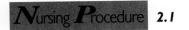

Nursing Process/Plan of Care Preparation

 EQUIPMENT

- Pencil or pen (if plan of care is permanent part of chart)
- Client Kardex or plan of care
- Appropriate reference books

Purpose

Provides a guiding foundation for individualized client care
Facilitates continuity of nursing care

Assessment

Assessment should focus on the following:

Data gathered from client environment
Client history
Physical and mental status
Social supports

Nursing Diagnoses

Will vary, depending on client's circumstances (see individual procedures)

Outcome Identification and Planning

Desired Outcomes (sample)
Individualized client care is planned and implemented.
Client receives consistent, continuous care as designed in the plan of care.

Special Considerations
When planning and implementing care, always consider safety and privacy needs of the client.
Involve client/family as much as possible in all stages of the nursing process.

23

Home Health

In the home setting, a plan of care acts as physician's orders for the client. The nurse must be able to complete the plan of care and turn it in to the agency for mailing to the physician in a timely manner. In the home setting, the plan of care reflects client condition, need for skilled care, schedule of visits, functional limitations, care needs, and general living situation. The plan includes all necessary information to meet agency policy, regulatory requirements, and payor source needs. Supplies needed should be noted on the plan of care to meet the requirement of some reimbursement agencies.

IMPLEMENTATION

Action	Rationale
Assessment includes gathering and analyzing client data and involves appraising areas in which client might require nursing care or assistance to meet basic or higher level needs.	
Data Gathering	
1. Systematically gather data: assess client status from admission history, physical examination, and diagnostic tests (may use body systems or basic needs areas).	*Organizes data*
2. Underline any abnormal data or note on separate pad.	*Designates areas of concern and probable causes*
3. Interview client regarding perceptions of condition and need priorities.	*Determines what needs client believes are of highest priority and how those needs might be met*
Data Analysis	
4. Organize and group areas of concern.	*Facilitates clear definition of needs or problems*
5. Determine client abilities and inabilities to meet identified needs; match client strengths and supports to needs.	*Determines level of nursing care needed—teaching, guidance, or direct nursing intervention*

Action	Rationale

Developing Nursing Diagnoses

6. Determine nursing diagnoses centering on needs requiring nursing intervention or teaching. Write diagnoses with two parts and a connector:

Part One—actual or potential client problem (Example: noncompliance to diet therapy)

Part Two—probable cause of problem (Example: knowledge deficit)

Connector—connecting phrase such as *related to* or *associated with* (Example: impaired skin integrity related to immobility)

Serves as guide for individualizing plan of care
Clearly communicates problems

Outcome Identification

Involves the establishment of the priorities of client needs and the establishment of key goals of care with criteria for evaluating if goals have been met. A goal is a statement of behavior that would reflect measurable progress toward resolution of the problem.

Guides selection and implementation of care measures
Promotes involvement of the client and support person in the plan of care

7. Prioritize diagnoses according to critical nature of problem and client's perceptions of need priority; life-threatening needs take first priority.
   Potential problems can often be addressed under a major actual concern (see goals).

Determines priorities for plan of care

8. Develop goals using these key elements:
   - Statement of what client is expected to accomplish

Expresses goals in concrete terms

Action	Rationale
(Example: demonstrates adequate tissue perfusion)	
- Goal criteria, in terms of measurable behaviors (Example: evidenced by capillary refill of 5–10 sec, 2+ or greater pulses, and warm skin)	
- Specific time/date at which expectation should be met (Example: by discharge or by third postoperative day)	
- Conditions or special circumstances associated with meeting goal (Example: with the assistance of vasodilator therapy)	
9. Use the following guidelines when writing goals:	*Develops clear, concise, realistic goals*
- Goals should be client-centered (Example: "The client will . . . ").	
- Goals should be written in active and measurable terms (Example: "The client will walk . . . ").	
- Establish realistic goals of health care and or maintenance.	
- Set realistic time limits, including short- and long-term goals.	
- Set one goal at a time.	
- Avoid terms like *understand, realize,* and so forth.	*Decreases measurability of goal*
Sample goal: By discharge, the client will demonstrate knowledge of diabetic self-care by giving own insulin and planning a 1500-calorie ADA diet without assistance or coaching.	

Action	Rationale

Planning

Involves developing strategies to help the client meet goals and attain desired outcomes

Promotes the delivery of individualized, effective, outcome-focused nursing care

- Special consideration should be given to circumstances that might impact on care strategies, such as age, transcultural, or economic issues.

Allows for tailoring of strategies to accommodate special circumstances

10. List actions needed to reach goals. Nursing actions may include supervising, teaching, assisting, monitoring, or direct intervention.

Identifies actions to meet goals

11. Determine who will perform actions to resolve problem.
Consult client and support persons to determine ability and willingness to perform actions.

Designates locus of control of nursing interventions as:
- ***client-centered**—actions performed by client*
- ***shared**—client and nurse jointly perform actions*
- ***nurse-centered**—actions performed by nurse*

12. State actions clearly, including the following elements:
- **Who** will perform the action (eg, client, nurse, assistant)
- **How often** or to what extent the action will be performed (Examples: three times daily; three out of four foods will be named)
- **Under what conditions** action will be performed (eg, with assistance, after instruction, with supervision)

Clearly communicates planned interventions

13. State actions singularly. Explain or clarify as needed.

Action	Rationale

Implementation
Involves carrying out actions/
nursing orders designed to
help client meet goals
14. Perform action (nurse or
   designated health care
   team member).

Evaluation
An ongoing step of reassessment and interpretation of
new data to determine if
goals are being met fully,
partially, or not at all
15. Assess client in view of
   goals and criteria.

*Identifies extent of progress
toward goal*

16. If some behaviors are
   noted, determine if
   desired outcomes were
   achieved.
17. Review behaviors and
   criteria.
18. Revise plan as needed:
   - Continue effective
     actions.

*Maintains good behaviors or
progress toward goal*

   - Determine factors hin-
     dering the meeting of
     goal and remove or
     minimize them.

Makes goal more reachable

   - Modify goal, if needed,
     by expanding time limits
     or lowering expectations.

*Makes goal more realistic for the
client*

   - Modify actions and
     eliminate those no
     longer indicated.

Maintains current, relevant plan

   - Add new actions, if
     needed.
   - If indicated, shift locus
     of control.
   - Continuously assess
     client status using data-
     gathering process.

Action	Rationale

Documentation

19. Documentation should be placed on appropriate temporary or permanent forms.
20. For samples of documentation, see examples in text.

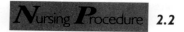

Nursing **P**rocedure 2.2

Nurses' Progress Notes

EQUIPMENT

- Small pad and pencil (for client summary notes)
- Client Kardex or plan of care
- Pen (black, blue, or per agency policy)
- Client-specific progress note or nurses' note sheets

Purpose

Facilitates comprehensive communication of relevant client data from one nursing caregiver to other nurses or members of health care team

Assessment

Assessment should focus on the following:

Previous notes from nurses, physicians, and other team members for an update on client status
Current status, as indicated by:
- Vital signs
- Intake (infusion rates and amount remaining in tube feedings, IVs, and other infusions)
- Output (drainage amounts); indicate locations of tubes and drains
- Dressings (degree and type of soiling, frequency of changes, and status of underlying skin/wound)
- Treatments (number of times performed, duration, and client response)

Outcome Identification and Planning

Desired Outcome (sample)
The client receives continuity of care through dissemination of information in an accurate, comprehensive, and brief form.

Special Considerations
Assessment data should be obtained at beginning of and throughout shift and should be recorded in small notebook until needed. Health care agencies may require that client data be recorded in a

specialized format using the following categories: Subjective, Objective, Assessment, Planning, Implementation, and Evaluation. These categories may be used in whole (SOAPIE), in part (SOAP, APIE), or in other variations. You may organize data into this format in your notebook so they are collected by indicating the type with an initial (eg, A for Assessment or Pl for Planning).

If routine client care flow sheets or checklists are used, do not duplicate data. Use nurses' notes to record data not covered on flow sheets and to elaborate, if needed.

Home Health

Notations should be made for each care visit regarding home-bound status of client.

Content of notes should address how sick client is. Report findings in objective and specific terminology.

Notes should be directed toward justifying reason for a home health visit.

IMPLEMENTATION

Action	Rationale
1. Designate body systems requiring detailed assessment and documentation.	*Provides framework for concise charting addressing only pertinent areas in great detail*
2. Assess client in an orderly manner (see Procedure 3.5), and record findings in small notebook.	*Organizes notes and facilitates accuracy through minimum dependence on memory*
3. When time allows, record initial client assessment in chart (Table 2.1 lists guidelines).	*Provides other health care team members with an update on pertinent client data*
4. As day progresses, record in small notebook or bedside activity flow chart, if available, time of, precise details of, and client response to treatments or teaching. Also record occurrences pertinent to client's physical or mental state.	*Indicates possible changes in client's status requiring update in documentation* *Facilitates prompt and accurate recording of client data*
5. Record pertinent observations in chart in an organized manner. USE ACTIVITY FLOW SHEETS, IF AVAILABLE. Or use	*Promotes problem-oriented charting and organized, thorough documentation* *Eliminates repetition and shortens notes*

Action	Rationale

SOAPIE categories (in whole or in part) or other formats.
- Subjective and Objective data with Assessment (interpretation of data in reference to identified client problems)
- Plan with goals to address noted client problems
- Implementation of actions
- Evaluation of implementation to determine degree to which goals were met

6. Document any changes from initial assessment, or the absence of any changes, at least every 4 hr.

Indicates ongoing nursing assessment and care

7. Use final note to highlight major shift events or progress toward goals.

Emphasizes priority shift occurrences and facilitates rapid review of notes

8. Document p.r.n. medication (medication given as necessary) in nurses' notes as per hospital policy.

Demonstrates adherence to established policy

9. Adhere to the following legalities in documentation:

Decreases indications of falsification or deception

- Never erase or scratch out errors in charting (draw a line through the sentence[s] and indicate the error).

- Check for and correct small errors (eg, wrong time or date).

Minimizes errors in charting that may decrease total credibility

- When recording events not witnessed or performed by you, use following form: " <u>name</u> reported administering or witnessing. . . . "

Clarifies that recorder did not personally perform or view action

- Draw a line through space at end of completed notes.

Prevents addition of information by someone else

- Sign notes before chart leaves your possession.

Avoids confusion of authorship should other people write on same form

Action	Rationale
- Chart actions on completion, not before performing - Use complete words or acceptable abbreviations only (see Appendix D)	*Avoids charting error due to delays in or cancellation of action* *Eliminates miscommunication*

TABLE 2.1	**Guidelines for Initial Assessment Notes**

Assessment Area	*Criteria*
Neurologic	Level of consciousness, orientation, verbal response, pupil size and reaction, incisions or head dressings, intracranial pressure monitor, sensory or mobility deficits (if applicable, expand musculoskeletal–mobility limitations, cast or traction, and extremity status). **Safety measures**—side rails, restraints (skin status and care)
Respiratory	Rate, depth, character, dyspnea, symmetry of chest movement, breath sounds, secretions, cough, incisions, dressings, oxygen therapy, and chest tubes
Circulatory	Skin color, temperature, capillary refill, heart sounds, pulse rate, rhythm, ECG pattern (if available), heart sounds, pulse assessment (absent to 4+), skin turgor, edema, neck vein distention, hemodynamic pressures (if available), intravenous therapy (with counts), and incisions/dressings
Gastrointestinal	Bowel sounds, shape and feel of abdomen, tenderness, nausea, emesis, diet and intake, dysphagia, bowel movements, nasogastric tube/tube feeding, ostomy site, stoma, drainage and care, and incision/dressings
Genitourinary	Urinary output, continence, appearance of urine, and Foley catheter status
Support therapy	Wound drains, irrigations, invasive lines, pain-control measure (transelectrical nerve stimulation unit, patient-controlled analgesia pump)

Evaluation

Were desired outcomes achieved?

Documentation (see documentation throughout text)

SAMPLE DOCUMENTATION

DATE	TIME	NARRATIVE CHARTING
1/23/03	1330	Alert, oriented ×3. Family at bedside. Skin warm and dry, with capillary refill of less than 5 sec. Respirations even and nonlabored, with faint expiratory wheezes noted. Cough strong with scant, thin, yellow secretions produced. Pillow pressed to chest by client to splint incision site during cough. Abdomen soft with active bowel sounds. Voiding without difficulty. Chest tubes intact on right chest wall, with dressing clean and dry. Drainage serous and moderate—30 to 40 ml/hr.
		NARRATIVE CHARTING
		TENS unit intact at settings of 45 and 30. No complaints of severe pain.
DATE	TIME	CHARTING BY EXCEPTION
1/23/03	1330	(Graphic sheet and assessment flow sheet or checklist are used to validate normal findings.) Faint expiratory wheezes noted bilaterally in lower lobes. Thin, yellow secretions produced with coughing. Moderate serous drainage—30 to 40 ml/hr noted from chest tubes. TENS unit in place at settings of 45 and 30.
DATE	TIME	SOAPIE CHARTING
1/23/03	1330	S—"I don't have any pain."
		O—Skin warm and dry with capillary refill less than 5 sec; respirations even with expiratory wheezes;
		(continued)

(*continued*)

cough strong with scant, thin, yellow secretions produced; chest tubes intact with clean, dry dressing. Drainage is serous and moderate—30 to 40 ml/hr. TENS unit intact at settings of 45 and 30.

A—Pain free.

P—Continue supportive care with TENS unit. Encourage use of pillow to splint chest incision site when coughing.

I— Pillow pressed to chest by client during deep breathing and cough exercise

E—Verbalized lack of pain after coughing.

DATE	TIME	FOCUS CHARTING
1/23/03	1330	
Incisional pain or	D (Data)	Grimacing during and 15 min after deep breathing and cough
Pain related to chest incision	A (Action) R (Response)	exercises. Instructed to hold pillow to chest to splint incision when coughing, return demonstration from patient received. Verbalized decrease in discomfort when coughing.

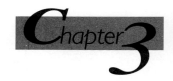

Basic Health Assessment

OVERVIEW

▶ Time spent in planning and organizing visits allows more concentration on care during visits and more efficient use of resources. When entering the home, have all needed supplies and documentation materials available and well organized.

▶ Detailed initial assessment of the client, the environment, and the support system contributes to an effective individualized plan of care.

▶ The nurse is a guest in the client's home and must be aware of cultural patterns and family dynamics and make adjustments accordingly. The nurse should explain every action taken and, if uncertain of the client's or family's reaction, ask permission.

▶ Because home health care is delivered on an intermittent or part-time basis, it is essential to have support systems in place for each client so care is consistent and adequate when home health care personnel are not present.

▶ In most situations, the TREND of vital sign reading is more relevant than any individual reading.

▶ Some experts consider pain as a fifth vital sign. Pain assessment should be thorough and regular.

▶ To obtain a true assessment of client status when using mechanical equipment, correlation of data with clinical findings is essential.

▶ Generally, the more acute the client and setting, the more frequently and more in-depth assessment must be performed.

▶ A thorough clinical assessment provides the foundation for competent and complete follow-up care.

▶ Assessment consists of objective and subjective data related to the client's present or past mental and physical status.

▶ Assessment performed in a systematic manner helps eliminate errors and oversights in data collection.

▶ Measuring the client's weight provides data about health state and cues for direction of treatment.

▶ Blood pressure and pulse may be obtained by a variety of methods to determine cardiac or vascular status. One method may be more appropriate in certain clinical situations than in others; however, each method requires precision.

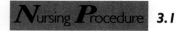

Preplanning and Organizing for Home Health Care

 EQUIPMENT

- Client case record
- Area map
- Medical supplies
- Scheduling notebook

Purpose

Organizes, to the extent possible, a plan for caring for clients scheduled to be seen the next day.

Assessment

Assessment should focus on the following:

Special needs of the client
Problems detected at prior visits

Nursing Diagnoses

The nursing diagnoses may include the following:

Health maintenance, altered related to knowledge deficit

Outcome Identification and Planning

Desired Outcome (sample)
All scheduled clients will be seen, and appropriate care will be given.

Special Considerations
If the client's culture is unfamiliar, check within the agency and community for people with specific knowledge of the culture, and obtain as much information as possible before making the visit.

HINTS

Always carry a list of local physicians' phone numbers and the name of a contact person in each office in case there are questions about care.

Know where the laboratories are in your area, what requisitions and specimen containers are used by each lab, and how quickly specimens need to get to the lab.

IMPLEMENTATION
BASIC IMPLEMENTATION

Action	Rationale
1. Review chart of clients to be seen the next day.	*Allows an opportunity to obtain missing or unclear information*
2. Determine special client needs (eg, timed specimens to be obtained, IV meds to be administered at a certain time).	
3. Use an area map to determine location of each client.	*Assists in reducing travel time between clients*
4. Determine approximate time frame for each visit (ie, 60–90 min for an initial visit, 30–60 min for a follow-up visit). If a specimen is to be obtained and taken to a lab, include the travel time to the lab in the total time for the visit.	*Allows for realistic scheduling of appointments, reduces chance of being late and keeping a client waiting*
5. Contact each client and set an approximate time for each visit. Remind each client that the time is approximate and is affected by travel conditions, emergencies, etc.	*Increases nurse flexibility and eliminates the need to rush through one visit to get to another by allowing a "time window" for each visit*
6. To the extent possible, take into account the client's preference for time of day, other appointments that the client may have, and the scheduling of other home health care providers.	*Increases client compliance by considering client wishes and helps avoid the scheduling of multiple providers on the same day, which could exhaust the client*
7. List the day's scheduled visits, with client names	*Enables the supervisor to reach the nurse if new client*

Action	Rationale

and approximate times of visits in the scheduling notebook. Follow agency policy regarding advising the supervisor of the visit schedule.

information needs to be passed on

8. For each client to be seen, assemble the needed documentation, including admission documentation, if applicable, appropriate lab requisitions, visit notes, and client education materials. Complete the demographic portion of each form as completely as possible before the visit. (If using a computerized system, be sure that all pertinent information is downloaded into the laptop.)

Organizes the materials before the visit, which allows for efficient use of actual visit time and better concentration on the client during the actual visit

9. Assemble any needed supplies and equipment for each client to be seen. Estimate and provide enough supplies for the client to use until the next scheduled visit. Do not overstock the home.

Ensures that proper supplies are available for each client
An adequate stock of supplies in the home reduces the need for extra visits to bring in supplies.

10. If scheduling visits for a week or more for multiple clients, take note of the clients' physician appointments, and total number of visits scheduled for any one day of the week.

Evens the nurse's caseload for the week, and allows the scheduling of clients in a certain area to be grouped on certain days to decrease travel time

PERSONAL SAFETY

Action	Rationale
1. On area map, pinpoint location of each client to be seen.	Determines if any client lives in an area previously considered unsafe (Check with agency supervisor to determine which areas are considered unsafe.)
2. Determine if any clients are to be seen at specific times.	Allows the nurse to schedule visits during the day because some areas may be unsafe at night
3. Be aware of agency policy concerning the use of escorts or law enforcement officers when making visits in unsafe area.	Permits time for advance notice and coordination if escorts are needed
4. Be sure to let the client know when you plan to arrive.	Allows the client to watch for the nurse's arrival and facilitates quick entry into the home
5. At all times, if using a car, be sure it is in good working order. If using public transportation, have all schedules with you.	Reduces the risk of being stranded in an unsafe area
6. Always lock the car. Avoid leaving anything in the car in plain sight.	Reduces the risk of theft
7. Be observant. Survey the area when approaching the client's home. Drive at a normal rate of speed, and, if illegal or dangerous activity appears to be occurring, keep driving to a safe area and notify the agency and client.	Avoids driving through unfamiliar neighborhoods at a very slow rate of speed, which could indicate that the nurse does not belong in the area and could attract unwanted attention
8. When entering a home, observe for exits, weapons, dangerous situations.	Allows the nurse to be aware of situations that may pose a threat to personal safety

Action	Rationale
9. Before making any visits to clients in unsafe areas, be sure the supervisor knows where you are going, and how long the visit is expected to take. Do not hesitate to terminate a visit if you believe that your personal safety is at risk.	*Promotes safety by providing agency backup and support*

Evaluation

Were desired outcomes achieved?

Documentation

According to agency policy and procedure

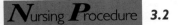
Supplies and Equipment

 EQUIPMENT

- Nursing bag
- Paper towels
- Handwashing soap
- Waterless handwashing solution
- Gloves—sterile and nonsterile
- Sterile dressing supplies
- Venipuncture supplies
- Blood pressure cuff
- Stethoscope
- Alcohol wipes
- Antiseptic solutions
- Tape
- Syringes
- Supplies specific to area of practice

Purpose

Maintains an adequate stock of needed medical supplies

Assessment

Assessment should focus on the following:

Types and amounts of items needed frequently
Specific supplies needed for area of practice or current caseload
Expiration dates, shelf life, and integrity of packaging of supply
  materials

Nursing Diagnoses

The nursing diagnoses may include the following:

Skin integrity, impaired related to surgical wound

Outcome Identification and Planning

Desired Outcomes (sample)

Needed supplies will be available in clean, usable condition.
Supplies will be restocked and rotated on a regular basis.
There will be minimal wastage of supplies due to soiling, loss of
package integrity, or deterioration.

Special Considerations

HINTS

Supplies carried in the car are subject to extremes of temperature
that may cause deterioration. Examples are urinary catheters
that become brittle, hydrocolloid dressings that dry out, and
vacuum tubes for blood collection that lose vacuum at high
temperatures. Supplies in the car are also subject to dust and
water contamination. When stocking supplies, the nurse must
consider exactly what supplies are needed and how the cleanliness and integrity of each item can best be maintained.

Carry a supply of plastic bags that may be used for disposal of
used supplies that are not considered biohazardous waste.
When possible, adapt items commonly kept in the home to provide client care (Appendix I).

IMPLEMENTATION

Nursing Bag Supplies

Action	Rationale
1. Keep paper towels, hand-washing soap, and water-less handwashing solution in the outside pocket of the nursing bag.	*Adheres to the principle that the outside of the bag is considered contaminated*
2. Carry items in the nursing bag that may be needed unexpectedly, or are used frequently for a number of clients. These may include sterile gauze pads, veni-puncture supplies, tape, syringes, blood pressure cuff, stethoscope, gloves, alcohol wipes, and antiseptic solutions.	*Allows for frequently needed supplies to be accessible and easily located* *Reduces the weight of the nursing bag*
3. Any item that is removed from the inside of the nursing bag must be cleaned before it is returned to the bag.	*Adheres to the principle that the inside of the nursing bag is considered "clean"*

Action	Rationale

4. The bag should be checked and restocked at intervals. The specific items carried will depend on the nurse's area of practice and typical client caseload.

Allows the nurse to have needed supplies available and in good condition
Allows for checking of expiration dates, soiling, or damage

5. For all supplies, a written note should be made when the last item is used, and the item should be restocked as soon as possible.

Eliminates extra trips to the agency office for needed supplies by giving a nurse a written reminder of needed replacements

6. The stock supplies in the nursing bag should not be used to meet a specific client's ongoing supply needs. Supplies provided for any particular client should be kept separate from the nurse's stock.

Reduces the risk of running out of supplies
Eliminates forgetting to charge supplies used for a specific client

7. When in a home, place the nursing bag on a clean, dry surface. If necessary, place a paper towel under the bag. If there is no suitable area in the home to place the bag, take into the home only those items needed for the visit.

Helps to avoid contamination of clean supplies

CAR SUPPLIES

1. For supplies carried in the car, assign specific areas for clean, sterile, and contaminated items.

Maintains cleanliness and avoids contamination

2. Place supplies in washable plastic containers, such as file bins with lids. Do not place supplies directly onto the trunk carpet. Label bins with type of supplies stored in each.

Maintains cleanliness, allows for easy removal of supplies
Covered bins prevent water and dust contamination.

3. Depending on the nurse's area of practice, supplies kept in the car may include Foley catheters, extra dressing supplies, drainage bags,

Ensures that supplies carried in the car will be used quickly
Reduces the risk of deterioration of supplies due to extremes of temperature and water and

Action	Rationale
paper towels, antiseptic solutions, etc. The nurse should carry the smallest amount possible of each item (Fig 3.1).	*dust contamination*
4. All supplies maintained in the car should be checked on a regular schedule. Soiled or outdated supplies should be discarded, and all dated supplies should be rotated.	*Maintains sterility, cleanliness, material integrity, and proper condition of supplies*

Evaluation

Were desired outcomes achieved?

Documentation

Agency policies vary as to how the use of supplies is to be documented. Be sure to record the use of materials for client care to facilitate charging for those items. Check the agency policy and procedure for documentation needs.

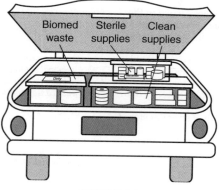

FIGURE 3.1

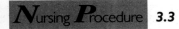

Environmental Assessment and Management

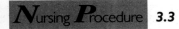 **EQUIPMENT**

- Pen
- Comprehensive assessment form (agency specific)
- Client history
- Completed physical assessment
- Client problem list or plan of care
- Physician's orders for care

Purpose

Determines strengths and weaknesses of client environment in relation to client's capabilities, physical condition, and care required

Assessment

Assessment should focus on the following:

Safety of the client in the current environment

Status and adaptability of the environment to accommodate client's functional limitations

Adequacy of environment for delivery of care ordered and indicated

Nursing Diagnoses

The nursing diagnoses may include the following:

Injury, risk for, related to environmental clutter

Self-care deficit related to lack of wheelchair access to bathroom facilities

Outcome Identification and Planning

Desired Outcomes (sample)

The client will function and receive care in a safe and supportive physical environment.

The client will actively participate in the adaptation of the environment to current needs.

Special Considerations

Before performing an environmental assessment, all nurses working in the home should be knowledgeable about the procedures and resources available to immediately remove a client from an unsafe environment.

Once the need for adaptation of the environment is determined, it may be necessary to enlist the help of the social worker, community resources, volunteer groups, and client family and friends to implement adaptations.

 Transcultural

The culture and belief system of the client is reflected in the home environment. Assess the environment in the context of the client's culture, not the nurse's. If you are unfamiliar with possible cultural implications, check within the agency for a resource person, or consult a text on cultural differences.

HINTS

Economic: Adaptations of the home environment may require structural changes or additions. Items in the home may be adapted for client care (Appendix I). The nurse must be aware of community or other resources, as partially listed above, for help that is available without cost or on a minimal cost basis.

Certain items needed for care, such as oxygen concentrators that operate on electricity, may increase the client's monthly electric bill. Consider these factors when assessing the suitability of the environment for care. Use social services and other resources, if indicated, to assist the client in meeting the expense of adaptation when necessary.

IMPLEMENTATION

Action	Rationale
1. Review the client physical assessment, the care ordered, client history, and community assessment (Display 3–1).	*Provides a basis for determining if the environment can support the needs of the client*

DISPLAY 3.1	Sample Assessment Form

NAME _____ DATE _____

ENVIRONMENTAL ASSESSMENT

NEIGHBORHOOD

Appears safe ___ Avoid after dark ___ Escort needed ___

Comments _____

PHYSICAL SETTING

Adequate space _____ Barriers to entry _____

Stairs inside home _____ Narrow doorways or halls _____

Inadequate floor, roof, or windows _____ Pets _____

Possible substance abuse by client/family _____

Comments _____

SAFETY

Inadequate lighting ___ Unsafe gas/electrical appliance ___

Inadequate heating ___ Inadequate cooling ___

Lack of fire safety devices ___ Unsafe floor covering ___

Inadequate stair railing ___ Lead-based paint ___

Unsafe wiring _____

Comments _____

SANITATION

No running water ___ No toileting facilities ___

Inadequate sewage disposal ___ Inadequate food storage ___

No cooking facilities ___ No refrigeration ___

Cluttered/soiled living area ___ No trash pickup ___

Insect infestation ___ Rodents present ___

Comments _____

SIGNATURE _____

Action	Rationale
2. Explain that a "walk-through" of the home is necessary to ensure that client needs can be met. Ask permission to look around the home.	*Increases client cooperation and enhances client control*
3. Assess barriers to entrance and exit from the home, such as steps or stairs that must be climbed. If needed, suggest ramps or alternative exits.	*Promotes client safety; alerts client that current physical limitations may hinder his or her ability to get in and out of the home*
4. Assess internal barriers to client mobility, such as stairs that must be climbed to reach bedroom or other essential living areas, narrow hallways, or uneven floors. If needed, work with client to find paths through the home that avoid or overcome these barriers, (eg, set up temporary bedroom downstairs, or obtain narrow walker or wheelchair, if indicated).	*Enhances client safety and mobility* *Promotes client participation in making needed changes.*
5. Assess electrical safety— how electricity is supplied (power company, generator, no electricity in the home). Assess electrical cords and outlets for fire hazards, and cord locations for hazards to ambulation. Assess adequacy of electrical system to support equipment needed for care, such as infusion or feeding pumps.	*Allows for adaptation of environment to promote safety* *Allows nurse and client to consider alternative methods of care delivery, if needed (eg, if electricity is unreliable, consider manually controlled infusion without pump)*
6. Assess adequacy of heating and cooling systems in the home. If needed, advise on safe heating units or fans. Assist client in using community resources to obtain needed equipment.	*Evaluates possible adverse effect of excessive heat or cold on client's physical condition and medical progress*

Action	Rationale
7. Assess adequacy of plumbing system and availability of running water.	*Identifies obstacles to good hygiene and infection control*
8. Assess fire safety, presence of smoke detectors, and client's plan for exit in case of fire.	*Promotes safety*
9. Assess general cleanliness and adequacy of lighting for provision of care. Assess capability for refrigeration.	*Optimizes setting for provision of care*
10. Assess kitchen environment for safety, cleanliness, possible safety hazards, adequacy of food storage, and preparation areas. Assess client ability to function in kitchen setting. Consider providing home health aide to assist with kitchen upkeep and food preparation. If client has new physical limitation, consider occupational therapy referral to instruct in skills for independent and safe use of the kitchen.	*Promotes infection control and good nutrition*
11. Considering client's current functional limitation, assess bathroom for safety and accessibility of tub, shower, and toilet. Obtain an order for adaptive equipment, and consider physical therapy for client instruction in safe techniques.	*Promotes client safety*
12. Assess for presence of insect infestation, presence of rodents. Assist in arranging for treatment of environment, if needed.	*Impacts on client hygiene, ability of nurse and client to perform clean or sterile procedures*

Action	Rationale
13. Assess communication devices (eg, telephone, intercom system, or presence of emergency call system).	*Determines client ability to contact help in an emergency*
14. Assess presence, habits, and care of pets in the home.	*Alerts home health care providers to presence of pets* *Evaluates possible impact of pets on client health*
15. With client assistance, assess ability to move through the home, get in and out of chairs, bed, etc. Suggest use of blocks to elevate furniture, use of suitable chairs, etc. Consider physical therapy referral for transfer training, and obtain order, if training is indicated.	*Determines client ability to safely perform activities of daily living in current home situation*
16. Ask client if he or she feels comfortable and secure in the home.	*Determines client comfort level and desire to stay in home setting*
17. Review suggested alterations to the home setting, and set a timetable for completion.	*Assists client in setting goals* *Enhances client independence*

Evaluation

Were desired outcomes achieved?

Documentation

The following should be noted on the client assessment:

- Safety hazards noted and actions taken to resolve
- Adaptations needed to ensure safe and adequate care
- Client ability to assist with environmental assessment
- Client response to assessment, feelings about remaining in the home, and response to suggestions for adaptations
- Contact with other disciplines and resources regarding adaptations

SAMPLE DOCUMENTATION

DATE	TIME	
05/29/02	1250	Environmental assessment completed with client cooperation. See assessment form.
		Suggestions to client re: need for smoke alarms, removal of scatter rugs in hallway, and need for shower grab bars, and elevated toilet seat.
		Client agreeable to adaptations; has concerns about financial factors. Client will contact family in regard to assistance with finances, and wishes to stay in the home. Nurse to assess progress in making adaptations next visit and contact social worker if additional community resources are needed.

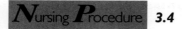

Support System Assessment

EQUIPMENT

- Pen
- Comprehensive assessment form (agency specific)
- Client history
- Completed physical assessment
- Client problem list or plan of care
- Physician's orders for care

Purpose

Determines extent of emotional support, physical assistance, and assistance with care that can be provided to the client by others

Assessment

Assessment should focus on the following:

Client relationship with family, friends, and others in the community

Client wishes regarding information given to others

Availability, willingness, and ability of others to assist with client care

Nursing Diagnoses

The nursing diagnoses may include the following:

Therapeutic regimen, ineffective management of, related to extensive physical injury

Self-care deficit, bathing/hygiene

Outcome Identification and Planning

Desired Outcomes (sample)

The client will be emotionally and physically supported.

The client will have sufficient support to meet care needs when home health care personnel are not present.

Special Considerations

Transcultural

Cultures vary widely in response to illness and to support of a person who is ill. In some cultures, offering assistance is considered insulting. In other cultures, everyone is involved with the client and is expected to know all details of care and the disease process. In still other cultures, certain disease processes are considered "shameful" and the client may be reluctant to risk any possibility of disclosure to another person. It is the responsibility of the nurse to be aware of cultural factors that influence the client, to assess the support system in a nonjudgmental manner, and to make every effort to provide resources that may support the client both emotionally and physically.

HINTS

When assessing client support systems, provide the client with privacy to enable him or her to answer questions honestly. In some instances, the nurse will be unable to accurately assess the support systems until the client has developed trust in the particular nurse.

Indications of abuse or neglect may be noted during an assessment of support systems. All nurses working in home health care settings should take classes in recognizing signs of abuse, and should be knowledgeable in actions to take.

IMPLEMENTATION

Action	Rationale
1. During any visit, observe the interaction between the client and others in the home.	*Provides insight into client relationships with others*
2. Initially, and on an ongoing basis, ask the client who is to be notified in an emergency and with whom information concerning the client may be discussed.	*Preserves the client's right to confidentiality and control of personal and medical information*
3. Explain to the client that it is necessary to know who is available to assist with care, run errands, etc.	*Enhances client cooperation*

Action	Rationale
4. If the client lives with others, inquire as to who can help with care, be responsible for decisions, provide emotional support, etc. Questioning must be done in a nonjudgmental manner, and questions about personal relationships, family matters, etc., must be avoided unless there will be an impact on care.	*Elicits information without violating the client's right to privacy*
5. Assess for indications of abuse—client appears fearful, appears to be restricted to one room in home, has bruising or injuries that cannot be explained; family members will not allow client to be alone with nurse, or appear very hostile to nurse's presence. Suspicions of abuse must be reported to the appropriate agency. Check agency policy and procedure.	*Identifies problem that will impact client safety; allows for interventions necessary to protect client*
6. If client lives alone, inquire about available friends, neighbors, or family members who could provide assistance and note on the assessment form.	*Determines the existence of extended support*
7. Once support people have been identified, ask the client what information may be shared with them.	*Protects client confidentiality*
8. Ask support people what help they can provide. Ask about help with care, errands, transportation, meals, and emotional support. Approach support individuals in a nonjudgmental manner to elicit honest responses.	*Determines if support people are able, willing, and available*

Action	Rationale
9. If no support system is identified, refer to social worker for assistance with use of community resources. Provide client with information on transportation services, grocery delivery, housekeeping services, etc. Assist client in use of services, including use of computer and Internet services. Advise client of local groups that may provide help. Consider using home health aides to assist with care, if appropriate.	*Provides a basis of support if no specific individuals can be identified*
10. Review the results of the support system assessment with other agency personnel involved in the care of the client.	*Prevents breach of client confidentiality, and provides consistency of care*

Evaluation

Were desired outcomes achieved?

Documentation

The following should be noted on the client assessment:

- Whom to notify in case of emergency
- Who has access to client information
- The availability, willingness, and ability of support people
- The name, address, phone number, and relationship to the client of each support person

SAMPLE DOCUMENTATION

DATE	TIME	
02/19/02	1050	Support system assessment completed. Client lives alone, has several friends and neighbors willing to help with care. Client has daughter out of state who is to be kept informed of care and condition. See assessment form for specific names and information.

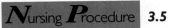

Basic Health Assessment

EQUIPMENT

- Pen
- Appropriate assessment form
- Gown
- Drape or sheet
- Blood pressure cuff
- Stethoscope
- Penlight
- Sphygmomanometer
- Thermometer
- Scales
- Watch with second hand
- Measurement tape
- Cotton balls
- Nonsterile gloves

Purpose

Determines strengths and weaknesses of physical and mental health status

Assessment

Assessment should focus on the following:

Medical diagnosis
Source of information
Information obtained on health history
Need for partial versus in-depth assessment

Nursing Diagnoses

The nursing diagnoses may include the following:

Altered physiologic and mental status related to drug overdose
Decreased tissue perfusion related to low blood cell level

Outcome Identification and Planning

Desired Outcome (sample)

Signs and symptoms of underlying mental or physical alterations do not go undetected.

Special Considerations

Clients with acute conditions may require a more in-depth assessment of specific systems.

Assessment in acute situations should be prioritized to address life-threatening areas immediately, with assessment of other areas undertaken as soon as possible thereafter.

After initial detailed assessment is obtained for baseline data, an abbreviated assessment of problem areas noted from initial assessment may be performed each shift. A detailed assessment may then be performed periodically (every 24 to 72 hr, depending on agency policy and client state of health).

Pediatric and Geriatric

Normal developmental stage and physiologic changes must be taken into consideration when assessing the client.

Although most of the information in the history may be obtained from the parent(s), the child's perspective regarding illness and care will be valuable throughout treatment plan.

Home Health

A complete assessment must be completed on the client initially, with abbreviated updates on each visit.

 Transcultural

- When interviewing clients for whom English is not their native language, secure an interpreter to reduce the potential for mistaken interpretations of client responses.
- Biocultural norms should be determined before judging whether findings are pathologic (eg, mongolian spots are a normal skin variation in children of African, Asian, or Latin cultural background but may be pathologic in Caucasian children).
- Color changes in persons of color may be best observed in areas of minimal pigmentation—sclera, conjunctiva, nailbeds, palms and soles, and mucosal areas. Consider, however, that a bluish hue may be normal for persons of Mediterranean or African descent.

Delegation Issues

RN or LPN (as specified by agency policy) should perform general assessment appropriate for client and setting. Significant abnormal findings may warrant a follow-up or more detailed assessment by the RN when the initial assessment is performed by the LPN.

Reports by unlicensed staff of indicators of acute changes such as patient complaints of pain, abnormal vital signs, or other findings should be promptly addressed.

IMPLEMENTATION

Action	Rationale
1. Wash hands, and organize equipment.	*Reduces microorganism transfer* *Promotes efficiency*
2. Explain procedure to client, emphasizing importance of accuracy of data.	*Decreases anxiety* *Increases compliance*
3. Provide for privacy.	*Decreases embarrassment*

Health History

4. Obtain health history by interviewing client using therapeutic communication techniques (see Nursing Procedure 1.3—Therapeutic Communication). Include the following areas:	*Provides baseline data for future reference when providing care*
- Biographic information (name, age, sex, race, marital status, informant)	*Identifies client*
- Chief complaint (as stated in client's own words)	*Explains why client sought health care and what problem means to client*
- History of present problem (date of onset; detailed description of problem nature, location, severity, and duration; as well as associating, contributing, and precipitating factors)	*Defines details of manifestations of problems* *Helps define diagnosis*
- Past medical and surgical history (date and description of problems, previous hospitalizations, doctor's name, allergies, as well as current medications and time of last dose)	*Serves as baseline and guide for treatment decisions* *Identifies potential problems related to present complaints*
- Family history of mental and physical conditions	*Identifies hereditary factors that may affect health status*

Action	Rationale

- Psychosocial history (occupation; educational level; abuse of alcohol and other drug substances; tobacco use; religious preference; cultural practices)

Identifies psychosocial, spiritual, and educational factors that may contribute to state of health

- Nutritional information (diet, food likes and dis-likes, special requirements, and compliance to diets)

Identifies nutritional factors related to present state of health

- Review of body systems (client's self-report of conditions or problems)

Detects subjective cues that may further define problem

Physical Assessment

5. Assess general appearance.

Provides objective cues about overall health state

6. Obtain vital signs, height, and weight.

Provides objective data about health state

7. Assess the following in relation to neuromuscular status:

Detects cues to abnormalities of neurologic or muscular status

Level of Consciousness
- Awake, alert, drowsy, lethargic, stuporous, or comatose

Orientation
- Oriented to person, time, and place or disoriented

Sensory Function
- Able to distinguish vari-ous sensations on skin surface (eg, hot/cold, sharp/dull, and aware of when and where sensation occurred)

Motor Function
- Muscle tone (as deter-mined by strength of extremities against resis-tance), gait, coordination hands and feet, and reflex responses

Action	Rationale

Range of Motion
- Structural abnormalities, such as burns, scarring, spinal curvatures, bone spurs, contractures

8. While proceeding from head to toe, inspect skin of head, neck, and extremities. — *Detects skin abnormalities*
- Note color, lesions, tears, abrasions, ulcerations, scars, degree of moisture, edema, vascularity
- Measure size of all abnormal lesions and scars with tape measure — *Provides baseline data for comparison*

9. Palpate skin, lymph nodes, pulses, capillary refill, and joints of head, neck, and extremities. — *Detects skin abnormalities and lymph enlargement*
  Note temperature, turgor, raised skin lesions, or lumps:
  - Lymph node tenderness and enlargement (Fig. 3.2 identifies lymph node areas)
  - Pulse quality, rhythm, and strength (Fig. 3.3 identifies pulse sites) — *Determines quality and character of pulses*
  - Crepitus, nodules, and mobility

10. Complete assessment of head and neck including eye, ear, nose, mouth, and throat: — *Detects cues to pathophysiologic abnormalities of eye, ear, nose, mouth, and throat*

Eye
- Pupillary status (size, shape, and response to light and accommodation)
- Visual acuity
- Using adequate lighting, have patient stand 20 feet from chart (glasses may be worn and should be noted in documentation) — *Snellen chart assesses visual acuity at a distance*

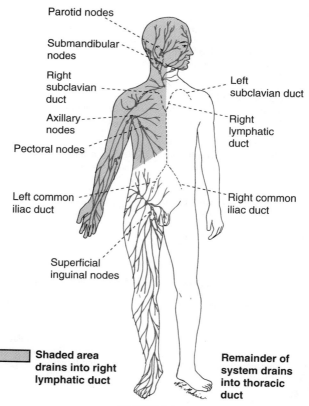

Parotid nodes

Submandibular nodes

Right subclavian duct

Axillary nodes

Pectoral nodes

Left common iliac duct

Superficial inguinal nodes

Left subclavian duct

Right lymphatic duct

Right common iliac duct

Shaded area drains into right lymphatic duct

Remainder of system drains into thoracic duct

FIGURE 3.2

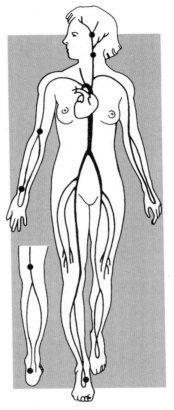

FIGURE 3.3

Action	Rationale

or
- Have patient read news or other small print
- Condition of cornea, conjunctival sac
- Abrasions, discharge, discoloration

Reading small print determines acuity of vision within close proximity

Ear
- External ear structure (shape, presence of abnormalities on inspection and palpation)
- Hearing acuity (ability of client to respond to normal sounds)
- Presence of ear discharge and degree of wax buildup

Nose
- External and internal structure
- Presence of unusual or excessive discharge
- Ability to inhale and exhale through each nostril
- Ability to identify common odors correctly

Mouth
- Presence of internal or external lesions
- Color of mucous membranes
- Abnormalities of teeth
- Unusual odor

Throat
- Presence of swelling, inflammation, or abnormal lesions
- Ability to swallow without difficulty

11. Inspect skin status of anterior and posterior trunk and extremities, including the feet.

Detects skin abnormalities

Action	Rationale
12. Palpate chest, breasts, axillary tail of Spence, and back, noting: - Raised lesions on any area, tenderness on palpation - Symmetry of breasts and nipples; skin status; lymph nodes; presence of discharge, lumps, or nodules	*Detects abnormal masses and lesions*
13. Assess cardiac status for the following: - Unusual pulsations at precordium - Character of first (S_1) and second (S_2) heart sounds - Presence or absence of third (S_3) or fourth (S_4) heart sounds - Presence of murmurs or rubs - Auscultate heart sounds in the following areas (Fig. 3.4): *Aortic*—at second or third intercostal space just to right of sternum *Pulmonic*—at second or third intercostal space just to left of sternum *Tricuspid*—at fourth intercostal space just to left of sternum *Mitral*—in left midclavicular line at fifth intercostal space	*Detects cues related to pathologic cardiac abnormalities*
14. Assess respiratory status. Note character of respirations and of anterior and posterior breath sounds in the following areas: *Bronchial*—over trachea *Bronchovesicular*—on each side of sternum between first and second intercostal spaces	*Determines if adventitious breath sounds (rales, rhonchi, or wheezes) are present, indicating abnormal pathophysiologic alterations. Side-to-side comparison approach increases possibility of detecting abnormalities in a given client.*

Action	Rationale

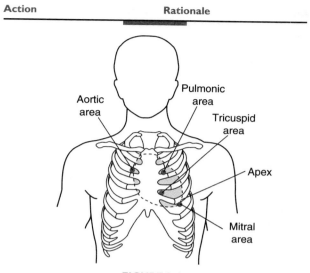

Aortic area

Pulmonic area

Tricuspid area

Apex

Mitral area

FIGURE 3.4

Vesicular—peripheral areas of the chest
Note: When auscultating breath sounds, use side-to-side sequence to compare breath sounds on each side (Fig. 3.5). Avoid auscultating over bone or breast tissue.

15. Assess abdomen.
PERFORM AUSCULTA-
TION BEFORE PALPA-
TION AND PERCUSSION
OF ABDOMEN.
  - Inspect size and contour.
  - Auscultate for bowel sounds in all quadrants.
  - Palpate tone of abdomen and check for underlying abnormalities (masses, pain, tenderness) and bladder distention.

Detects masses, abnormal fluid retention, or decrease or absence of peristalsis. Palpation and percussion set underlying structures in motion, possibly interfering with character of bowel sounds.

Action	Rationale

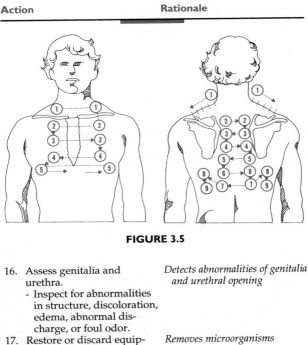

FIGURE 3.5

16. Assess genitalia and urethra.
    - Inspect for abnormalities in structure, discoloration, edema, abnormal discharge, or foul odor.

    Detects abnormalities of genitalia and urethral opening

17. Restore or discard equipment properly.

    Removes microorganisms

18. Wash hands.

    Prevents spread of microorganisms

Evaluation

Were desired outcomes achieved?

Documentation

The following should be noted on the client's chart:

- Time of assessment
- Informant
- Chief complaint
- Information from client history
- Detailed description of assessment area related to chief complaint
- Detailed description of abnormalities
- Reports of abnormal subjective data (pain, nausea, etc.)
- Priority areas of assessment
- Assessment procedures deferred to a later time
- Ability of client to assist with assessment

SAMPLE DOCUMENTATION

DATE	TIME	
4/29/02	0830	A 44-year-old black man presented with nagging chest pain in center of chest that started 24 hr ago.
		Denies nausea, headache, or radiation of pain to arms or back. No abnormal heart sounds detected. Vital signs: blood pressure, 130/90; pulse, 82; temperature, 98.8°F; respirations, 22. Bedside oscilloscope displays normal sinus rhythm. No jugular vein distention. Pulses in upper and lower extremities weak (1+). Skin slightly moist but warm. No jugular vein distention or lower extremity edema noted.

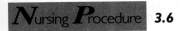

Electronic Vital Signs Measurement

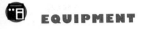 **EQUIPMENT**

- Electronic blood pressure monitor with appropriate-sized cuff for size and age
- Noninvasive blood pressure printer (optional)
- Flow sheet for frequent readings (if printer is not used)
- Watch with second hand

Purpose

Provides objective data for determining client's blood pressure status

Allows frequent monitoring of blood pressure electronically through noninvasive means

Assessment

Assessment should focus on the following:

Ordered frequency of readings, if any

Conditions that might indicate need for frequent readings (eg, head injury, trauma, surgery)

Skin integrity of arm (or extremity being used)

Initial and previous blood pressure recordings

Circulation in extremity in which readings are obtained (skin color and temperature, pulse volume, capillary refill)

Presence of shunt, fistula, or graft in extremity

History of mastectomy or lymph node removal from extremity

Choice of extremity to use to obtain blood pressure (eg, if arm cannot be used for brachial blood pressure, use leg for popliteal pressure)

Nursing Diagnoses

The nursing diagnoses may include the following:

Decreased peripheral tissue perfusion related to hypotension or dehydration

Altered cardiopulmonary perfusion related to dehydration or decreased venous return

Outcome Identification and Planning

Desired Outcomes (sample)

Blood pressure is within normal limits.

Skin is warm and dry, mucous membranes are pink, and capillary refill is brisk.

Special Considerations

Readings reflecting a 20-mmHg change in blood pressure, or pulse below 60 or above 100 beats per minute, should be reported. For clients at significant risk for fluid or blood loss, such as those at risk for gastrointestinal bleeding, a 10-mmHg blood loss may be considered significant. Frequently assess clients who show any of these changes.

Assess frequently clients in immediate postoperative or post-trauma states, or clients with acute neurologic deficits.

If client has had a mastectomy, do not take pressure in affected extremity.

Avoid placing cuff on extremity in which hemodialysis shunt, fistula, graft, or IV infusion is being maintained.

Ensure that blood pressure cuff falls within range parameters when wrapped around extremity to verify adequacy of cuff size. A cuff too small will result in elevation of blood pressure; a large cuff will excessively decrease blood pressure (Fig. 3.6.).

Pediatric

Use games to encourage cooperation and decrease anxiety.

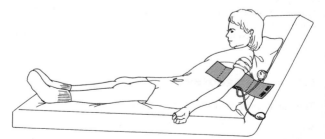

FIGURE 3.6

Delegation Issues

Unlicensed assistants or technicians may obtain vital signs. Significant changes or abnormal findings may warrant a follow-up or more detailed assessment by the RN or LPN. Trends should be addressed by the nurse.

IMPLEMENTATION

Action	Rationale
1. Explain procedure to client.	*Reduces anxiety*
2. Wash hands and organize equipment.	*Reduces microorganism transfer* *Promotes efficiency*

Electronic blood pressure and pulse measurement

3. Check the cuff and tubing of automated vital signs machine for air leaks and kinks.	*Facilitates accurate readings*
4. Attach noninvasive blood pressure printer to blood pressure module, if available, and turn both machines on.	*Activates equipment* *Allows continuous recording of vital signs*
5. Place arm at level of heart in straight position (see Fig. 3.6).	*Facilitates correct reading—if arm is below the level of the heart, the blood pressure will be elevated; if above, the blood pressure will be decreased*
6. Palpate brachial pulse.	*Determines most accurate position for cuff placement*
7. Assess client's pulse and blood pressure manually, using the arm you will use for automated vital signs readings.	*Provides baseline vital signs for comparison to determine the accuracy of automated readings*
8. Remove manual cuff and place cuff of automated machine snugly around extremity (artery arrow) above brachial pulse.	*Places cuff pressure directly over artery*
9. Press MANUAL, STAT, or START button (Fig. 3.7). Turning the machine on will often result in a manual reading.	*Obtains initial reading*

Action   **Rationale**

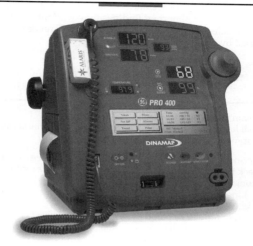

FIGURE 3.7

10. Obtain reading(s) from   *Provides baseline data*
    digital display panel:
    - Systolic pressure
    - Diastolic pressure
    - Arterial mean pressure
    - Heart rate
11. Compare manual blood   *Assesses accuracy of monitor*
    pressure and pulse   *function*
    readings to those obtained
    from the automated vital
    signs machine.
12. Check cuff for full   *Prevents prolonged obstruction*
    deflation.   *of blood flow in extremity*
13. Set timer for recheck of   *Assesses accuracy of timing*
    readings in 1 to 2 min, and   *device*
    check time interval with a
    reliable watch.
14. Check new data readings   *Assesses accuracy of machine*
    and time elapsed since last   *functioning and verifies range*
    reading.   *of current blood pressure*

Action	Rationale

15. Set timer for frequency of readings as desired. (Method may vary, but time is usually set by increasing or decreasing minutes until desired time intervals are obtained.)

Regulates frequency of readings

16. Set alarm limits with appropriate controls.

Alerts nurse to readings that require immediate attention

17. Reassess circulation status of extremity and cuff deflation with each reading.

Prevents inadvertent compromise of circulation

Electronic temperature measurement

a. Obtain disposable probe cover. Cover thermometer probe and slide cover over probe until it snaps into place.

Prevents contamination of the thermometer probe

b. Place covered probe into appropriate body orifice:
* Note additional preparation when indicated by route.
Oral—place probe in the posterior sublingual pocket and ask the client to close lips around the probe

Promotes contact with mucous membranes or skin for accurate reading

Axillary—place probe in the axilla and hold the arm down securely at the client's side
Rectal—lubricate probe, then gently insert lubricated probe past the outer rectal sphincter
Tympanic—some units require you to push the "on" button and await the "ready" signal on the unit first. Then insert the probe snugly in the external ear canal and aim it toward the tympanic membrane

Action	Rationale
(pull the pinna of the ear up and back)	*Promotes visualization of tympanic membrane by straightening the ear canal for accurate reading*
c. For oral, axillary, and rectal thermometers, hold the probe in place until an audible signal is noted indicating that the reading is complete. For tympanic thermometer, activate unit by pushing trigger button (located on top of some units), then remove the probe from the ear. The reading will be immediate.	
d. Note the temperature reading, then discard the probe cover.	
e. Replace the thermometer in its charger/holder.	*Recharges thermometer for future use*

Evaluation

Were desired outcomes achieved?

Documentation

The following should be noted on the client's chart:

- Vital sign readings (record in nurses' notes only if reading is significantly different from previous readings)
- Summary of trends of readings
- Condition of extremity from which pressure was taken
- Need for increase or decrease in frequency of readings

SAMPLE DOCUMENTATION

DATE	TIME	
2/24/02	1500	Oral temperature elevated at 100°F, pulse 102. Left arm BP 120/80. Left hand remains pink with brisk capillary refill.

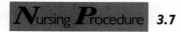

Blood Pressure by Palpation

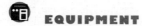 **EQUIPMENT**

- Blood pressure cuff
- Sphygmomanometer
- Flow sheet for reading of frequent assessments

Purpose

Obtains blood pressure measurement by palpation for pulse return (systolic pressure) when blood pressure cannot be obtained by auscultation

Assessment

Assessment should focus on the following:

Ordered frequency of readings, if any, or conditions that might indicate need for frequent readings (eg, cardiac failure, trauma, postoperative hemorrhage)

Extremity being used to obtain blood pressure (eg, if arm cannot be used for brachial blood pressure, use leg for popliteal pressure)

Skin integrity of extremity being used

Initial and previous blood pressure recordings

Circulation in extremity in which readings are being obtained (skin color and temperature, color of mucous membranes, pulse volume, capillary refill)

Nursing Diagnoses

The nursing diagnoses may include the following:

Decreased peripheral tissue perfusion related to dehydration

Outcome Identification and Planning

Desired Outcomes (sample)

Significant changes in blood pressure are detected at early stages.
Client shows signs of adequate tissue perfusion (brisk capillary refill; normal heart rate; warm, pink, dry skin).

Special Considerations

If blood pressure was audible previously and becomes palpable only, notify the physician and continue to monitor the client closely with blood pressure, pulse, and respirations every 5 to 10 min.

Readings reflecting a 20-mmHg change in blood pressure should be reported.

Systolic readings in popliteal area are usually 10 to 40 mmHg above brachial readings.

Although a diastolic pressure can be obtained by palpation, frequent errors occur in obtaining results.

If you are unable to palpate blood pressure, try using Doppler (see Nursing Procedure 3.8—Doppler Pulse Assessment).

If client has had a mastectomy or has a hemodialysis shunt or IV infusion, avoid taking blood pressure in the affected extremity.

Pediatric

In the young pediatric client, the flush method frequently is used to obtain blood pressures rather than the palpation method. Consult a nursing fundamentals text or agency policy manual for instructions.

Geriatric

Avoid leaving blood pressure cuff on elderly clients because skin may be thin and fragile.

Delegation Issues

Blood pressure may be delegated to skilled technician or performed by nurse.

IMPLEMENTATION

Action	Rationale
1. Explain procedure to client and family.	*Decreases anxiety* *Promotes cooperation*
2. Wash hands, and organize equipment.	*Reduces microorganism transfer* *Promotes efficiency*

Action	Rationale
3. Palpate for brachial or radial pulse.	*Finds pulse offering best palpable volume for procedure*
4. Place cuff on arm selected for blood pressure.	*Positions cuff for inflation*
5. Palpate again for pulse. Once pulse is obtained, continue to palpate.	*Relocates pulse for procedure*
6. Inflate cuff until unable to palpate pulse.	*Occludes arterial blood flow*
7. Inflate cuff until measurement gauge is 20 mmHg past the point at which pulse was lost on palpation.	*Clearly identifies point of pulse return*
8. Slowly deflate cuff at rate of 2 to 3 mmHg per second.	*Prevents missing first palpable beat*
9. Note reading on measurement gauge when pulse returns.	*Identifies systolic blood pressure reading*
10. Repeat steps 5 through 9.	*Confirms readings*
11. Remove cuff (or leave on if readings are being obtained at frequent intervals).	*Promotes comfort*
12. Restore equipment.	*Prepares for next use*
13. Wash hands.	*Reduces microorganisms*

Evaluation

Were desired outcomes achieved?

Documentation

The following should be noted on the client's chart:

- Systolic blood pressure measurement upon palpation
- Extremity from which blood pressure was obtained
- Circulatory indicators (capillary refill, color of skin and mucous membranes, skin temperature, quality of pulses)
- Level of consciousness

SAMPLE DOCUMENTATION

DATE	TIME	
3/4/02	0830	Blood pressure by palpation, 80 mmHg systolic from right arm. Client slightly lethargic at times. Skin cool to touch. Nailbeds and mucous membranes slightly blanched in color. Capillary refill, 5 sec.

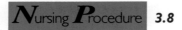

Doppler Pulse Assessment

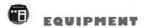 **EQUIPMENT**

- Doppler
- Coupling gel
- Washcloth
- Small basin of warm water
- Soap
- Towel

Purpose

Determines presence of arterial blood flow when pulse is not palpable

Assessment

Assessment should focus on the following:

Medical diagnosis
History of medical problems related to cardiovascular deficits
Quality of pulses in extremities
Circulatory indicators of extremities (color, temperature, sensation, and capillary refill)
Pulse rate and blood pressure

Nursing Diagnoses

The nursing diagnoses may include the following:

Decreased tissue perfusion related to decreased blood flow to lower extremities

Outcome Identification and Planning

Desired Outcome (sample)
Changes in pulse presence or quality are detected at an early stage, and early treatment (if needed) is facilitated.

Special Considerations

Delegation Issues

May be delegated to skilled technician or performed by nurse

IMPLEMENTATION

Action	Rationale
1. Explain procedure to client and family.	*Decreases anxiety* *Promotes cooperation*
2. Wash hands and organize equipment.	*Reduces microorganism transfer* *Promotes efficiency*
3. Squirt coupling gel over pulse area. (Inform client that gel will be cold.)	*Enhances transmission of vascular and pulse sounds*
4. If using portable manual Doppler, place eartips of Doppler scope in ears (similar to positioning stethoscope).	*Enables sound to be detected by nurse*
5. Place Doppler transducer over identified pulse area (Fig. 3.8).	*Places transducer over area that will transmit pulse sound*

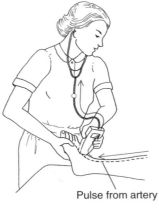

Pulse from artery

FIGURE 3.8

Action	Rationale
6. Turn Doppler on until faint static sound is audible.	*Activates system*
Adjust volume with control knob.	*Sets volume to suit listener's hearing range*
7. Identify pulse by listening for a hollow, rushing, pulsatile sound (a "swooshing" sound).	*Confirms presence of pulse*
8. If pulse is not audible within 4 to 5 sec, slowly slide Doppler over a 1- to 2-inch radius within same pulse area. If pulse still is not audible, continue this step, increasing radius by 1–2 inches until pulse is audible or until convinced that pulse is not present.	*Locates pulse*
9. Wash gel from skin, rinse, and pat dry.	*Prevents skin irritation*
10. If pulse was difficult to obtain, draw circle around pulse site.	*Outlines location of pulse for next assessment*
11. Restore equipment.	*Prepares for next use*
12. Wash hands.	*Promotes cleanliness*

Evaluation

Were desired outcomes achieved?

Documentation

The following should be noted on the client's chart:

- Area in which pulse was obtained
- Circulatory indicators in all extremities (capillary refill, color and temperature of skin, quality of pulses)
- Pulse rate and blood pressure

SAMPLE DOCUMENTATION

DATE	TIME	
3/3/02	0600	Right foot cool; nailbeds and sole of foot slightly bluish. Pedal pulse detectable only by Doppler. Left foot cool, with faint palpable pulse. Capillary refill, 6 sec in right foot and 3 sec in left foot.

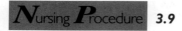

Apical–Radial Pulse Measurement

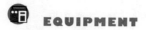 **EQUIPMENT**

- Stethoscope
- Watch with second hand

Purpose

Detects presence of pulse deficit that is related to poor ventricular contractions or dysrhythmias

Assessment

Assessment should focus on the following:

Ordered frequency of readings with follow-up orders
History of dysrhythmias, cardiac conditions
Pulse characteristics
Previous pulse recordings
Medication regimen for cardiac drugs

Nursing Diagnoses

The nursing diagnoses may include the following:
Decreased tissue perfusion related to irregular pulse

Outcome Identification and Planning

Desired Outcome (sample)
No undetected pulse irregularities or pulse deficit is experienced during immediate postoperative period.

Special Considerations
Clients with ventricular (pump) pathologies and cardiac dysrhythmias are particularly prone to pulse deficits.

Pediatric

Some infants and children experience occasional nonpathologic
dysrhythmias, such as premature ventricular contractions
(PVCs).

Obtain a baseline of pulse deficit occurrence, and note client response.

Monitor for change in frequency of occurrence or response.

Geriatric

Clients with such chronic conditions as diabetes and atheroscle-
rosis are particularly prone to pulse deficits and should be
checked every 24 hr for apical–radial pulse deficit.

Home Health

Because procedure requires two people, enlist and train a family
member to assist. Teach family members to perform the procedure between nurse visits.

Delegation Issues

May be performed by skilled technician or nurse.

IMPLEMENTATION

Action	Rationale
1. Explain procedure to client.	*Decreases anxiety*
2. Wash hands and organize equipment.	*Reduces contamination* *Promotes efficiency*
3. Have one nurse position himself or herself to take radial pulse (at radial artery).	
4. Have second nurse place stethoscope under gown at apex (fifth intercostal space at midclavicular line) to obtain apical pulse. Main-tain privacy.	*Locates apical pulse*
5. Place watch so both nurses can see second hand.	*Facilitates accuracy in beginning and ending*
6. State "begin" when ready to start (nurse counting apical pulse will state when to begin and end counting).	*Prevents error in count because nurse with stethoscope in ear cannot hear count call*
7. Both nurses should count pulse for 1 full minute AT THE SAME TIME.	*Ensures accuracy of reading*

Action	Rationale
8. Call out "stop" when minute has passed.	*Ends 1-min count*
9. Compare rates obtained. If a difference is noted between apical and radial rates, subtract the radial rate from the apical rate.	*Determines if pulse deficit exists* *Pulse deficit will be the number obtained by deducting radial from apical pulse*
10. Repeat steps 6 through 9.	*Verifies results*
11. Lower gown and adjust for comfort.	*Restores privacy*
12. Wash hands.	*Reduces microorganisms*
13. Notify physician if pulse deficit was noted.	*Initiates prompt medical intervention*

Evaluation

Were desired outcomes achieved?

Documentation

The following should be noted on the client's chart:

- Apical–radial pulse rate
- Quality of pulse
- Irregularities of pulse rhythm (if present)
- Calculated pulse deficit, if present
- Response to deficit
- Current cardiac drugs

SAMPLE DOCUMENTATION

DATE	TIME	
1/6/02	0830	Apical–radial pulse, 94 apical and 74 radial with pulse deficit of 20. Pulse irregular. Client states no dizziness, faintness, or chest discomfort. Dr. Britt notified.

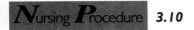

Obtaining Weight With a Sling Scale

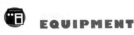 **EQUIPMENT**

- Sling scale with sling (mat)
- Disposable cover for sling (or disinfectant and cleaning supplies)
- Washcloth
- Pen
- Graphic sheet or weight record

Purpose

Obtains body weight when client is unable to stand or tolerate sitting position

Assessment

Assessment should focus on the following:

Doctor's orders regarding frequency and specified time of weighing
Medical diagnosis
Previous body weight
Rationale for bedscales (eg, client's weakness or inability to stand; standing contraindicated)
Type and amount of clothing being worn (client should always be weighed in same type and amount of clothing)
Adequacy of bedscale function

Nursing Diagnoses

The nursing diagnoses may include the following:

Alterated nutrition: more than body requirements related to poor dietary habits
Weight gain related to fluid volume excess

Outcome Identification and Planning

Desired Outcomes (sample)

A 1-kg weight loss per sling scale weight is noted after three series of dialysis exchanges.

Daily sling scale readings indicate weight loss of 3 kg per week.

Special Considerations

If the client is unable to turn independently or has drainage tubes that could become dislodged, obtain assistance to move client.

If client's weight possibly exceeds weight capacity of sling scale, seek alternative means for weighing client.

Figure 3.9 displays parts of the sling scale.

Pediatric

Infants and small toddlers should be weighed on pediatric scale for exactness.

Delegation Issues

May be performed by assistant, skilled technician, or nurse.

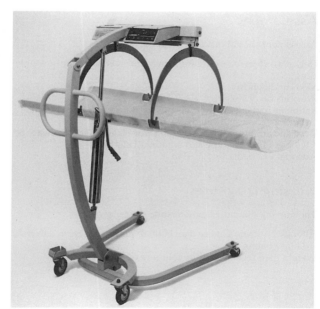

FIGURE 3.9

IMPLEMENTATION

Action	Rationale
1. Explain procedure to client.	*Decreases anxiety*
2. Wash hands and organize equipment.	*Reduces microorganism transfer* *Promotes efficiency*
3. Calibrate (zero balance) scales (with sling across stretcher frame) according to manufacturer's directions.	*Ensures accuracy of results*
4. Remove sling from stretcher frame and cover with disposable cover. Roll sling into tube and place in storage holder. Leave scale close to bed.	*Reduces transfer of microorganisms between clients*
5. Raise height of bed to comfortable working level.	*Promotes use of good body mechanics*
6. Secure all tubes so no pulling occurs during procedure. Have an assistant hold tubes, if necessary.	*Prevents dislodgment and subsequent client injury*
7. Lower head of bed.	*Places client in position to roll onto sling*
8. Remove sling from storage holder.	
9. Lower bed rail on side of bed with clearest access or from which most tubing originates. Be sure opposite side rail is in raised position.	*Facilitates placement of base under bed without disrupting tubing or other equipment* *Prevents accidental falls*
10. To place client on sling: - Roll client to one side of bed. - Place rolled sling on other side of bed and unroll partially. - Assist client to turn to opposite side of bed (over rolled portion of sling to flat portion) - Unroll entire sling until flat - Turn client supine on sling	*Positions client on sling with minimal disturbance*

Action	Rationale
- Position top sheet over client	*Maintains privacy*
BE SURE BED RAILS ARE UP ON UNATTENDED SIDE OF BED.	*Prevents accidental falls*
11. Roll scale to bedside, lower bed rail, and roll caster base under bed.	
12. Center stretcher frame over client.	*Ensures centering of body*
13. Widen stance of base with shifter handle of caster base.	*Provides support base for weight*
14. Slowly release control valve and lower stretcher frame. Tighten valve when frame reaches mattress level.	*Enables proper placement of hooks in holes*
15. Place rings (hooks) on end of stretcher frame into sling holes.	*Attaches sling to weighing portion of scale*
16. Have client fold arms across chest.	*Prevents injury to arms*
17. Raise client up with hydraulic pump handle until body is clear of bed.	*Places weight of body and attached tubing on scale*
18. Hold all tubing, wires, and equipment above client's body.	*Removes weight from equipment*
19. Press button on readout console.	*Obtains weight (in pounds or kilograms)*
20. Lower client onto bed by slowly releasing control valve.	*Returns client to bed gently*
21. Remove client from sling, rolling from side to side, as in step 10. Remove sling cover, roll sling, and place in storage holder (or place sling in holder for cleaning of sling cover at later time).	
22. Remove caster base from under bed.	

Action	Rationale
23. Lift side rails.	*Ensures safety*
24. Raise head of bed and lower height of bed. Place client in comfortable position.	*Restores bed to position of safety and comfort*
25. Replace covers.	*Ensures privacy*
26. Restore or discard all equipment appropriately.	*Reduces transfer of microorganisms between patients and prepares equipment for future use*
27. Wash hands.	*Reduces microorganisms*
28. Record weight immediately.	*Avoids loss of data and reweighing of client*

Evaluation

Were desired outcomes achieved?

Documentation

The following should be noted on the client's chart:

- Weight obtained in pounds or kilograms
- Type (and number or location) of scale used for weighing (eg, sling bedscale on unit)
- Client's tolerance of procedure

SAMPLE DOCUMENTATION

DATE	TIME	
3/9/02	0600	Weight after third dialysis exchange: 82 kg on sling scale. Weight loss of 1 kg from predialysis weight. Client reported slight shortness of breath in flat position, although respirations were smooth and nonlabored during weighing process. Client resting quietly in semi-Fowler's position.

Chapter 4

Oxygenation

OVERVIEW

▶ One key to successful chest drainage and oxygen therapy is tube patency. Tubing must remain free of clots, kinks, or other obstructions to ensure proper equipment function.

▶ Agency policy and physician protocols vary regarding milking or stripping of chest tubes. Consult policy before intervening.

▶ Increasing restlessness or decreased level of consciousness is a characteristic sign of hypoxia. Note associated signs or symptoms: elevated respiratory rate, tachycardia, or dysrhythmia.

▶ Improperly maintained artificial airway or tube cuff can cause trauma to mucous membranes, edema, and obstruction.

▶ High oxygen levels can be LETHAL to certain clients.
▶ **Remember "NO SMOKING" signs—OXYGEN IS HIGHLY COMBUSTIBLE.**
▶ Some major nursing diagnostic labels related to oxygenation are ineffective airway clearance, ineffective breathing pattern, and anxiety.

 Transcultural

- The assessment of skin color is subjective and depends on the sensitivity of the observer to color.
- For clients of African, Mediterranean, American Indian, Spanish, or Indian descent:
  - When caring for patients with highly pigmented skin, the nurse must first establish the baseline skin color.
  - Daylight is the best light source for this assessment, but, when not available, a lamp with at least a 60-watt bulb should be used.
  - Observation of skin surfaces with the least amount of pigmentation may be helpful. These include the palms of the hands, the soles of the feet, the abdomen and buttocks, and the volar (flexor surface) of the forearm.
  - The nurse should look for an underlying red tone, which is typical of all skin, regardless of how dark or light its pigment. An absence of this red tone may indicate pallor.
  - Nailbeds may be highly pigmented, thick, or lined and may contain melanin deposits. Nonetheless, for baseline assessment, it is important to evaluate how rapidly the color returns to the nailbed after pressure has been released from the nail.

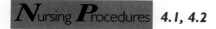

 Chest Drainage System Preparation (4.1)

 Chest Tube Maintenance (4.2)

EQUIPMENT

- Chest drainage system
- Suction source and setup (wall cannister or portable)
- Nonsterile gloves
- Sterile irrigation saline or sterile water (500-ml bottle)
- Funnel (optional)
- 2-inch tape
- Sterile gauze sponges

Purpose

Removes fluid or air from chest cavity
Restores negative pressure, facilitating lung reexpansion

Assessment

Assessment should focus on the following:

Doctor's orders for type of drainage system (water-seal or suction) and amount of suction
Purpose and location of chest tube(s)
Type of drainage systems available
Agency policy regarding use of saline or water in drainage system
Baseline data: breath sounds; respiratory rate, depth, and character; pulse rate and rhythm; temperature; pulse oximetry reading, blood gases; and chest drainage type and amount

Nursing Diagnoses

The nursing diagnoses may include the following:

Ineffective breathing pattern related to decreased lung expansion

Outcome Identification and Planning

Desired Outcome (sample)

The client ventilates effectively, as evidenced by smooth, non-labored respirations and a respiratory rate within client's normal limits

Client demonstrates lung re-expansion by breath sounds audible in all lobes

Special Considerations

Rules regarding clamping or not clamping chest tubes vary greatly among facilities and doctors. Investigate agency's policy BEFORE an emergency occurs.

Geriatric and Pediatric

Prolonged immobility can result in joint stiffening in geriatric clients and in increased frustration for hospitalized pediatric clients. Obtain rolling cart for drainage system, and encourage ambulation as soon as it is allowed.

IMPLEMENTATION

Action	Rationale

Procedure 4.1 Chest Drainage System Preparation

Action	Rationale
1. Wash hands and organize equipment.	*Decreases microorganism transfer* *Promotes efficiency*
2. Open saline or water container.	
3. Unwrap drainage system and stand it upright.	
4. Fill chambers to appropriate level:	*Establishes proper amount of water-seal pressure*
- Place funnel in tubing or port leading to suction-control chamber.	
- Pour fluid into suction-control port until designated amount is reached—per doctor's orders, or to specific line marked on bottle—usually indicating the 20-cm water pressure level.	*Level of water controls amount of suction pressure*

Action	Rationale
Fill water-seal chamber of drainage system to the 2-cm level.	*Allows air to escape chest while preventing air reflux into chest*
5. Don gloves, and connect drainage system to chest tube and suction source, if suction is indicated.	
- Connect tubing from client to tubing entering drainage collection chamber. MAINTAIN STERILITY OF CONNECTOR ENDS.	
- If changing drainage systems, ask client to take a deep breath, hold it, and bear down slightly while tubing is being changed quickly. Some systems have an easy snap-out and snap-in connection for system tubing changes; others require disconnecting tubing nearer chest tube insertion site.	*Prevents air influx into chest while water seal is broken*
- If indicated, connect tubing from suction-control chamber to the suction source.	
6. Adjust suction-flow regulator until quiet bubbling is noted in suction-control chamber.	*Regulates flow of suction, not pressure; vigorous flow is unnecessary unless large air leak is present*
7. Discard gloves and disposable materials.	
8. Position client for comfort with call button within reach.	

Procedure 4.2 Chest Tube Maintenance

1. Observe water-seal chamber for bubbling. Suspect air leak if bubbling is present and client has no known pneumothorax. Also suspect air leak if bubbling is noted	*Indicates air entering system (from client or air leak)* *Determines if air is entering system through loose tube connections*

Action	Rationale

and chest tube is clamped
or if bubbling is excessive.
Check security of tube
connections.
2. Every 1 to 2 hr (depending
on amount of drainage or
orders):
- Mark drainage in
  collection chamber.
- Monitor the drainage
  system for bubbling in
  suction-control chamber.
- Check for fluctuation in
  water-seal chamber with
  respirations.
3. If drainage slows or stops,
consult agency policy and,
if allowed, gently milk chest
tube (or strip as last resort
unless against policy):

Detects hemorrhage or increased or decreased drainage
Indicates that suction is intact

Indicates patent tubing (may not fluctuate if lung re-expanded)

Stripping tubes causes extreme pain and can cause hemorrhage.

Milking
- Grasp tube close to chest
  and squeeze tube between
  fingers and palm of hand
  (Fig. 4.1*A*).
- Move other hand to next
  lower portion of tube and
  squeeze.
- Release first hand, and
  move to next portion of
  tube.
- Continue toward drainage
  container.

Pushes clotted blood toward drainage system

Exerts gentle increased suction to facilitate drainage

Stripping
- Place lubricant on fingers
  of one hand and pinch
  chest tube with fingers of
  other hand (Fig. 4.1*B*).
- Squeeze tubing below
  pinched portion with
  lubricated fingers and
  slide fingers down tube
  toward drainage system.

Decreases pulling on tube while stripping
Stabilizes tube to prevent dislodging
Exerts increased suction to facilitate drainage (may disrupt tissue healing and cause hemorrhage, so perform with caution)

Action	Rationale

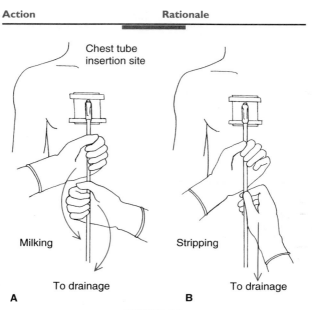

FIGURE 4.1

- Slowly release pinch of
  nonlubricated fingers,
  then release lubricated
  fingers.
- Repeat one to two times.   *Facilitates prompt tube replace-*
  Notify doctor if unable to   *ment and avoids development*
  clear clots from tubing.   *of hemothorax*
  Monitor for tension
  pneumothorax/hemothorax.

4. Every 2 hr (more frequently   *Determines possible source of air*
   if changes are noted)   *leak, hemorrhage, or tube*
   monitor: *obstruction and leakage at*
                                                tube insertion site

   - Chest tube dressing for
     adequacy of tape seal and
     amount and type of soiling
   - Breath sounds   *Indicates progress toward lung*
                                                reinflation

Action	Rationale

5. Every 2 to 4 hr, monitor vital signs and temperature. Use the following trouble-shooting tips in maintaining chest tube drainage.

Facilitates detection of such complications as hemorrhage tension pneumothorax/ hemothorax, and infection

Troubleshooting Tips
If:
- *Drainage system is turned over and water seal is disrupted,* reestablish water seal and assess client.

Prevents additional air reflux and determines presence of pneumothorax

- *Drainage decreases suddenly,* assess for tube obstructions (ie, clots or kinks), and milk tubing.

Determines if drainage has been blocked and reestablishes tube patency

- Check that gravity drainage systems and suction systems are below level of client's chest. WATCH FOR TENSION PNEUMOTHORAX AND HEMOTHORAX.

Ensures proper gravitational pull and negative water seal

Indicates air or blood is entering chest cavity, increasing pres-sure on structures in chest cavity

- *Drainage increases suddenly or becomes bright red,* take vital signs, observe respiratory status, and notify doctor.

Indicates possible hemorrhage

- *Dressing becomes saturated,* reinforce with gauze, and tape securely. If permitted, remove soiled dressings without disturbing petroleum jelly gauze seal and apply new gauze pads.

Retains original seal around chest tube

- *Drainage system is broken,* clamp tube with Kelly clamp or hemostat and replace system immediately OR place end of tube in sterile saline bottle, place bottle below level of chest, and replace drainage system immediately.

Prevents entrance of air into chest
Establishes temporary water seal

Action	Rationale
CLAMP CHEST TUBES FOR NO MORE THAN A FEW MINUTES (SUCH AS DURING SYSTEM CHANGE).	*Air can enter pleural cavity with inspiration and, if not able to escape, will cause tension pneumothorax.*

Evaluation

Were desired outcomes achieved?

Documentation

The following should be noted on the client's chart:

- System function (type and amount of drainage)
- Time suction was initiated or system changed
- Client status (respiratory rate, breath sounds, pulse, blood pressure, skin color and temperature, mental status, and core body temperature)
- Chest dressing status and care done

SAMPLE DOCUMENTATION

DATE	TIME	
6/8/02	1100	Client alert and oriented; skin warm and dry. Chest tubes intact, with dressing dry and intact. Disposable drainage system changed, with no signs of air leak noted. Suction maintained at 20 cm. Drainage scant, with 10 ml serous fluid this hour. Respirations, 12; nonlabored, with breath sounds in all lobes. Pulse and blood pressure within client's normal range.

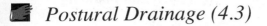

Postural Drainage (4.3)

Chest Percussion (4.4)

Chest Vibration (4.5)

EQUIPMENT

- Large towel (optional)
- Suctioning equipment
- Emesis basin or tissues and paper bag

Purpose

This three-part regimen, often referred to as *chest physiotherapy*, achieves the following:

- Loosens secretions in airways
- Uses gravity to drain and remove excessive secretions
- Decreases accumulation of secretions in unconscious or weakened clients

Assessment

Assessment should focus on the following:

Bilateral breath sounds
Respiratory rate and character
Doctor's orders regarding activity/position restrictions
Tolerance of previous physiotherapy
Current chest radiographs

Nursing Diagnoses

The nursing diagnoses may include the following:

Ineffective airway clearance related to excessive secretions

Outcome Identification and Planning

Desired Outcomes (sample)

The client's respirations are 14 to 20, of normal depth, smooth, and symmetric.

Breath sounds are clear in target areas; chest radiograph reveals clear lung fields.

Arterial blood gases are within normal limits for client.

Special Considerations

Postural drainage should be omitted in clients with poor tolerance to lying flat (ie, clients with increased intracranial pressure or those with extreme respiratory distress).

Length of time of therapy or degree of head elevation should be altered for client tolerance.

Therapy should not be initiated until 2 or more hours after solid food intake (1 hour after liquid diet intake).

Performance of therapy before meals and at bedtime opens airways for easier breathing during meals and at night.

Do not percuss or vibrate over areas of skin irritation or breakdown, soft tissue, the spine, or wherever there is pain.

Always have suction equipment available (particularly with pediatric clients) in case of aspiration.

Geriatric and Pediatric

Pressure used in percussion or vibration must be modified to prevent fracture of the brittle bones of elderly or pediatric clients.

Home Health

Pillows and rolled linens may be used to achieve positions.

IMPLEMENTATION

Action	Rationale

Procedure 4.3 Postural Drainage

Action	Rationale
1. Explain and demonstrate procedure to client and family.	*Facilitates relaxation and cooperation*
2. Wash hands and organize equipment.	*Reduces microorganism transfer* *Promotes efficiency*
3. Administer bronchodilators, expectorants, or warm liquids, if ordered or desired.	*Loosens and liquefies secretions*
4. Encourage client to void.	*Prevents interruption of therapy*
5. Position client to drain specific lung area (Fig. 4.2A).	

Action	Rationale

To drain *upper lung segments/ lobes*, position client:
- Sitting upright in bed or chair; perform therapy to right and left chest (see Fig. 4.2*A*)

Drains anterior right and left apical segments

- Leaning forward in sitting position; perform therapy to back (Fig. 4.2*B*)

Drains posterior right and left apical segments

- Lying flat on back; perform therapy to right and left chest (Fig. 4.2*C*)

Drains anterior segments

- Lying on abdomen, tilted to right or left side; perform therapy to right or left back (Fig. 4.2*D*)

Drains posterior segments

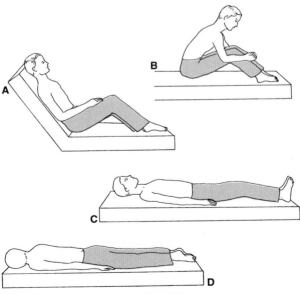

FIGURE 4.2

Action	Rationale

To drain *middle lobe*, position client:
- Lying on back, tilted to left side in Trendelenburg's position; perform therapy to right chest (Fig. 4.2*E*)
- Lying on abdomen, tilted to left side, with hips elevated; perform therapy to right back (Fig. 4.2*F*)

Drains middle anterior lobe

Drains middle posterior lobe

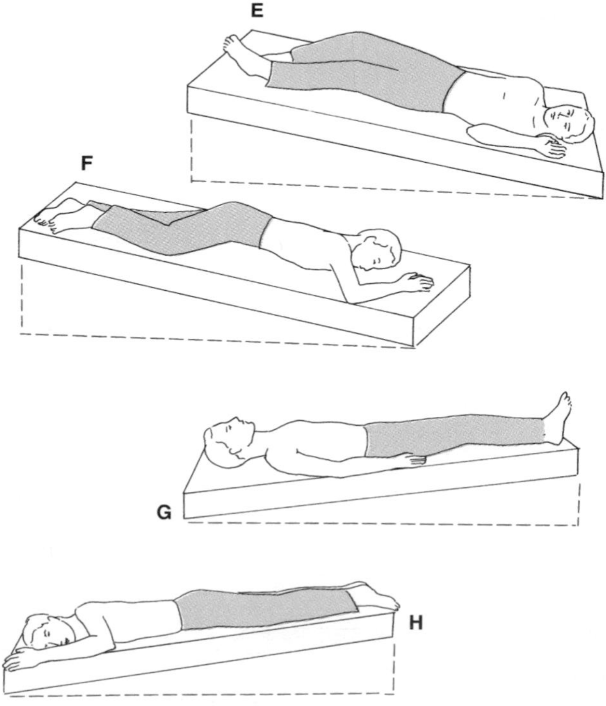

FIGURE 4.2 (cont.)

Action	Rationale

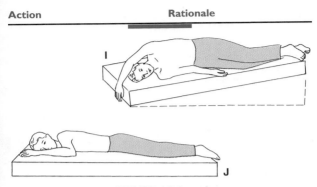

FIGURE 4.2 (cont.)

To drain *basal/lower lobes*,
position client:
- Lying in Trendelenburg's
  position on back; perform
  therapy to right and left
  chest (Fig. 4.2*G*)

Drains anterior basal lobes

- Lying in Trendelenburg's
  position on abdomen;
  perform therapy to right
  and left back (Fig. 4.2*H*)

Drains posterior basal lobes

- On right or left side, in
  Trendelenburg's position;
  perform therapy to back
  (Fig. 4.2*I*)

Drains lateral basal lobes

- Lying on abdomen,
  perform therapy to right
  and left back (Fig. 4.2*J*)

Drains superior basal lobes

6. Maintain client in position
   until chest percussion and
   vibration are completed
   (approximately 5 min).

Loosens secretions in target area

7. Assist client into position for
   coughing or position client
   for suctioning of trachea.

*Removes secretions from lungs
accumulating in trachea*

8. Position client to drain next
   target area and repeat
   percussion and vibration.

9. Continue sequence until
   identified target areas have
   been drained.

*Completes drainage of congested
lung fields*

Action	Rationale

Procedure 4.4 Chest Percussion

1. Place client in position to drain target lung field, and place towel over skin, if desired (see Procedure 4.3).

Decreases friction against skin

2. Close fingers and thumb together and flex them slightly, making shallow cups of your palms (Fig. 4.3).

Allows palms to be used to trap air and cushion blows to chest

3. Strike target area using palm cups, holding wrists stiff, and alternating hands (a hollow sound should be produced).

Delivers cushioned blows and prevents "slapping" of skin with flat palm or fingertips

4. Percuss entire target area, using a systematic pattern and rhythmic hand alternation.

Ensures loosening of secretions in entire target area

5. Continue percussion for 1 to 2 min per target area, if tolerated.

Facilitates maximum loosening of secretions from airway

6. Perform chest vibration to site (see Procedure 4.5), assist client to clear secretions, and position client for new target area (see Procedure 4.3).

7. Repeat percussion, vibration, and cough/suction sequence until identified lung fields have been drained.

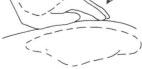

FIGURE 4.3

Action	Rationale

Procedure 4.5 Chest Vibration

1. Prepare and position client to drain target area.
2. Perform chest percussion to target area (see Procedures 4.3 and 4.4).

   Facilitates loosening of secretions

3. Instruct client to breathe in deeply and exhale slowly (may use pursed lip breathing).

   Uses air movement to push secretions from airways

4. With each respiration, perform vibration techniques as follows:
   - Place your hands on top of one another over target area (Fig. 4.4).
   - Instruct client to take deep breath.
   - As client exhales slowly, deliver a gentle tremor or shaking by tensing your arms and hands and making hands shake slightly.

     Provides gentle vibration to shake secretions loose

   - Continue tremor throughout exhalation phase.

     Moves secretions from lobes of lungs and bronchi into trachea

   - Relax arms and hands as client inhales.
5. Repeat vibration process for five to eight breaths, moving hands to different sections of target area.

   Facilitates loosening secretions over entire target area

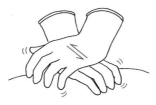

FIGURE 4.4

Action	Rationale
6. Assist client in clearing secretions (through coughing or suction).	*Removes secretions drained into trachea and pharynx from lungs*
7. Position client for drainage of next target area.	
8. Repeat steps 2 to 7 until all targeted lung fields have been drained.	*Clears secretions from obstructed lung fields and prevents obstruction of airways*
9. Assess breath sounds in targeted lung fields.	*Evaluates effectiveness of therapy and need for additional treatment*
10. Assist client with mouth care.	*Removes residual secretions from oral cavity and freshens mouth*
11. Position client in bed with head of bed elevated 45 degrees or more.	*Facilitates lung expansion and deep breathing*
12. Turn client to side with pillow at back.	*Facilitates movement of secretions*
13. Raise side rails and place call light within reach.	*Facilitates client safety and communication with nurse*
14. Wash hands and chart procedure.	

Evaluation

Were desired outcomes achieved?

Documentation

The following should be noted on the client's chart:

- Breath sounds before and after procedure
- Character of respirations
- Significant changes in vital signs
- Color, amount, and consistency of secretions
- Tolerance to treatment (eg, state of incisions, drains)
- Replacement of oxygen source, if applicable

SAMPLE DOCUMENTATION

DATE	TIME	
1/22/02	1200	Postural drainage with chest percussion and vibration performed to right upper, middle, and lower lobes of lungs. Cough productive with thick, yellow sputum. Positioned on left side with oxygen at 2 L per cannula.

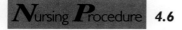

 Nasal Cannula/Face Mask Application

EQUIPMENT

- Oxygen humidifier (and distilled water, if needed for humidifier)
- Oxygen source (wall or cylinder)
- Oxygen flow meter
- Nasal cannula or appropriate facemask
- Nonsterile gloves
- "NO SMOKING" sign
- Cotton balls
- Wash cloth
- Petroleum jelly

Purpose

Provides client with additional concentration of oxygen to facilitate adequate tissue oxygenation

Assessment

Assessment should focus on the following:

Doctor's order for oxygen concentration, method of delivery, and parameters for regulation (blood gas levels)
Baseline data: level of consciousness, respiratory status (rate, depth, signs of distress), blood pressure, and pulse

Nursing Diagnoses

The nursing diagnoses may include the following:

Ineffective breathing pattern related to neuromuscular impairment
Anxiety related to inability to breathe

Outcome Identification and Planning

Desired Outcomes (sample)

Respirations are 14 to 20, of normal depth, smooth, and symmetric; lung fields are clear; no cyanosis.

Special Considerations

In most acute situations, placing client on oxygen is a nursing decision and does not require a doctor's order before initiation of therapy; check agency policy. Once oxygen is applied, notify doctor for further orders.

A face mask provides better control of inspired oxygen concentration than the nasal cannula.

The nasal cannula may be unsuitable for emergency oxygen delivery if high oxygen percentages are desired.

If client has history of chronic lung disease or extensive tobacco abuse, DO NOT PLACE ON MORE THAN 2 TO 3 L OF NASAL OXYGEN (30% FACE MASK) WITHOUT A DOCTOR'S ORDER.

Geriatric

Monitor for signs of chronic lung disease and take appropriate precautions.

Pediatric

An oxygen tent or canopy is the most suitable oxygen delivery method for infants and very young children.

Young children are very sensitive to high levels of oxygen. Be careful not to expose them to high percentage of oxygen for extended periods unless ordered.

Home Health

If problems are noted in oxygen equipment, contact medical equipment supplier for assistance.

"NO SMOKING" signs should be placed on door of client's home if oxygen is in use.

Clients may require extra-long tubing to permit movement from room to room without moving oxygen cylinder.

A pulse oximeter may be used to assess oxygenation instead of requiring blood samples for blood gases.

Transcultural

- Before touching the client's head, note ethnic/cultural background. Acknowledge related cultural taboos, and discuss alternatives (eg, have client or family member apply cannula/mask).
- With clients of African or Mediterranean descent, exercise caution when assessing for cyanosis, particularly around the mouth, because this area may be dark blue normally. Coloration varies from client to client and should be carefully evaluated on an individual basis.*

*Boyle and Andrews, *Transcultural Concepts in Nursing Care*, Philadelphia: Lippincott Williams & Wilkins, 1999

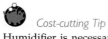

Cost-cutting Tip

Humidifier is necessary only for long-term oxygen therapy via nasal cannula or for rates over 3 to 4 liters/min or if client is dehydrated.

IMPLEMENTATION

Action	Rationale
1. Wash hands, and organize equipment.	*Decreases microorganism transfer* *Promotes efficiency*
2. Explain equipment and procedure to client.	*Decreases anxiety and facilitates cooperation*
3. Insert flow meter into outlet on wall, or place oxygen cylinder near client.	
4. Prepare humidifier: Add distilled water, if needed, or remove prefilled bottle from package and screw enclosed spiked cap to bottle (Fig. 4.5A).	*Delivers moistened oxygen to mucous membranes of airway*
5. Connect humidifier to flow meter (Fig. 4.5B).	*Controls flow of oxygen*
6. Connect humidifier to tubing attached to cannula or mask (Fig. 4.5C).	*Connects humidification to delivery mechanism*
7. Turn on oxygen flow meter until bubbling is noted in humidifier. If no bubbling is noted, check that flow meter is securely inserted, ports of humidifier are patent, and connections are tight. Contact respiratory therapist or supervisor if unable to correct problem.	*Determines if oxygen flow is adequate and connections are intact*
8. Regulate flow meter as ordered (with Venturi masks, attach oxygen percentage regulator to oxygen mask). Regulate flow as indicated.	*Regulates oxygen delivery*
9. Check oxygen flow rate and doctor's orders every 8 hr.	*Ensures correct level of oxygen administration*

Action	Rationale

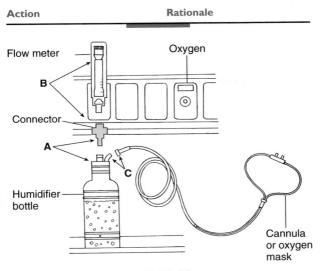

FIGURE 4.5

Action	Rationale
10. Don gloves.	*Avoids contact with secretions*
11. Place oxygen cannula or mask on client.	

Cannula

- Clear nares of secretions with moist cotton balls.	*Removes secretions*
- Place cannula prongs into client's nares.	
- Slip attached tubing around client's ears and under chin (Fig. 4.6). Cotton between tubing and ear may add comfort.	*Holds tubing in place*
- Tighten tubing to secure cannula but make sure client is comfortable.	

Mask

- Place mask over nose, mouth, and chin.	*Places mask correctly*

Action	Rationale

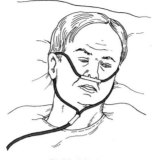

FIGURE 4.6

- Adjust metal strip at nose bridge of mask to fit securely over bridge of client's nose.	*Individualizes fit*
- Pull elastic band around back of head or neck.	*Secures mask*
- Pull band at sides of mask to tighten (Fig. 4.7). Cotton under bridge of face mask may decrease pressure on nose.	*Ensures secure fit*
12. Remove cannula each shift or every 4 hr to assess skin, apply petroleum jelly to nares, and clean away accumulated secretions. Remove mask every 2 to 4 hr, wipe away	*Provides opportunity to assess skin condition* *Promotes comfort* *Prevents infection*

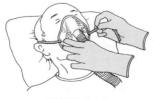

FIGURE 4.7

Action	Rationale
accumulated mist, and assess underlying skin.	
13. Position client for comfort with head of bed elevated.	*Facilitates lung expansion for gas exchange*
14. Dispose of or store equipment appropriately.	*Decreases spread of microorganisms*
15. Place "NO SMOKING" signs on door and over bed.	*Prevents contact of fire with combustible oxygen*
16. Evaluate respirations of client.	

Evaluation

Were desired outcomes achieved?

Documentation

The following should be noted on the client's chart:

- Time of initiation of oxygen therapy
- Amount of oxygen and delivery method
- Respiratory status before and after initiation
- Color of skin and mucous membranes
- Client teaching performed regarding therapy and client understanding of teaching
- Blood gas results

SAMPLE DOCUMENTATION

DATE	TIME	
1/15/02	1200	Client complained of chest pain and shortness of breath. Three L of O_2 begun per nasal cannula. Respiratory rate, 32/min before oxygen administration, decreased to 24/min within 10 min. Resting comfortably, states pain decreased.

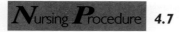

Oral Airway Insertion

EQUIPMENT

- Oral airway
- Equipment for suctioning
- Tape strips—one approximately 20 inches, one 16 inches (may use commercially manufactured airway holder)
- Tongue depressor
- Petroleum jelly
- Mouth moistener or swabs with mouthwash
- Nonsterile gloves

Purpose

Holds tongue forward and maintains open airway
Facilitates easy removal of secretions

Assessment

Assessment should focus on the following:

Level of consciousness, agitation, and ability to push airway from mouth
Respiratory status (respiratory rate, congestion in upper airways), blood pressure, pulse
Color, amount, and consistency of secretions
Alternative methods of maintaining airway

Nursing Diagnoses

The nursing diagnoses may include the following:

Ineffective breathing pattern related to airway blockage by tongue

Outcome Identification and Planning

Desired Outcomes (sample)
The client will attain and maintain clear airway passage, evidenced by nonlabored respirations and clear breath sounds.
Airway is patent and free of secretions.

Skin and mucous membranes of lips and oral area are intact, without dryness or irritation.

Special Considerations

If client is alert and agitated enough to push airway out or resist it, DO NOT INSERT. Airway could stimulate gag reflex and cause client to aspirate. Use another method of maintaining airway, if needed.

If goal is to prevent client from biting on endotracheal tube, use a bite block, preferably a dental bite block, and secure well to prevent block from sliding to back of throat.

IMPLEMENTATION

Action	Rationale
1. Explain procedure to client and family.	*Decreases anxiety and facilitates cooperation*
2. Wash hands and organize equipment.	*Reduces microorganism transfer Promotes efficiency*
3. Lay long strip of tape down with sticky side up and place short strip of tape over it with sticky side down, leaving equal length of sticky tape exposed on either end of long strip. Split either end of tape 2 inches (see Fig. 4.14 and Procedure 4.12). May substitute commercial holder.	*Prepares tape as holder for oral airway*
4. Don gloves.	*Avoids contact with secretions*
5. Rinse airway in cool water.	*Facilitates insertion*
6. Open mouth and place tongue blade on front half of tongue.	*Flattens tongue and opens mouth, facilitating airway insertion*
7. Turn airway on side and insert tip on top of tongue (Fig. 4.8).	*Promotes deeper insertion of airway without stimulating gag*
8. Slide airway in until tip is at lower half of tongue.	*Ensures accurate placement*
9. Remove tongue blade.	
10. Turn airway so tip points toward tongue, (outer ends of airway should be vertical).	*Places tongue under curve of airway, holding tongue forward and away from pharynx*

Action	Rationale

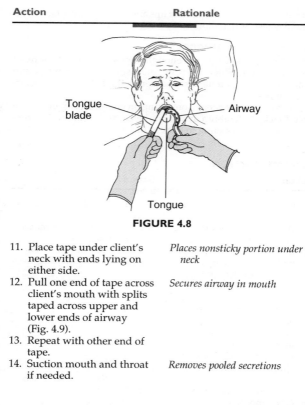

Tongue blade

Airway

Tongue

FIGURE 4.8

Action	Rationale
11. Place tape under client's neck with ends lying on either side.	*Places nonsticky portion under neck*
12. Pull one end of tape across client's mouth with splits taped across upper and lower ends of airway (Fig. 4.9).	*Secures airway in mouth*
13. Repeat with other end of tape.	
14. Suction mouth and throat if needed.	*Removes pooled secretions*

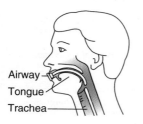

Airway
Tongue
Trachea

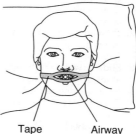

Tape   Airway

FIGURE 4.9

Action	Rationale
15. Swab mouth with moisturizer and mouth-wash.	*Freshens mouth and removes microorganisms*
16. Apply petroleum jelly to lips.	*Decreases dryness of lips*
17. Position client in good alignment and for comfort.	
18. Evaluate respirations of client.	
19. Raise side rails and place call light within reach.	*Ensures safety* *Permits communication*
20. Remove gloves and wash hands.	*Removes microorganisms*

Evaluation

Were desired outcomes achieved?

DOCUMENTATION

The following should be noted on the client's chart:

- Respiratory rate, quality, degree of congestion
- Status of lips and mucous membranes
- Time of airway insertion
- Suctioning and mouth care performed
- Tolerance of procedure

SAMPLE DOCUMENTATION

DATE	TIME	
3/4/02	0830	Client semicomatose, moves arms to painful stimuli. Upper airway congestion noted, with tongue at back of throat. Oral airway inserted, with no resistance. Suctioned clear secretions from mouth. Mouth swabs to oral area, petroleum jelly to lips. No broken skin noted on lips or in oral area.

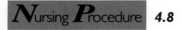 **Nursing Procedure** 4.8

 Nasal Airway Insertion

EQUIPMENT

- Nasal airway
- Equipment for suctioning
- Petroleum jelly
- Moist tissue/cotton balls
- Cotton-tipped swabs
- Nonsterile gloves
- Washcloth

Purpose

Facilitates easy removal of secretions

Assessment

Assessment should focus on the following:

Level of consciousness, agitation, and inability to tolerate oral airway
Available alternative methods of maintaining airway
Respiratory status (respiratory rate, congestion in upper airways)
Blood pressure, pulse
Color, amount, and consistency of secretions

Nursing Diagnoses

The nursing diagnoses may include the following:
Ineffective airway clearance related to excessive secretions

Outcome Identification and Planning

Desired Outcomes (sample)

The client will:

Attain and maintain clear airway passage, as evidenced by smooth, nonlabored respirations, and clear breath sounds
Maintain good skin integrity of nose and intact nasal mucous membranes without dryness or irritation.

Special Considerations

The decision to use continuous or intermittent nasal airway should be based on client's needs and the status of circulation to the underlying tissue. If circulation is poor, the nasal airway may need to be alternated between nares frequently or an alternate method of airway maintenance should be considered.

If airway is difficult to insert, it may be maintained continuously, but it will require frequent checks and care.

Geriatric

Tissue is often thin and fragile, requiring frequent checks and skin care.

Pediatric

The small airway diameter of pediatric clients can easily become obstructed by blood, mucus, vomitus, or the soft tissue of the pharynx; therefore, inspect airway every 1 to 2 hr.

Home Health

Teach family to insert airway and perform maintenance for care between nurse's visits.

IMPLEMENTATION

Action	Rationale
1. Explain procedure to client and family.	*Decreases anxiety* *Facilitates cooperation*
2. Wash hands, and organize equipment.	*Reduces microorganism transfer* *Promotes efficiency*
3. Don gloves.	*Avoids contact with secretions*
4. Ask client to breathe through one naris while the other is occluded.	*Determines patency of nasal passage*
5. Repeat step 4 with other naris.	*Determines patency of nasal passage*
6. Have client blow nose with both nares open (if client is comatose, proceed to next step).	*Facilitates removal of excess mucus and dried secretions*
7. Clean mucus and dried secretions from nares with wet tissue or cotton-tipped swab.	*Clears nasal passage*
8. Lubricate airway.	*Facilitates insertion*
9. Insert airway into naris in a smooth downward arch (Fig. 4.10).	*Decreases trauma to nasal tissue*

Action	Rationale

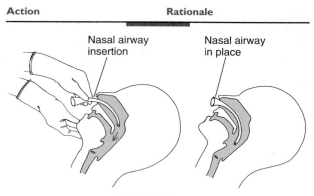

Nasal airway insertion

Nasal airway in place

FIGURE 4.10

Action	Rationale
10. Roll airway from side to side while gently pushing down.	*Promotes deeper insertion of airway without tissue damage*
11. Slide airway in until horn of airway fits against outer naris.	*Ensures accurate placement*
12. Remove excess lubricant.	
13. Suction pharynx and mouth if needed (see Procedure 4.9).	*Removes pooled secretions*
14. Apply petroleum jelly to nares.	*Decreases dryness of nares*
15. Reposition client.	
16. Evaluate client's respirations.	*Determines airway is patent*
17. Discard gloves.	*Decreases spread of organisms*
18. Raise side rails and place call light within reach.	*Facilitates client safety and permits communication*

Maintenance Techniques

Action	Rationale
19. At least once each shift, don gloves, slide airway slightly outward, and inspect underlying tissue.	
20. Lubricate naris with petroleum jelly and massage gently.	*Keeps tissue moist* *Promotes skin circulation*

Action	Rationale
21. Alternate nares (if both are unobstructed) if airway is to be maintained for extended periods or inserted and removed for each suctioning episode.	

Cleaning and Storage

Action	Rationale
22. Remove tube by: - Donning gloves - Gently pulling airway out using a side-to-side twisting motion - Covering tube with wash-cloth as it is withdrawn	*Prevents client from seeing dirty tube*
23. Clean nares with moist cotton ball, and apply petroleum jelly to nares.	*Decreases dryness of nares*
24. Place tube in warm, soapy water, and soak for 5 to 10 min; pass water through tube several times.	*Loosens thick and dried secretions*
25. Use cotton and cotton-tipped swabs to clean lumen of tube.	*Removes secretions*
26. Rinse tube with clear water.	*Removes soap and secretions*
27. Dry lumen with cotton-tipped swabs.	*Removes remaining water*
28. Cover in clean, dry cloth and store at bedside.	*Keeps airway clean and dry for future use*
29. Remove gloves and discard soiled equipment appropriately.	*Removes microorganisms*

Evaluation

Were desired outcomes achieved?

Documentation

The following should be noted on the client's chart:

- Time of airway insertion
- Client's tolerance of procedure

- Suctioning and skin care performed
- Respiratory rate, quality, degree of congestion
- Status of nares

SAMPLE DOCUMENTATION

DATE	TIME	
3/4/02	0830	Client alert, restless, moves arms to painful stimuli. Upper airway congestion noted with tongue at back of throat. Nasal airway inserted with no resistance. Suctioned clear secretions from pharynx. Lemon-glycerin swabs to oral area, petroleum jelly to nasal entrance. No broken skin on nares.

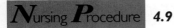 **4.9**

Oral Airway Suctioning

EQUIPMENT

- Suction source (wall suction or portable suction machine)
- Large towel
- Nonsterile gloves
- Irrigation saline or sterile water
- Oral moisturizer swabs
- Mouthwash (optional)
- Petroleum jelly
- Suction catheter (adult, size 14 to 16 French; pediatric, 8 to 12), or oral suction (Yankauer)

Purpose

Clears oral airway of secretions
Facilitates breathing
Decreases halitosis and anorexia

Assessment

Assessment should focus on the following:

Respiratory status (respirations, breath sounds)
Lips and mucous membranes (dryness, color, amount and consistency of secretions)
Ability or desire of client to perform own suctioning

Nursing Diagnoses

The nursing diagnoses may include the following:

Ineffective airway clearance related to weak cough
Altered nutrition: less than body requirements related to excess oral secretions

Outcome Identification and Planning

Desired Outcomes (sample)
The client will:

Attain and maintain a patent upper airway, as evidenced by respiratory rate of 14 to 20 breaths per minute (or within normal limits for client), with clear upper airway and no pooling of oral secretions

Special Considerations
If a client, adult or child, is capable and wishes to manage suctioning independently, provide instruction in the use of the suction catheter or Yankauer.

Pediatric

Suctioning of infants may require two people. Parents may be particularly helpful in assisting and in allaying the infant's fears.

Home Health

A bulb syringe may be purchased at a pharmacy and used.

IMPLEMENTATION

Action	Rationale
1. Explain procedure to client.	*Reduces anxiety*
2. Wash hands and organize equipment.	*Reduces microorganism transfer* *Promotes efficiency*
3. Check suction apparatus for appropriate functioning.	*Maintains safety*
4. Position client in semi-Fowler's or Fowler's position.	*Facilitates forward draining of secretions in mouth*
5. Turn suction source on and place finger over end of attached tubing.	*Tests suction apparatus (use 50- to 120-mmHg pressure)*
6. Open sterile irrigation solution and pour into sterile cup.	*Allows for sterile rinsing of catheter*
7. Open mouthwash and dilute with water (optional).	*Freshens mouth and decreases oral microorganisms*
8. Don gloves.	*Prevents contact with secretions*
9. Open suction catheter package.	*Facilitates organization*

Action	Rationale
10. Place towel under client's chin.	*Prevents soiling of clothing*
11. Attach suction-control port of suction catheter to tubing of suction source.	*Ensures correct attachment of catheter to suction source*
12. Lubricate 3 to 4 inches of catheter tip with irrigating solution.	*Prevents mucosal trauma when catheter is inserted*
13. Ask client to push secretions to front of mouth.	*Facilitates secretion removal*
14. Insert catheter into mouth along jawline and slide to oropharynx until client coughs or resistance is felt. BE SURE FINGER IS NOT COVERING OPENING OF SUCTION PORT.	*Promotes removal of pooled secretions* *Prevents application of suction as catheter is inserted*
15. Withdraw catheter slowly while applying suction. AVOID DIRECT CONTACT OF CATHETER WITH IRRITATED OR TORN MUCOUS MEMBRANES.	*Facilitates removal of secretions from oropharynx* *Prevents additional trauma to oral tissue*
16. Place tip of suction catheter in sterile solution and apply suction for 1 to 2 sec.	*Clears secretions from tubing*
17. Ask client to take three to four breaths while you auscultate for bronchial breath sounds and assess status of secretions.	*Permits reoxygenation* *Determines need for repeat suctioning*
18. Repeat steps 13 to 17 once or twice if secretions are still present.	*Promotes adequate clearing of airway*
19. When secretions are adequately removed, irrigate mouth with 5 to 10 ml of mouthwash and ask client to rinse out mouth.	*Removes microorganisms and thick secretions* *Freshens breath and improves taste sensation*
20. Suction mouth; repeat irrigation and suctioning.	*Removes secretions and residual mouthwash*
21. Disconnect suction catheter from machine tubing, turn off suction source, and discard catheter.	

Action	Rationale
22. Apply petroleum jelly to lips, and mouth moistener to inner lips and tongue, if desired.	*Prevents cracking of lips and maintains moist membranes*
23. Dispose of or store equipment properly.	*Decreases spread of micro-organisms*
24. Position client for comfort with head of bed elevated 45 degrees.	*Lowers diaphragm and promotes lung expansion*
25. Raise side rails and leave call light within reach.	*Promotes safety* *Permits communication*

Evaluation

Were desired outcomes achieved?

DOCUMENTATION

The following should be noted on the client's chart:

- Breath sounds after suctioning
- Character of respirations after suctioning
- Color, amount, and consistency of secretions
- Tolerance to treatment
- Replacement of oxygen equipment on client after treatment

SAMPLE DOCUMENTATION

DATE	TIME	
2/30/02	1400	Suctioned moderate amount of thick, cream-colored secretions from mouth and oropharynx. Mouth care given. Upper airway clear; respirations nonlabored. Ventimask reapplied at 40% FIO_2.

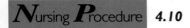

*N*ursing *P*rocedure 4.10

Nasopharyngeal/ Nasotracheal Suctioning

EQUIPMENT

- Suction machine or wall suction setup
- Large towel or linen saver
- Sterile irrigation saline or water
- Suction catheter (adults, size 14 to 16 French; pediatrics, 8 to 12 French)
- Sterile gloves
- Cotton-tipped swabs
- Moist tissue/cotton swabs
- Goggles and mask (optional) or face shield

Purpose

Clears airway of secretions
Facilitates breathing

Assessment

Assessment should focus on the following:

Chart for doctor's order
Respiratory status (respiratory character, breath sounds)
Circulatory indicators (skin color and temperature, capillary re-
  fill, blood pressure, pulse)
Nasal skin and mucous membranes
Color, amount, and consistency of secretions
Facility policy regarding use of irrigation in suctioning

Nursing Diagnoses

The nursing diagnoses may include the following:

Ineffective airway clearance related to weak cough
Anxiety related to inability to breathe effectively

Outcome Identification and Planning

Desired Outcomes (sample)

The client's respirations are 14 to 20 breaths per minute, of normal depth, smooth, and symmetric.

Upper lung fields are clear; no cyanosis.

Special Considerations

Clients sensitive to decreased oxygen levels should be suctioned for shorter durations, but more frequently, to ensure adequate airway clearance without hypoxia.

Whenever possible, an assistant should be secured to minimize unnecessary tube manipulation and to facilitate bagging with less risk of contamination.

Pediatric

Two people may be required to suction infants and children to minimize trauma.

Proper length for insertion of suction catheter should be determined by measuring from the tip of the child's nose to the ear lobe, then to the midsternum. The premeasured length should be used, *not* the stimulated cough, to prevent tracheal trauma.

 Cost-cutting Tip

Depending on brand used, suction catheter kits are less expensive than the items gathered individually.

IMPLEMENTATION

Action	Rationale
1. Explain procedure to client.	*Reduces anxiety*
2. Wash hands and organize equipment.	*Reduces microorganism transfer* *Promotes efficiency*
3. Apply nonsterile gloves.	*Prevents contact with secretions*
4. Position client in semi-Fowler's position.	*Facilitates maximal breathing during procedure*
5. Turn suction machine on and place finger over end of tubing attached to suction machine.	*Tests suction pressure (use 60 mmHg for children and up to 120 mmHg for adults for normal secretions)*
6. Open sterile irrigation solution and pour into sterile cup.	*Allows for sterile rinsing of catheter*
7. Open sterile gloves and suction catheter package.	*Maintains aseptic procedure*

Action	Rationale
8. Place towel under client's chin.	*Prevents soiling of clothing*
9. Ask client to breathe through one naris while the other is occluded.	*Determines patency of nasal passage*
10. Repeat step 9 with other naris.	*Determines patency of nasal passage*
11. Have client blow nose with both nares open.	*Clears nasal passage without pushing microorganisms into inner ear*
12. Clean mucus and dried secretions from nares with moist tissues or cotton-tipped swabs.	*Clears nasal passage*
13. Don sterile glove on dominant hand.	*Maintains sterile technique*
14. Holding suction catheter in sterile hand, attach suction-control port to tubing of suction source (held in nonsterile hand).	*Maintains sterility while establishing suction*
15. Slide sterile hand from control port to suction catheter tubing (wrap tubing partially around hand).	*Facilitates control of tubing*
16. Lubricate 3 to 4 inches of catheter tip with irrigating solution.	*Prevents mucosal trauma when catheter is inserted*
17. Ask client to take several deep breaths—with oxygen source nearby.	*Provides additional oxygen to body tissues before suctioning*
18. Insert catheter into an unobstructed naris, using a slanted downward motion. BE SURE FINGER IS NOT COVERING OPENING OF SUCTION PORT.	*Facilitates unrestricted insertion of catheter* *Prevents trauma to membranes due to suction from catheter*
19. As catheter is being inserted, ask client to open mouth.	*Allows for visibility of tip of catheter once inserted*
20. Proceed to step 21 for pharyngeal suctioning or to step 26 for nasotracheal suctioning.	

Action	Rationale

Nasopharyngeal Suctioning

21. Once catheter is visible in back of throat or resistance is felt, place thumb over suction port (Fig. 4.11).

Applies suction

22. Withdraw catheter in a circular motion, rotating it between thumb and finger. SUCTION SHOULD NOT BE APPLIED FOR MORE THAN 10 SEC.

Promotes cleaning of large area and sides of lumen

Prevents unnecessary hypoxia

23. Place tip of suction catheter in sterile solution and apply suction for 1 to 2 sec.

Clears secretions from tubing

24. Allow client to take about five breaths while you listen to bronchial breath sounds and assess status of secretions.

Determines if repeat suctioning is needed

25. Repeat steps 18 to 24 once or twice if assessment indicates that secretions have not cleared well. Proceed to step 34 for completion of procedure.

Promotes adequate clearing of airway

Nasotracheal Suctioning

26. Once catheter is visible in back of throat or resistance is felt, ask client to pant or cough.

Opens trachea and facilitates entrance into trachea

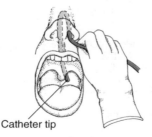

Catheter tip

FIGURE 4.11

Action	Rationale
27. With each pant or cough, attempt to insert the catheter deeper.	*Decreases resistance to catheter insertion*
28. Place thumb over suction port.	*Initiates suction of secretions*
29. Encourage client to cough.	*Facilitates loosening and removal of secretions*
30. Withdraw catheter in a circular motion, rotating it between thumb and finger.	*Minimizes adherence of catheter to the sides of the airway*
SUCTION SHOULD NOT BE APPLIED FOR MORE THAN 10 SEC.	*Prevents unnecessary hypoxia*
31. Place tip of suction catheter in sterile solution and apply suction for 1 to 2 sec.	*Clears clogged tubing*
32. Allow client to take about five breaths while you listen to bronchial breath sounds and assess status of secretions.	*Determines if repeat suctioning is needed*
33. Repeat steps 18 to 32 once or twice if assessment indicates that secretions have not cleared well.	*Promotes adequate clearing of airway*
34. To complete the suctioning procedure:	
- Perform oral airway suctioning.	*Clears secretions from oral airway*
- Disconnect suction catheter from suction tubing and turn off suction machine.	
- Properly dispose of or store all equipment.	*Prevents spread of micro-organisms*
35. Assess incisions and wounds for drainage and approximation.	*Detects complications, such as bleeding or weakened incisions, from coughing and straining*
36. Position client for comfort.	*Facilitates slow, deep breathing*
37. Raise side rails and leave call light within reach.	*Promotes safety* *Permits communication*
38. Wash hands.	*Removes microorganisms*

Evaluation

Were desired outcomes achieved?

DOCUMENTATION

The following should be noted on the client's chart:

- Breath sounds after suctioning
- Character of respirations
- Significant changes in vital signs
- Color, amount, and consistency of secretions
- Tolerance to treatment (eg, state of incisions, drains)
- Replacement of oxygen equipment on patient after treatment

SAMPLE DOCUMENTATION

DATE	TIME	
12/3/02	0400	Suctioned moderate amount of thick, cream-colored secretions via nasopharynx (nasotrachea). Lungs clear in all fields after suctioning. Client slightly short of breath after procedure. Deep breaths with 100% O_2 taken. Respirations are 22, smooth and nonlabored. O_2 per nasal cannula reapplied at 3 L/min. Chest dressing dry and intact.

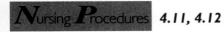

 Endotracheal Tube Suctioning (4.11)

 Endotracheal Tube Maintenance (4.12)

🖥 EQUIPMENT

- 5-ml syringe
- Nonsterile gloves
- Suction machine or wall suction setup
- Sterile gloves (in kit)
- Large towel (or linen saver, possibly in kit)
- Sterile irrigation saline in sterile container
- Suction catheter or kit (adult, 14 to 16 French; pediatric, 6½ to 12 French)
- Irrigation saline (prefilled tubes or a filled 3- to 10-ml syringe)
- Wrist restraints (optional)
- Goggles or protective glasses
- Gown or protective apron
- Face mask
- Endotracheal tube holder, 1-inch tape, or Elastoplast
- Benzoin or skin preparation (optional)
- Nasal/oral care items (eg, oral swabs or moistener, cotton swabs)
- Petroleum jelly
- Sphygmomanometer

Purpose

Maintains open airway for breathing assistance and continuous positive airway pressure
Facilitates maximum clearance of secretions

Assessment

Assessment should focus on the following:

Doctor's orders
Airway patency (clear inspiratory and expiratory breath sounds, absence of mucous plugs in tubing, consistency of secretions, absence of triggering of ventilator pressure alarm)

Ventilation adequacy (respiratory rate of 12–16 breaths per minute or within range of baseline rate; respirations even and nonlabored; mucous membranes and nailbeds pink)

Endotracheal (ET) tube stability (tube placed securely; cuff properly inflated with minimum or no leak audible; pressure in cuff at 14–18 mmHg or 20–25 cm H_2O)

Functioning of oxygen apparatus (chest rises with ventilator cycle, excursion symmetric, breath sounds audible bilaterally to bases, and respiratory rate not less than ventilator rate setting [with mandatory ventilation setting—intermittent mandatory ventilation (IMV)])

Apparatus settings: Oxygen level (FIO_2), type of setting (assist-control or mandatory ventilations), tidal volume, and positive end expiratory pressure (PEEP) or continuous positive airway pressure (CPAP)

Orientation of client (tendency to pull or disconnect tubing, resist ventilation, or resist suctioning)

Nursing Diagnoses

The nursing diagnoses may include the following:

Inadequate respiratory pattern related to muscle paralysis
Ineffective airway clearance related to weak cough
Anxiety related to inability to breathe effectively

Outcome Identification and Planning

Desired Outcomes (sample)
The client's:

Respirations are 14 to 20 breaths per minute, of normal depth, smooth, and symmetric.
Lung fields are clear; no cyanosis.
Nasal or oral passage is free of skin breakdown.

Special Considerations

Clients sensitive to decreased oxygen levels (eg, with head injury or with possibly increased intracranial pressure) must be well ventilated and oxygenated before beginning suctioning to prevent carbon dioxide buildup. Suction these clients briefly, and increase frequency of suctioning.

For maximum client safety and oxygenation during suctioning and tracheostomy care, an assistant should be secured before beginning the procedure.

Confused clients or pediatric clients may need to be restrained. Place them in soft wrist restraints to prevent ET tube dislodgment.

Geriatric

The skin is often thin and sensitive to pressure in the elderly; therefore, special care should be taken to avoid breakdown.

Pediatric

The head may need to be stabilized with sandbags to prevent extubation.

Use two people when performing suctioning or ET tube care.

Home Health

May substitute oxygen saturation per oximeter for blood gases.

An emergency power source must be available for ventilator-dependent clients.

 Cost-cutting Tip

In-line suction circuits are less expensive than items assembled individually; goggles, mask, and face shields are not needed.

IMPLEMENTATION

Action	Rationale

Procedure 4.11 Endotracheal Tube Suctioning

Action	Rationale
1. Explain procedure to client.	*Reduces anxiety*
2. Wash hands and organize equipment.	*Reduces microorganism transfer* *Promotes efficiency*
3. Perform any procedures that loosen secretions (eg, postural drainage, percussion, nebulization).	*Facilitates removal of secretions from all lobes*
4. If changing ET tube, prepare tape (see Procedure 4.12). To determine length of catheter to be inserted: - *Nasal tracheal*—measure distance from tip of nose to earlobe and along side of neck to thyroid cartilage (Adam's apple). - *Oral tracheal*—measure from mouth to mid-sternum.	*Maintains proper tube placement*

Action	Rationale
5. Don gloves, goggles, gown, and mask.	*Protects nurse from contact with secretions*
6. Position client on side or back with head of bed elevated.	*Facilitates maximal breathing during procedure*
7. Turn suction machine on and place finger over end of tubing attached to suction machine.	*Tests suction pressure (should range from 50 mmHg in infants to 120 mmHg in adults)*
8. Open sterile irrigation solution and pour into sterile cup.	*Allows for sterile rinsing of catheter*
9. Open sterile gloves and suction catheter package.	*Maintains sterility of procedure*
10. Place towel under client's chin.	*Prevents soiling of clothing*
11. Don sterile glove on dominant hand.	*Maintains sterile technique*
12. Pick up suction catheter with sterile hand and attach suction-control port to tubing of suction source (held with nonsterile hand).	*Maintains sterility* *Ensures correct attachment of catheter*
13. Slide sterile hand from control port to suction catheter tubing (may wrap tubing around hand).	*Facilitates control of tubing*
14. Lubricate 3 to 4 inches of catheter tip with irrigating solution.	*Facilitates passage of suction catheter into ET tube*
15. Set oxygen on Ambu breathing bag to 100% and turn on full flow.	
16. Have assistant deliver ventilations (Fig. 4.12): - Disconnect oxygen supply tubing, and attach Ambu bag. - Administer three to five deep ventilations, or allow client to take three to five deep breaths, if able. - Remove Ambu bag.	*Provides additional oxygen to body tissues before suctioning*

Action	Rationale

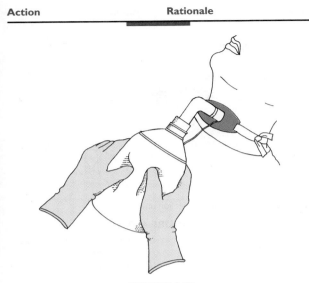

FIGURE 4.12

17. Perform suction
    maneuvers:
    - Insert catheter into ET
      tube using a slanted,
      downward motion
      (Fig. 4.13). BE SURE   *Prevents trauma to membranes*
      FINGER IS NOT   *due to suction from catheter*
      COVERING OPENING
      OF SUCTION PORT.
      Continue insertion until
      resistance is met or
      coughing is stimulated.
      If catheter meets resist-
      ance after being inserted
      the expected distance, it
      may be on the carina. If
      so, pull back 1 cm before
      advancing further or
      suctioning.
    - Place thumb over suction   *Applies suction*
      port.

Action	Rationale

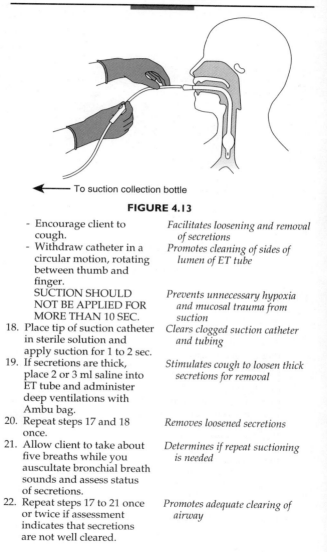

← To suction collection bottle

FIGURE 4.13

- Encourage client to cough.	*Facilitates loosening and removal of secretions*
- Withdraw catheter in a circular motion, rotating between thumb and finger.	*Promotes cleaning of sides of lumen of ET tube*
SUCTION SHOULD NOT BE APPLIED FOR MORE THAN 10 SEC.	*Prevents unnecessary hypoxia and mucosal trauma from suction*
18. Place tip of suction catheter in sterile solution and apply suction for 1 to 2 sec.	*Clears clogged suction catheter and tubing*
19. If secretions are thick, place 2 or 3 ml saline into ET tube and administer deep ventilations with Ambu bag.	*Stimulates cough to loosen thick secretions for removal*
20. Repeat steps 17 and 18 once.	*Removes loosened secretions*
21. Allow client to take about five breaths while you auscultate bronchial breath sounds and assess status of secretions.	*Determines if repeat suctioning is needed*
22. Repeat steps 17 to 21 once or twice if assessment indicates that secretions are not well cleared.	*Promotes adequate clearing of airway*

Action	Rationale
23. Deflate ET tube cuff and repeat suctioning (steps 17 and 18).	*Removes secretions pooled above tube cuff*
24. Reinflate cuff to appropriate pressure.	*Prevents trauma to tracheal tissue from excessive pressure*
25. Suction oral airway and perform oral care (see Procedure 4.9).	Removes pooled secretions
26. Disconnect suction catheter from suction tubing and turn off suction machine.	
27. Assess incisions and wounds for approximation and drainage.	*Promotes early detection of complications or bleeding*
28. Position client with head of bed at 45 degrees, side rails up, and call light within reach (restraints on, if ordered and required).	*Maximizes lung expansion* *Facilitates communication and client safety* *Prevents tube dislodgment*
29. Discard equipment appropriately.	*Promotes clean environment*
30. Proceed to Procedure 4.12 to perform routine maintenance or to change tube holder.	

Closed Tracheal or In-Line Suctioning

1—3. Follow steps 1, 2, and 3 of Procedure 4.11.	
4. Attach 10-cc unit dose saline to the lavage/rinse port.	*Prepares for lavage and rinse*
5. Attach suction connecting tube if not already attached.	*Prepares for the suctioning and removal of secretions from the client*
6. Turn on suction 15% to 20% higher than usual (120 mmHg).	*Adjusts for the extra length of the tracheal care catheter*
7. Advance catheter 1 to 2 inches down tracheal tube or 4 to 5 inches down ET tube.	*Begins to move catheter into position for secretion removal*
8. Instill 3 to 5 cc saline solution.	*Lubricates catheter and stimulates cough*
9. Turn on thumb port.	*Allows suction*

Action	Rationale
10. Stabilize the ET tube with the non-dominant hand while advancing the catheter 2 inches at a time until the carina is reached (at premeasured point for child).	*Avoids movement of the ET tube while advancing the catheter*
11. Pull back 1 cm and begin withdrawing slowly, using continuous suction.	*Prevents trauma to membranes due to suction from catheter*
12. Repeat as necessary.	
13. Withdraw the catheter until the black line can be seen through the bag.	*Ensures that catheter is out of airway*
14. Depress the thumb port and hold it down while gently squeezing in the remaining saline from the unit dose syringe.	*Allows for rinsing of catheter*
15. Lock thumb port.	*Prevents inadvertent application of suction*
16. Close lavage/rinse port.	*Closes potential entry port into catheter*
17. Position catheter in secure area.	*Prevents inadvertent displacement of the catheter*
18. Then follow steps 21 to 30 of Procedure 4.11.	

Procedure 4.12 Endotracheal Tube Maintenance

Action	Rationale
1. Don nonsterile gloves.	
2. Every 2 hr, assess client for:	
- Level of consciousness, respiratory status, vital signs, and temperature.	*Determines whether client is adequately oxygenated*
IF CLIENT IS CONFUSED, USE SOFT WRIST RESTRAINTS (obtain doctor's order, if required).	*Prevents client from dislodging ET tube*
- Symmetry of chest excursion with inspiration and presence of breath sounds bilaterally.	*Determines correct tube placement (main stem bronchus)*
3. Inspect ET tube every 2 to 4 hr to determine if obstructed by kinks, mucous plugs, secretions, or client's bite.	*Indicates need for suctioning, tube repositioning, or bite block to maintain patency*

Action	Rationale
Check ventilator, if applicable, for high or increasing ventilation pressures.	*Indicates resistance to flow of air*
4. Check tube holder or tape for severe odor, soiling, and stability. IF ET TUBE HOLDER/TAPE REQUIRES REPLACEMENT, ENLIST AN ASSISTANT TO HOLD TUBE STABLE.	*Indicates need for adjustment or replacement of holder/tape* *Maintains placement of tube during manipulation*
5. Replace tape/holder only when needed. To replace holder, see vendor's instructions. To prepare tape to secure tube:	
- Tear two long strips of tape (one 14 inches, the other 24 inches).	
- Lay 24-inch strip of tape down with sticky side up.	
- Place short strip of tape (sticky side down) on center of 24-inch strip.	*Prepares nonsticky area of tape for neck*
- Split each end of 24-inch strip 4 inches (Fig. 4.14).	*Facilitates secure taping of ET tube*
- Place nonsticky tape under client's neck.	

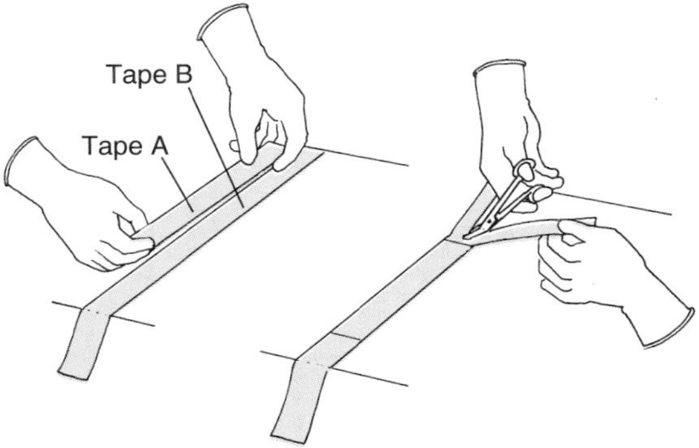

Tape B

Tape A

FIGURE 4.14

Action	Rationale

- For oral tube, position tube in corner of mouth, grasp one sticky tape end, press half of split tape end across upper lip, and wrap other half around the tube (Figure 4.15). Repeat steps with other end of tape.
- For nasal tube, press half of split tape end across upper lip and wrap other half around tube. DO NOT OCCLUDE NARIS. Repeat steps with other end of tape.
  (Use of Elastoplast or application of benzoin may provide a secure holder.)

Resists perspiration and skin oils

6. With *nasal ET tube*, inspect naris for redness, drainage, ulcer, or pressure area around tube.

Constant pressure to tissue due to immobility of nasal tube compromises blood flow

With *oral ET tube*, inspect oral cavity and lips for irritation, ulcer, or pressure areas. Rotate tube position to opposite side of mouth every 24 to 48 hr.

Detects development of skin breakdown

Prevents continuous pressure on one area of lips

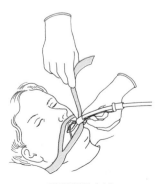

FIGURE 4.15

Action	Rationale
7. Perform oral care every 2 to 4 hr (suctioning, swabs, petroleum jelly to lips).	*Removes pooled secretions and moistens lips and mucous membranes*
8. Assess cuff status (see Procedure 4.16).	*Prevents tracheal tissue damage from cuff overinflation*
9. Properly dispose of or store supplies or equipment.	*Prevents spread of micro organisms*
10. Position client for comfort with head of bed at 45 degrees, side rails up, call light within reach (and restraint on, if needed).	*Facilitates lung expansion* *Permits communication* *Ensures client safety*
11. Wash hands.	*Decreases spread of organisms*

Evaluation

Were desired outcomes achieved?

Documentation

The following should be noted on the client's chart:

- Breath sounds after suctioning
- Character of respirations
- Significant changes in vital signs
- Color, amount, and consistency of secretions
- Status of oral or nasal passage
- Tolerance of treatment (eg, state of incisions, drains)
- Replacement of oxygen equipment after treatment

SAMPLE DOCUMENTATION

DATE	TIME	
12/3/03	0400	Suctioned moderate amount of thick, cream-colored secretions via ET tube. Lungs clear in all fields after suctioning. Respirations smooth and non-labored. Ventilator resumed with IMV 6, FIO_2 40%; spontaneous respirations 10 to 14/min. Lips and mucous membranes pink and without irritation. Right chest incision line dry and intact.

Tracheostomy Suctioning (4.13)

 Tracheostomy Cleaning (4.14)

 Tracheostomy Dressing and Tie Change (4.15)

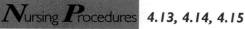

EQUIPMENT

- Tracheostomy care kit
  - sterile bowls or trays (two)
  - cotton-tipped swabs
  - pipe cleaners
  - nonabrasive cleaning brush
  - tracheostomy ties
  - gauze pads
- Normal saline (500-ml bottle)
- Hydrogen peroxide
- Equipment for suctioning:
  - suction machine or wall suction setup
  - suction catheter (size should be half of the lumen of the trachea; adult, 14 to 16 French)
- Pair of nonsterile gloves
- Pair of sterile gloves (often in suction catheter kit)
- Towel or waterproof drape
- Goggles or protective glasses
- Face mask (optional)
- Gown or protective apron (optional)
- Irrigation saline (prefilled tubes or filled 3-, 5-, or 10-ml syringe)
- Hemostat

Purpose

Clears airway of secretions
Facilitates tracheostomy healing
Minimizes tracheal trauma or necrosis

Assessment

Assessment should focus on the following:

Agency policy regarding tracheostomy care
Status of tracheostomy (ie, time since immediate postoperative period)
Type of tracheostomy tube (ie, metal, plastic, cuffed)
Respiratory status (respiratory character, breath sounds)
Color, amount, and consistency of secretions
Skin around tracheostomy site

Nursing Diagnoses

The nursing diagnoses may include the following:

Ineffective airway clearance related to weak cough
Risk of infection related to impaired skin integrity

Outcome Identification and Planning

Desired Outcomes (sample)
The client's:

Respirations are 14 to 20 breaths per minute, of normal depth, smooth, and symmetric.
Upper lung fields are clear; no cyanosis.
Tracheostomy site remains intact without redness or signs of infection.

Special Considerations
For maximum client safety and oxygenation during suctioning and tracheostomy care, an assistant should be secured before beginning procedure.
Clients sensitive to decreased oxygen levels should be suctioned for shorter durations but more frequently to ensure adequate airway clearance without hypoxia or carbon dioxide buildup.
If client has nasogastric (NG) tube and cuffed tracheostomy, monitor closely for signs of pharyngeal trauma.
Client participation in tracheostomy care provides opportunity to teach home care.

Home Health
Clean technique may be substituted for sterile technique in home health care, extended care, and care in other facilities.

Family members should be taught to perform care and assist nurse in care.

Tape hemostat to head of bed or wall above bed for emergency use if tracheostomy tube becomes dislodged.

IMPLEMENTATION

Action	Rationale
1. Explain procedure to client.	*Reduces anxiety*
2. Wash hands and organize equipment.	*Reduces microorganism transfer* *Promotes efficiency*
3. Perform any procedure that loosens secretions (eg, postural drainage, percussion, nebulization)	*Facilitates removal of secretions from all lobes of lungs*

Procedure 4.13 Tracheostomy Suctioning

Action	Rationale
4. Don nonsterile gloves, goggles, gown, and mask.	*Protects nurse from contact with secretions*
5. Position client on side or back with head of bed elevated.	*Facilitates maximal breathing during procedure*
6. Turn suction machine on and place finger over end of tubing attached to suction machine.	*Tests suction pressure (should not exceed 120 mmHg)*
7. Open sterile irrigation solution, and pour into sterile cup.	*Allows for sterile rinsing of catheter*
8. Draw 10 ml sterile saline into syringe and place back into sterile holder (or place 3-ml saline containers on table).	*Provides fluid for irrigation of lungs to loosen secretions during suctioning*
9. If performing tracheostomy care, set up tracheostomy care equipment (see Fig. 4.17 and Procedure 4.14). If not, proceed to step 10.	
10. Increase oxygen concentration to tracheostomy collar or Ambu bag to 100%.	*Increases oxygen level inspired before suctioning*
11. Open sterile gloves and suction catheter package.	*Ensures aseptic procedure*

Action	Rationale
12. Place towel or drape on client's chest under tracheostomy.	*Prevents soiling of clothing*
13. Place sterile glove on dominant hand.	*Maintains sterile technique*
14. Pick up suction catheter with sterile hand and attach suction-control port to tubing of suction source (held with non-sterile hand).	*Maintains sterility* *Ensures correct attachment of catheter*
15. Slide sterile hand from control port to suction catheter tubing (may wrap tubing around hand).	*Facilitates control of tubing*
16. Lubricate 3 to 4 inches of catheter tip with irrigating solution.	*Prevents mucosal trauma when catheter is inserted*
17. Ask client to take several deep breaths with tracheostomy collar intact (Fig. 4.16) or Ambu bag at tracheostomy tube entrance. If necessary,	*Provides additional oxygen to body tissues before suctioning*

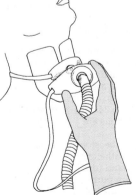

FIGURE 4.16

Action	Rationale
	have assistant deliver four to five deep breaths with Ambu bag.	
18.	Remove tracheostomy collar or Ambu bag.	*Allows entrance into tracheostomy*
19.	Insert catheter approximately 6 inches into inner cannula (or until resistance is met or cough reflex is stimulated). BE SURE FINGER IS NOT COVERING OPENING OF SUCTION PORT.	*Places catheter in upper airway and facilitates clearance* *Prevents trauma to membranes due to suction from catheter*
20.	Encourage client to cough.	*Facilitates loosening and removal of secretions*
21.	Place thumb over suction port.	*Initiates suction of secretions (often catheter stimulates cough)*
22.	Withdraw catheter in a circular motion, rotating catheter between thumb and finger. Intermittent release and application of suction during withdrawal is recommended. APPLY SUCTION FOR NO MORE THAN 10 SEC.	*Facilitates removal of secretions from sides of the airway* *Prevents unnecessary hypoxia* *Minimizes trauma to mucosa*
23.	Place tip of suction catheter in sterile solution, and apply suction for 1 to 2 sec.	*Clears clogged tubing*
24.	Allow client to take about five breaths while you auscultate bronchial breath sounds and assess status of secretions.	*Assesses if repeat suctioning is needed* *Permits reoxygenation*
25.	Repeat steps 19 to 24 once or twice if secretions are still present.	*Promotes adequate clearing of airway*
26.	If performing tracheostomy cleaning, wrap catheter around sterile hand (do not touch suction port) and proceed to step 4 of Procedure 4.14.	*Maintains sterility and control*

Action	Rationale

27. If not performing tracheostomy cleaning or dressing/tie change, discard materials. — *Completes procedure*

28. Position client for comfort and place call light within reach. — *Provides for client safety and communication*

29. Wash hands. — *Prevents spread of micro-organisms*

Procedure 4.14 Tracheostomy Cleaning

1. If tracheostomy cleaning is to follow tracheostomy suctioning, leave suction catheter around sterile hand (see Procedure 4.13) and proceed to step 4. — *Clears secretions / Maintains sterility*

2. If suctioning is not required, set up tracheostomy care equipment (Fig. 4.17):
   - Open tracheostomy care kit and spread package on bedside table. — *Provides sterile field*

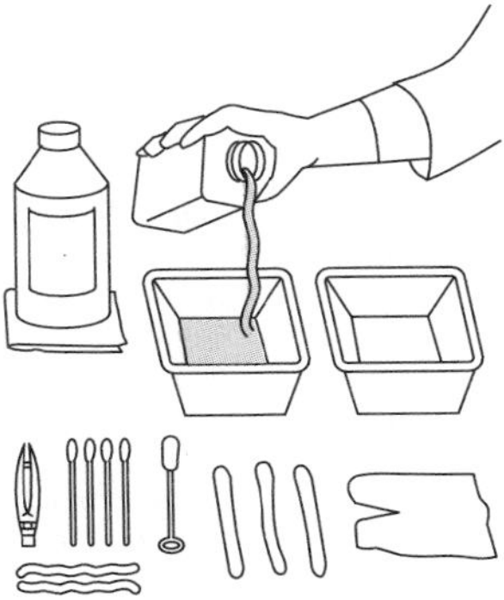

FIGURE 4.17

Action	Rationale
- Maintaining sterility, place bowls and tray with supplies in separate locations on paper.	*Arranges equipment for easy access without contamination*
- Open sterile saline and peroxide bottles, and fill first bowl with equal parts of peroxide and saline (do not touch container to bowl).	*Provides half-strength peroxide mixture for tracheostomy cannula cleaning*
	Maintains sterility of supplies
- Fill second bowl with saline.	*Provides rinse for cannula*
- Don sterile gloves.	
3. Place four cotton-tipped swabs in peroxide mixture, then place across tracheal care tray.	*Provides moist swabs for cleaning skin*
4. Pick up one sterile gauze with fingers of sterile hand.	*Allows nurse to touch nonsterile items while maintaining sterility*
5. Stabilize neck plate with nonsterile hand (or have assistant do so).	*Decreases discomfort and trauma during removal of cannula*
6. With sterile hand, use gauze to turn inner cannula counterclockwise until catch is released (unlocked).	*Separates inner and outer cannulas*
7. Gently slide cannula out using an outward and downward arch (Fig. 4.18).	*Follows curve of tracheostomy tube*
8. Place cannula in bowl of half-strength peroxide.	*Softens secretions*
9. Discard gauze.	*Avoids contaminating sterile items*
10. Unwrap catheter and suction outer cannula of tracheostomy.	*Removes remaining secretions*
11. Have client take deep breaths or use Ambu bag to deliver 100% oxygen.	*Provides oxygenation after suctioning*
12. Disconnect suction catheter from suction tubing and discard sterile glove and catheter.	*Prevents spread of micro-organisms*

Action	**Rationale**

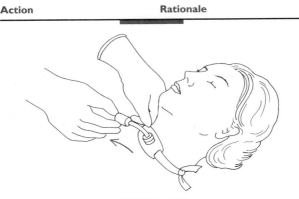

FIGURE 4.18

13. Remove tracheostomy dressing.

Exposes skin for cleaning

14. Using gauze pads, wipe secretions and crustation from around tracheostomy tube.

Removes possible airway obstruction and medium for infection

15. Use moist swabs to clean area under neck plate at insertion site.

Decreases possible infection

16. Discard gloves.

Prevents spread of micro-organisms

17. Don sterile gloves.

18. Pick up inner cannula and scrub gently with cleaning brush.

Removes crustation and secretions from outside and inside of cannula

19. Use pipe cleaners to clean lumen of inner cannula thoroughly.

Decreases accumulation of mucus in lumen

20. Run inner cannula through peroxide mixture.

Removes remaining debris

21. Rinse cannula in bowl containing sterile saline.

Rinses away peroxide mixture and residual debris

22. Place cannula in sterile gauze and dry thoroughly; use dry pipe cleaner to remove residual moisture from lumen.

Prevents introduction of fluid into trachea

Action	Rationale
23. Slide inner cannula into outer cannula (keeping inner cannula sterile), using smooth inward and downward arch and rolling inner cannula from side to side with fingers.	*Facilitates insertion and reduces resistance*
24. Hold neck plate stable with other hand and turn inner cannula clockwise until catch (lock) is felt and dots are in alignment.	*Ensures that inner cannula is securely attached to outer cannula*
25. If performing tracheostomy dressing or tie change, proceed to Procedure 4.15.	
26. If not performing dressing or tie change, discard materials, wash hands, and position client for comfort.	*Completes procedure and prevents spread of micro-organisms*

Procedure 4.15 Tracheostomy Dressing and Tie Change

1. Have assistant hold tracheostomy by neck plate while you clip old tracheostomy ties and remove them.	*Prevents accidental dislodgment of tracheostomy during tie replacement*
2. Slip end of new tie through tie holder on neck plate, and tie a square knot 2 to 3 inches from neck plate (Fig. 4.19).	*Facilitates removal of tie while holding tracheostomy tube firm*
3. Place tie around back of client's neck and repeat above step with other end of tie, cutting away excess tie.	
4. Apply tracheostomy dressing: - Hold ends of tracheostomy dressing (or open gauze and fold into V shape).	*Places dressing in position to catch secretions from tracheostomy or surrounding insertion site*

Action **Rationale**

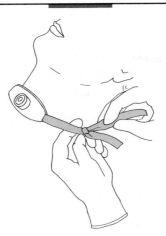

FIGURE 4.19

- Gently lift neck plate
  and slide end of dressing
  under plate and tie.
- Pull other end of
  dressing under neck
  plate and tie.
- Slide both ends up
  toward neck, using a
  gentle rocking motion,
  until middle of dressing
  (or gauze) rests under
  neck plate (Fig. 4.20).
5. Position client for comfort.
6. Discard materials and   *Reduces spread of infection*
   wash hands.
7. Raise side rails and leave   *Facilitates client safety*
   call light within reach.   *Permits communication*

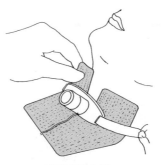

FIGURE 4.20

Evaluation

Were desired outcomes achieved?

Documentation

The following should be noted on the client's chart:

- Breath sounds after suctioning
- Character of respirations
- Status of tracheostomy site
- Significant changes in vital signs
- Color, amount, and consistency of secretions
- Tolerance to treatment (ie, state of incisions, drains)
- Replacement of oxygen equipment after treatment

SAMPLE DOCUMENTATION

DATE	TIME	
7/3/02	0400	Suctioned moderate amount of thick, cream-colored secretions via trachea. Lungs clear in all fields after suctioning. Tracheostomy care done. Stoma site dry, with no redness or swelling. Client slightly short of breath after procedure. Respirations smooth and nonlabored after deep breaths with 100% O_2 taken. O_2 per tracheostomy collar reapplied at 30%. Client tolerated procedure with no pain or excess gagging. Client observed procedure with mirror to learn care procedure.

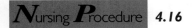 **4.16**

 Tracheostomy/Endotracheal
Tube Cuff Management

EQUIPMENT

- 10-ml syringe
- Blood pressure manometer
- Three-way stopcock
- Mouth-care swabs, moistener, and mouthwash
- Suctioning equipment
- Nonsterile gloves

Purpose

Maintains minimum amount of air in cuff to ensure adequate
ventilation without trauma to trachea

Assessment

Assessment should focus on the following:

Size of cuff
Maximum cuff inflation pressure (check cuff box)
Bronchial breath sounds
Respiratory rate and character
Agency policy or doctor's orders regarding cuff care

Nursing Diagnoses

The nursing diagnoses may include the following:

Ineffective airway clearance related to thick secretions

Outcome Identification and Planning

Desired Outcomes (sample)
The client's respirations are 14 to 20 breaths per minute, of nor-
mal depth, smooth, and symmetric.
The client's lung fields are clear; no cyanosis.
Minimum occlusive pressure is maintained while cuff is inflated.
The client experiences no undetected tracheal damage.

Special Considerations

Some cuffs are low-pressure cuffs and require minimum manipulation; however, client should still be monitored periodically
to ensure proper cuff function.

Pediatric

Tracheal tissue is extremely sensitive in pediatric clients.
Smaller cuffs require lower inflation pressures: be very careful
not to overinflate them.

IMPLEMENTATION

Action	Rationale

Cuff Pressure Check (for long-term cuff inflation)

Action	Rationale
1. Wash hands and organize equipment.	*Reduces microorganism transfer* *Promotes efficiency*
2. Check cuff balloon for inflation by compressing between thumb and finger (should feel resistance).	*Indicates cuff is inflated*
3. Attach 10-ml syringe to one end of three-way stopcock. Attach manometer to another stopcock port. Close remaining stopcock port.	*Establishes connection between syringe and manometer*
4. Attach pilot balloon port to closed port of three-way stopcock (Fig. 4.21).	
5. Instill air from syringe into manometer until 10-mmHg reading is obtained.	*Prevents rapid loss of air from cuff*
6. Auscultate tracheal breath sounds, noting presence of smooth breath sounds or gurgling (cuff leak).	*Determines if cuff leak is present*
7. If smooth breath sounds are noted: - Turn stopcock off to manometer. - Withdraw air from cuff until gurgling is noted with respirations.	

Action	Rationale

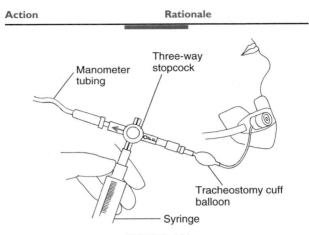

FIGURE 4.21

8. Once gurgling breath sounds are noted, insert air into cuff until gurgling is noted only on inspiration.

Provides minimum leak and minimizes pressure on trachea (airway is larger on inspiration)

9. Turn stopcock off to syringe.

Allows reading of pressure in cuff

10. Note manometer reading as client exhales. Record reading. (Note if pressure exceeds recommended volume. Do not exceed 20 mmHg). Notify physician if excessive leak persists or if excess pressure is needed to inflate cuff.

Expiratory cuff pressure indicates minimum occlusive volume (cuff pressure on tracheal wall)

11. Turn stopcock off to pilot balloon and disconnect.

Intermittent Cuff Inflation

12. Auscultate tracheal breath sounds, noting presence of smooth breath sounds (cuff inflated), or vocalization/hiss (cuff deflated).

Determines if cuff leak is present

Action	Rationale

13. If smooth breath sounds are noted, withdraw air from cuff until faint gurgling is noted with respirations. If vocalization or hiss is noted, insert air into cuff until faint gurgling is noted with respirations.

14. Once gurgling breath sounds are noted, insert air into cuff until gurgling is noted only on inspiration.

Provides minimum leak and minimizes pressure on trachea (airway is larger on aspiration)

15. Monitor breath sounds every 2 hr until cuff is deflated.

Determines that minimum leak remains present

Cuff Maintenance Principles

16. Every 2 to 4 hr, check tracheal breath sounds (more frequently if indicated) and note pressure of pilot balloon between fingers.

Determines if minimum or excessive cuff leak is present

17. Every 8 to 12 hr or per agency policy, check cuff pressure and note if minimum occlusive volume increases or decreases.

Indicates if tracheal tissue damage or softening is occurring or if tracheal swelling is present

18. If oral or tube feedings are being received, assess secretions for tube feeding or food particles.

Indicates possible tracheoesophageal fistula

19. To perform cuff deflation:

Prepares for removal of secretions pooled on top of cuff
Facilitates oxygenation

   - Obtain and set up suctioning equipment.
   - Enlist assistance and perform oral or nasopharyngeal suctioning.

Removes secretions pooled in pharyngeal area

   - Set up Ambu bag (if client is not on ventilator and long-term cuff inflation has been used).

Provides for deep ventilations to move secretions

Action	Rationale
- Have assistant initiate deep sigh with ventilator, or administer deep ventilation with Ambu bag as you remove air from cuff with syringe.	*Pushes pooled secretions into oral cavity as cuff is deflated*
- Suction pharynx and oral cavity again.	*Removes remaining secretions*
20. Perform mouth care with swabs and mouthwash.	*Freshens mouth and moistens mucous membranes*
21. Apply lubricant to lips.	
22. Dispose of supplies appropriately.	
23. Position client for comfort with call light within reach.	*Promotes comfort and safety* *Permits communication*

Evaluation

Were desired outcomes achieved?

Documentation

The following should be noted in the client's chart:

- Cuff pressures noted and tracheal breath sounds
- Suctioning performed and nature of secretions
- Tolerance to procedure (changes in respiratory status and vital signs)

SAMPLE DOCUMENTATION

DATE	TIME	
1/2/02	1800	Tracheal tube cuff checked, with 15-mmHg minimum occlusive pressure noted. Suctioned scant, thin secretions via nasopharynx, then cuff deflated fully. Client remains in bed with head of bed elevated. Respirations even and nonlabored.

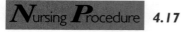

Suctioned Sputum Specimen Collection

EQUIPMENT

- Gown and mask
- Goggles
- Sterile sputum trap
- Suctioning equipment (see procedure for specific type of suctioning)
- Sterile saline in sterile container and prefilled tubes for irrigation
- Specimen bag and labels
- Sterile gloves
- Nonsterile gloves

Purpose

Obtain sputum specimen for analysis while minimizing risk of contamination

Assessment

Assessment should focus on the following:

Doctor's orders for test to be done and method of obtaining specimen

Breath sounds indicating congestion and need for suction

Previous notes of nurses and respiratory therapists to determine if secretions are thick or if catheter insertion (nasotracheal or nasopharyngeal) was difficult

Nursing Diagnoses

The nursing diagnoses may include the following:

Risk of infection related to pooled secretions

Outcome Identification and Planning

Desired Outcomes (sample)

The client's airway is clear of secretions before discharge.
An uncontaminated sputum specimen is obtained.

Special Considerations

Home Health

Time home visits to coincide with scheduled suctioning and specimen collection. Deliver specimen to laboratory immediately.

IMPLEMENTATION

Action	Rationale
1. Explain procedure to client.	*Reduces anxiety*
2. Wash hands and organize equipment.	*Reduces microorganism transfer* *Promotes efficiency*
3. Don clean gloves, goggles, gown, and mask.	*Protects nurse from contact with secretions*
4. Prepare suction equipment for type of suction to be performed (see appropriate procedure in this chapter).	*Promotes efficiency*
5. Open sputum trap package.	
6. Remove sputum trap from package cover and attach suction tubing to short spout of trap.	*Establishes suction for secretion aspiration*
7. Place sterile glove on dominant hand.	*Maintains sterility of process*
8. Wrap suction catheter around sterile hand.	*Maintains control of catheter*
9. Holding catheter suction port in sterile hand and rubber tube of sputum trap with nonsterile hand, connect suction to sputum trap (Fig. 4.22).	*Maintains sterility of procedure*

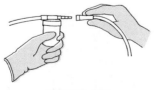

FIGURE 4.22

Action	Rationale
10. Suction client until secretions are collected in tubing and sputum trap. (If secretions are thick and need to be removed from catheter, suction small amount of sterile saline until specimen is cleared from tubing.)	*Obtains specimen* *Facilitates collection of thick sputum specimen*
11. If insufficient amount of sputum is collected, repeat suction process.	*Ensures adequate specimen*
12. Using nonsterile hand, disconnect suction from sputum trap.	
13. Disconnect suction catheter and sputum trap, maintaining sterility of suction catheter control port, trap tubing, and sterile glove.	*Maintains catheter sterility for further suctioning, if needed*
14. Reconnect suction tubing to catheter, and continue suction process, if needed.	*Clears remaining secretions from airway*
15. Discard suction catheter and sterile glove when suctioning is complete.	*Prevents spread of micro-organisms*
16. Connect rubber tubing to sputum trap suction port (Fig. 4.23).	*Seals specimen closed*

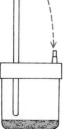 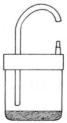 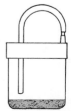

FIGURE 4.23

Action	Rationale
17. Place specimen in plastic bag (if agency policy) and label with client's name, date, time, and nurse's initials.	*Ensures proper identification of specimen* *Prevents spread of micro-organisms*
18. Discard equipment.	
19. Position client for comfort with side rails up and call light within reach.	*Facilitates client comfort and safety*
20. Wash hands.	*Reduces spread of infection*

Evaluation

Were desired outcomes achieved?

Documentation

The following should be noted on the client's chart:

- Date, time, and type of specimen collection
- Type of suction done
- Amount and character of secretions
- Client's tolerance of process

SAMPLE DOCUMENTATION

DATE	TIME	
1/6/02	1415	Sputum specimen obtained by naso-tracheal suctioning. Large amounts of thick, white mucus obtained; cough reflex stimulated, with strong cough noted. Respirations even and non-labored; breath sounds clear. Specimen sent to lab.

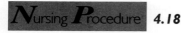 **4.18**

Pulse Oximetry

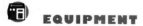 **EQUIPMENT**

- Pulse oximeter
- Sensor (permanent or disposable)
- Alcohol wipe(s)
- Nail polish remover

Purpose

Noninvasive monitoring of the oxygen saturation of arterial blood

Assessment

Assessment should focus on the following:

Other signs and symptoms of hypoxemia (restlessness; confusion; dusky skin, nailbeds, or mucous membranes)
Quality of pulse and capillary refill proximal to potential sensor application site
Respiratory rate and character
Amount and type of oxygen administration, if applicable

Nursing Diagnoses

The nursing diagnosis may include the following:

Impaired gas exchange related to excessive secretions

Outcome Identification and Planning

Desired Outcomes (sample)

Client's arterial oxygen saturation (SaO_2) remains between 90% and 100%.
Client exhibits signs or symptoms of adequate gas exchange evidenced by respirations 18–20, nailbeds pink, capillary refill less than 3 seconds.
Client demonstrates knowledge of exogenous factors affecting pulse oximeter readings (ie, movement-restrictive probe placement, outside light, and anemia)

Special Considerations

Geriatric

Be sensitive to probe placement. This includes tension on probe site, as well as tape applied to dry, thin skin.

Pediatric

Choose appropriate sensor.

Stabilization of sensor may be accomplished only by safely immobilizing the monitoring site. An acceptable alternative monitoring site may be the shaft of the penis.

 Transcultural

- When choosing the earlobe as a site for pulse oximetry in clients of African descent, be sensitive to the presence of keloids. These ropelike scars, which are the result of an exaggerated wound-healing process, may occur as a result of ear piercing.
- These scars may not allow accurate SaO_2 readings.

IMPLEMENTATION

Action	Rationale
1. Wash hands and organize equipment.	*Reduces microorganism transfer Promotes efficiency*
2. Explain procedure to conscious client.	*Decreases anxiety and facilitates cooperation*
3. Choose sensor.	*Sensor types may vary according to weight of client and site considerations*
4. Prepare site (see Pediatric Considerations for alternative site). Use alcohol wipe to cleanse site gently. Remove nail polish or acrylic nails, if needed, when using finger as monitoring site.	*Alcohol wipes aid in ensuring that site is clean and dry* *Frosted or colored nail polish and acrylic nails may interfere with pulse oximetry reading*
5. Check capillary refill and pulse proximal to the chosen site.	*Compromised peripheral circulation, caused by restriction (probe applied too tightly) or poor circulation due to medications or other conditions, may yield false readings*

Action	Rationale

6. Ascertain the alignment of the light-emitting diodes (LEDs) and the photo detector (light-receiving sensor). These sensors should be directly opposite each other (Fig. 4.24).

Sensors that are not properly aligned will not yield an accurate SaO_2 reading via the pulse oximeter

7. Turn the pulse oximeter to the ON position.

   REMEMBER: DISPOSABLE SENSORS NEED TO BE ATTACHED TO THE PATIENT CABLE BEFORE TURNING THE PULSE OXIMETER ON.

The emitting sensors (LEDs) will transmit red and infrared light through the tissue

The receiving sensor (photodetector) will measure the amount of oxygenated hemoglobin (which absorbs more infrared light) and deoxygenated hemoglobin (which absorbs more red light)

SaO_2 will be computed by the pulse oximeter using these data

8. Listen for a beep and note waveform or bar of light on front of pulse oximeter.

Each beep indicates a pulse detected by the pulse oximeter

The light or waveform changes and indicates the strength of the pulse. A weak pulse may not yield an accurate SaO_2

9. Check alarm limits. Reset if necessary. Always make certain that both high and low alarms are on before leaving the patient's room.

Alarm limits for both high and low SaO_2 and high and low pulse rate are preset by the manufacturer but can be easily reset in response to doctor's orders

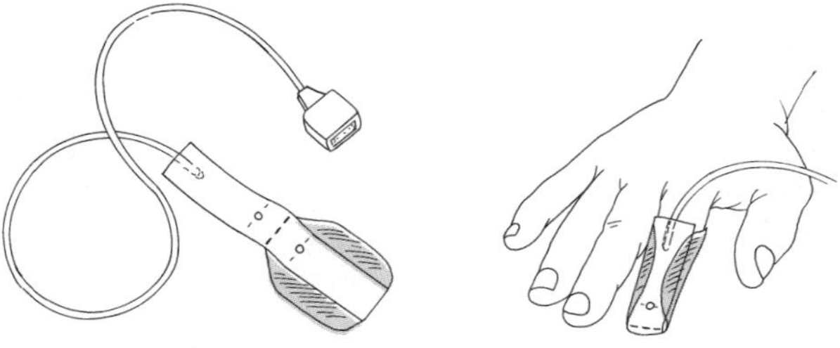

FIGURE 4.24

Action	Rationale
10. Teach patient common position changes that may trigger the alarm, such as bending the elbow or gripping the side rails or other objects.	*Patient participates in care, thus decreasing anxiety*
11. Relocate finger sensor at least every 4 hr. Relocate spring tension sensor at least every 2 hours.	*Prevents tissue necrosis*
12. Check adhesive sensors at least every shift.	*Irritation may occur because of the adhesive*

Evaluation

Were desired outcomes achieved?

Documentation

The following should be noted on the client's chart:

- Type and location of sensor
- Presence of pulse proximal to sensor and status of capillary refill
- Percentage of oxygen saturated in arterial blood (SaO_2)
- Rotation of sensor according to guidelines
- Percentage of oxygen (or room air) client is receiving
- Interventions as a result of deviations from the norm

SAMPLE DOCUMENTATION

DATE	TIME	
7/26/02	1800	Finger sensor (probe) applied to left index finger, capillary refill brisk, radial pulse present. Pulse oximeter yielding SaO_2 of 96% on room air.
	2200	Finger probe applied to right index finger, capillary refill brisk, radial pulse present. Pulse oximeter yielding SaO_2 of 97% on room air.

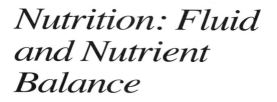

Chapter 5

Nutrition: Fluid and Nutrient Balance

OVERVIEW

▶ Initiation of intake and output measurement is an appropriate nursing decision any time the potential for fluid imbalance is present.

▶ Malnourished clients have a high susceptibility to infection, and nutrition support substances provide a medium for possible microorganism growth; thus, good asepsis is a crucial concern.

▶ Careful monitoring and regulation of fluid administration are essential to prevent a potentially lethal fluid overload.

▶ Intake and output and daily weights are crucial in assessing nutritional support and fluid balance.

▶ Infusion of hyperosmotic solutions into the thoracic cavity or aspiration into the pulmonary tree could result in major respiratory compromise; thus, verification of feeding tube or central line placement is a primary concern in nutritional support.

▶ To prevent possible exposure to infectious organisms, nurses should wear gloves when contact with body fluids is probable.

▶ Some major nursing diagnostic labels related to fluid and nutrient balance are fluid volume excess, fluid volume deficit, risk of decreased cardiac output, and altered nutrition.

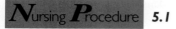

Intake and Output Measurement

EQUIPMENT

- Graduated 1000-ml measuring container
- Graduated water pitcher
- Graduated cups
- Scale
- Nonsterile gloves
- Felt pen or fine-tip marker

Purpose

Facilitates control of fluid balance
Provides data to indicate effects of diuretic or rehydration therapy

Assessment

Assessment should focus on the following:

Doctor's orders for frequency of intake and output (I & O; hourly, every shift, 24-hourly)
Client status indicating need for I & O: edema, poor skin turgor, severely low or high blood pressure, congestive heart failure, dyspnea, reduced urinary output, intravenous infusion
Medications being taken that alter fluid status

Nursing Diagnoses

The nursing diagnoses may include the following:

Fluid volume excess related to excess IV fluid intake
Fluid volume deficit related to anorexia

Outcome Identification and Planning

Desired Outcomes (sample)

Blood pressure, pulse, and respirations are within normal limits.
Skin turgor is normal (ie, pinched skin returns to position immediately before discharge).

Edema is reduced from pitting to nonpitting type within 48 hr.
Client demonstrates an output equal to intake (plus or minus insensible loss).

Special Considerations

Strict I & O involves accounting for incontinent urine, emesis, and diaphoresis, if possible. Weigh soiled linens to determine fluid loss or estimate it.

Family members could be important allies in obtaining accurate I & O measurement. Explain procedure and enlist their assistance.

When measuring output, gloves should be worn to protect the caregiver from exposure to contaminated body fluids.

Pediatric and Geriatric

For pediatric, geriatric, or other incontinent clients without bladder control, weigh diapers as a rough estimate of output (1 g is equal to 1 ml).

Home Health

If the homebound client has difficulty understanding units of measure or seeing calibration lines, make an I & O sheet including columns of drinking glasses, cups of ice, bowls of Jello and soup, and so forth, to represent intake and for client to cross off. Have client measure output by number of voidings.

Delegation

INTAKE AND OUTPUT IS OFTEN DELEGATED TO UNLICENSED PERSONNEL. HOWEVER IV INTAKE MUST BE ADDED TO INTAKE TOTALS, AND THE NURSE MUST ALWAYS CHECK THE INFORMATION GATHERED AND REPORT ANY EVIDENCE OF FLUID OVERLOAD OR DEFICIT.

IMPLEMENTATION

Action	Rationale
1. Wash hands, and organize equipment.	*Reduces microorganism transfer* *Promotes efficiency*
2. Post pad on door or in room, and instruct team members to record intake or output; instruct client and family on use of I & O record, with return demonstration. (If calorie count is in progress, list type of food and fluid consumed as well.)	*Ensures complete, accurate record of I & O* *Allows dietary department to calculate caloric intake correctly based on standard institutional serving sizes*

Action	Rationale

Intake

3. Place graduated cups in room, and request that all fluids be measured in the cups before consumption.

   Ensures common units of measurement
   Minimizes error of measurement

4. Semisolid substance intake should be recorded in percentage or fraction of amount. Most institutions use standard portions.

   Facilitates accurate calculation of intake

5. Measure all oral intake:

   Takes into account the wide variety of fluids consumed orally

   - Water: note volume in pitcher at shift's beginning, plus any fluid added, and subtract fluid remaining in pitcher at shift's end.
   - Ice chips: multiply volume by 0.5.

     When melted, the volume of ice is approximately half its previous volume

   - All liquids (juice, beverage, broth) should be measured in graduated container.
   - Soup: indicate kind; measure volume or obtain standard volume measurement from food services.
   - Jello, ice cream, sherbet: use institution's standard volume or volume on container.

6. Measure nasogastric (NG) or gastric tube feedings:

   Maintains accurate record by including gastrointestinal (GI) intake in addition to oral intake

   - Note volume in bottle hanging at beginning of shift (amount left from previous shift) plus any feeding added during shift. (Allow prior feeding to infuse almost totally before adding new solution.)

     Indicates volume infusing during current shift

     Prevents feeding from hanging for more than 8 hr

Action	Rationale
- Subtract fluid remaining in bag at end of shift (or read infusion total from pump if previous shift has cleared pump total).	*Maintains complete I & O measurement*
- Liquid, oral, or NG medications should be mixed with a measured volume of water.	
7. Measure all IV intake using same methodology as that of step 6. Volume of each type of intake is often designated on flow sheet (eg, colloids, blood products).	*Maintains complete I & O measurement*
8. If NG irrigation is performed and irrigant is left to drain out with other gastric contents, enter irrigant in intake section of flow sheet (or subtract irrigant amount from total output; see step 13).	

Output

Action	Rationale
9. Place one or more (depending on amount of drainage) large, graduated containers in room.	*Maintains accurate output measurement*
	Standardizes measurement units (some containers vary slightly)
For small amounts of drainage (wound drains or scant NG drainage), place graduated cups in room with clearly marked labels.	*Prevents inadvertent use of cup for use of intake*
For drainage measurement, designate if urine measurement from urinals will be used or if urine should be poured into containers.	*Standardizes measurement units (some containers vary)*
10. At end of each shift, or hourly if needed, don gloves and empty drainage into graduated container.	*Minimizes exposure to body fluids*

Action	Rationale
An alternate method of measuring output draining into a graduated container is to mark the level of drainage on a tape strip on the container. Mark drainage level with date and time of each shift, or calibrate in intervals of desired number of hours (Fig. 5.1). When container is nearly full, empty or dispose of container and replace with new container.	*Allows monitoring on a more frequent basis*
11. Record amount and source of drainage, particularly with drains from different sites.	*Identifies abnormal drainage and source*
12. Measure output from:	*Takes into account output from all sources*

- NG or gastrostomy tubes
   - Ostomy drainage
   - Wound drains
   - Chest tube drainage
   - Urinary drainage or voidings
   - Emesis
   - Liquid stool	

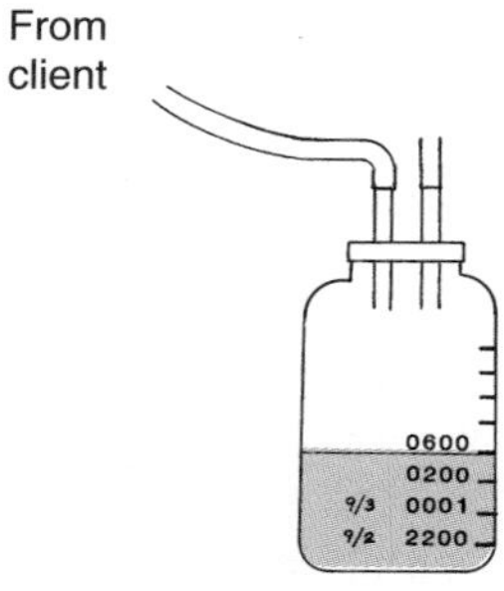

FIGURE 5.1

Action	Rationale
- Blood or serous drainage and extreme diaphoresis (weigh soiled pads or linens and subtract dry weight to estimate output)	
13. If intermittent or ongoing irrigation is performed, calculate true output (urinary or NG) by measuring total output and subtracting total irrigant infused (record only true output or indicate calculations on forms).	*Eliminates the double counting of output*
14. At end of 24-hr period, usually at end of evening or night shift, add total intake and total output. Report extreme I/O discrepancy to doctor (eg, if input is 1 to 2 L more than output). Correlate weight gains with fluid intake excesses.	*Indicates I & O status over 24-hr period*
15. Clean containers, and store in client's room. Discard gloves, and wash hands.	*Prevents spread of infection*

Evaluation

Were desired goals achieved?

Documentation

The following should be noted on the client's chart:

- Intake from all sources on appropriate graphic sheet
- Output from all sources on appropriate graphic sheet
- Medication or fluid given to improve fluid balance and immediate response noted (eg, diuresis, blood pressure increase)
- Vital signs and skin status indicating fluid balance or imbalance

SAMPLE DOCUMENTATION

DATE	TIME	
6/9/02	0600	Client excreted 1200 ml urine after Lasix administration. Ankle diameter measurement remains 6 inches with 2+ pitting edema. D_5W infusing into right wrist angiocath at 10 ml/hr by infusion pump.

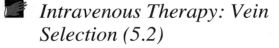

 Intravenous Therapy: Vein Selection (5.2)

 Intravenous Therapy: Solution Preparation (5.3)

 Intravenous Therapy: Catheter/IV Lock Insertion (5.4)

EQUIPMENT

- Nonsterile gloves
- Over-the-needle catheter or butterfly catheter/needle
- IV fluid (if continuous infusion) or infusion plug and heparin flush solution (if IV lock)
- Armboard (optional)
- Infusion tubing (vented for IV fluid bag, unvented for IV bottles)
- IV pole (bed or rolling) or IV pump/controller
- IV insertion kit or supplies:
  - tourniquet (or blood pressure cuff)
  - tape—1 inch wide (or 2-inch tape, cut)
  - alcohol pads
  - povidone pad (optional)
  - ointment (optional)
  - dressing—2 × 2-inch gauze, transparent dressing (Opsite)
  - adhesive bandage
  - adhesive labels
- Razor and soap (optional)
- Towel or linen saver

Purpose

Provides venous route for administration of fluids, medications, blood, or nutrients

Assessment

Assessment should focus on the following:

Reason for initiation of IV therapy for particular client
Orders for type and rate of fluid and/or specified IV site
Status of skin on hands and arms; presence of hair or abrasions; previous IV sites
Client's ability to avoid movement of arms or hands for duration of procedure
Allergy to tape, iodine, antibiotic pads, or ointment
Client knowledge of IV therapy

Nursing Diagnoses

The nursing diagnoses may include the following:

Fluid volume deficit related to poor oral intake
Risk of infection related to invasive procedure
Risk of decreased cardiac output related to systemic vasoconstriction

Outcome Identification and Planning

Desired Outcomes (sample)

The client obtains and maintains fluid and electrolyte balance, as evidenced by good skin turgor, brisk capillary refill, no edema.
IV intake is consistent with ordered rate.
Electrolyte levels are within normal limits.
Client performs self-care activities without disruption of IV assembly.
Verbalize understanding of movement limitations related to IV infusions and complications to be reported to the nurse
IV insertion site is clean and dry, with no pain, redness, or swelling.

Special Considerations

Gloves must be worn because contact with blood is likely.
Maintenance of aseptic technique is a prime concern for the nurse performing IV therapy.
Choose tubing and needle appropriate for solution to provide optimal fluid flow. Viscous solutions require larger needles.
Small catheters cause less vein wall irritation than large ones. Choose the smallest gauge needle that will meet the need.
When working with children, confused clients, or other clients who are restless, obtain an assistant to help hold extremities still.

Because venous blood runs upward toward the heart, attempt to enter a vein at its lower (distal) end so the same vein can be used later without leakage.

If it is difficult to insert catheter fully, wait until fluid infusion is initiated and then gently advance the catheter.

To facilitate accurate 24-hour management, each shift should report to oncoming shift: the amount of IV fluid remaining, the need for new bottle/bag, tubing or site change, or need for site care.

Geriatric

Veins are often fragile. When veins are elevated and clearly visible, needle insertion may be performed without tourniquet.

Pediatric

Microdrip tubing with volume control chambers should be used for strict volume control. Infusion devices are often used for additional safety.

Clear explanations should be given with a demonstration of the equipment (except needles), using a puppet or game. Explain need for a helper to assist client in holding extremity stable during needle insertion. Talk to child during procedure.

Scalp vein needles (butterfly catheters) may be used for infants.

Armboards may be used for stabilization of IV in an extremity.

Home Health

If nursing visits are intermittent and IV therapy is continuous, instruct client and family on rate regulation, signs and symptoms of infiltration, and method for discontinuing IV catheter.

Delegation

Unlicensed assistive personnel should not be designated to perform IV site care. Although the licensed practical nurse (LPN) does not commonly administer IV medication, the LPN can often provide site care to peripheral lines, check agency policy, and consider the skill level of the person to whom you might delegate site care.

IMPLEMENTATION

Action	Rationale

Procedure 5.2 Intravenous Therapy: Vein Selection

Action	Rationale
1. Wash hands and organize equipment.	*Reduces microorganisms* *Promotes efficiency*
2. Explain procedure, including client assistance needed during and after therapy initiation.	*Decreases anxiety and ensures cooperation*

Action	Rationale
3. Encourage client to use bedpan or commode before beginning.	*Avoids interruption during IV insertion process*
4. Help client into loose-fitting gown or IV gown.	*Promotes ease of gown changes during IV therapy*
5. Ask client which hand is dominant.	*Facilitates placement of needle in nondominant hand or arm*
6. Tie tourniquet on arm 3 to 5 inches below elbow.	*Facilitates assessment of distal arm veins and hand veins*
7. Ask client to open and close hand or hang arm at side of bed.	*Pumps blood to extremity* *Dilates vein*
8. Look for vein with fewest curves or junctions and largest diameter (puffiness).	*Allows more complete insertion of catheter and use of large-gauge catheters*
9. Find vein on lower arm, if possible. Check anterior and posterior surfaces.	*Lower arm has natural splint of radial and ulnar bones*
10. If lower arm veins are unsuitable, look at hand and wrist veins.	
11. Look for site with 2 inches of skin surface below it (Fig. 5.2). If a large vein is needed, tie tourniquet just above antecubital area and search upper arm for suitable vein. A doctor's order is usually required before a vein in the lower extremities can be used. *For PICC catheter, the basilic or cephalic veins are most appropriate.*	*Permits taping with greater stability* *Upper arm veins are large and support large needle gauges (18 or 16) often needed for blood or blood products* *Lower extremities are more prone to thrombophlebitis and other peripheral vascular problems*
12. Release tourniquet.	*Reestablishes blood flow*
13. Obtain supplies.	
14. Select smallest catheter size that meets infusion needs and is appropriate for vein size.	*Prevents irritation of vein lining, which causes phlebitis and infiltration*
15. Include two appropriately sized catheters and one smaller-gauge catheter with other supplies.	*Prevents delay if second attempt is needed or smaller vein must be used*

Action	Rationale

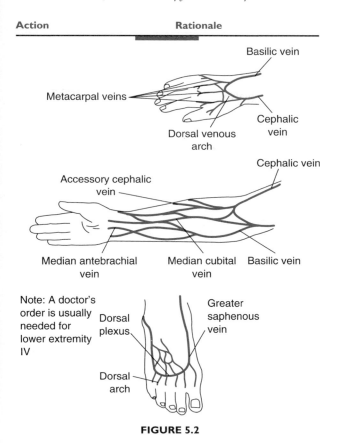

FIGURE 5.2

Procedure 5.3 Intravenous Therapy: Solution Preparation

1. Select vein (see Procedure 5.2).
2. Open tubing package and check tubing for cracks or flaws. Check ends for covers and verify that regulator clamp is closed (rolled down, clamped off, or screwed closed).

Ensures that no defective materials are used and that tubing remains sterile
Allows better fluid control, minimizing air in tubing

Action	Rationale

3. Open IV fluid container:
   - **Bottles:** With one hand, hold bottle firmly on counter; with other hand, lift, then pull metal tab down, outward, and around until entire ring is removed (Fig. 5.3); lift metal cap and pull flat rubber pad up and off.

   Prevents injury or bottle breakage

   MAINTAIN STERILITY OF BOTTLE TOP.

   Avoids introducing micro-organisms into client's vein

   - **Bags:** Remove outer bag covering; hold bag by neck in one hand; pull down on plastic tab with other hand and remove (see Fig. 5.3).

   Prevents squeezing of fluid or air from bag when spike is inserted, increasing accuracy of fluid measurement

4. To attach tubing, first remove cap from tubing spikes:
   - **Bottles:** Wipe top with alcohol; push spike into bottle port that is not attached to white tube.

   Prevents blockage of tube that provides air vent

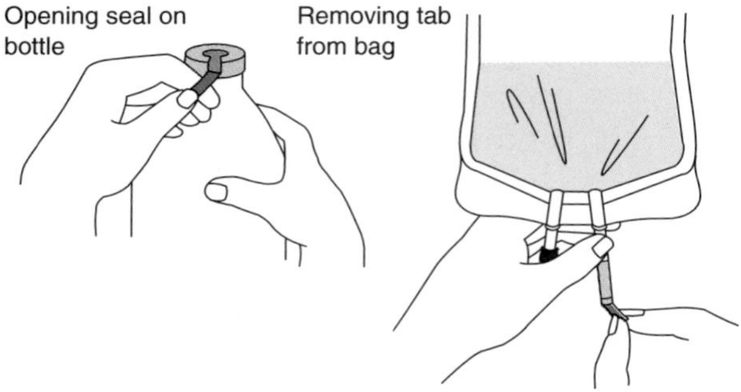

Opening seal on bottle

Removing tab from bag

FIGURE 5.3

Action	Rationale
- **Bags:** Push spike into port until flat end of tubing and bag meet.	*Ensures complete connection of bag and tubing*
5. Prime the tubing (remove air):	
- Hang bottle or bag on IV pole or wall hook; squeeze and release drip chamber until fluid level reaches ring mark.	*Eliminates introduction of air into tubing*
- Remove cap from end of tubing.	
- Open roller clamp and flush tubing until air is removed.	*Removes air from tubing*
- Hold rubber medication plugs and in-line filter (if present) upside down and tap while fluid is running.	*Forces air bubbles from plugs and filter*
- Close roller clamp.	
6. Replace cap on end of tubing.	*Maintains sterility*
7. Put tag on bag or bottle, stating client's name, room number, date and time initiated, rate of infusion, and your initials.	*Identifies when fluid should be replaced (24-hr maximum); prevents fluid contamination*
Apply time strip (see Procedure 5.6).	*Facilitates monitoring of infusion rate*
8. Tag tubing with date and time hung and own initials.	*Indicates when tubing replacement is due (every 24 to 48 hr or per agency policy)*
9. Proceed to bedside with equipment. Drape tubing over pole.	*Maintains sterility of tubing*

Procedure 5.4 Intravenous Therapy: Catheter/IV Lock Insertion

For Primary Infusion Line and IV Lock

1. Select vein (see Procedure 5.2) and prepare solution (see Procedure 5.3). Place IV tubing on bed beside client.	*Selects most appropriate vein* *Provides fluid for infusion* *Places tubing at easy access*
2. Lower side rail and assist client into a supine position. Raise bed to high position.	*Provides easier access to veins* *Promotes comfort during procedure* *Promotes use of good body mechanics*

Action	Rationale
3. Tear three 1-inch tape strips. Cut one piece down center.	*Narrow strip will secure catheter without covering insertion site*
4. Prepare needle/catheter for insertion:	
Over-the-needle catheter: Examine catheter for cracks or flaws. Rotate catheter and hold the needle securely.	*Ensures that catheter and needle are intact and plastic sheath will thread smoothly into vein*
Butterfly: Check needle tip for straight edge without bends or chips.	*Prevents shearing of vein by jagged needle*
5. Open several alcohol pads.	*Provides fast access to cleaning supplies*
6. Place towel under extremity.	*Prevents soiling of linens*
7. Place tourniquet on extremity.	*Restricts blood flow, distending vein*
8. Locate largest, most distal vein.	*Permits entrance of vein at higher point on future attempts without leakage*
9. Don gloves.	*Prevents contact with blood*
10. With alcohol pad, clean vein area, beginning at the vein and circling outward in a 2-inch diameter.	*Maintains asepsis*
11. Encourage client to take slow, deep breaths as you begin.	*Facilitates relaxation*
12. Hold skin taut with one hand while holding catheter with other (Fig. 5.4).	*Stabilizes vein and prevents skin movement during insertion*
Over-the-needle catheter: Hold the catheter by holding fingers on opposite sides of needle housing, not over catheter hub. (A needlestick protective over-the-needle catheter will have ribbed lines on the clear needle housing.)	*Facilitates viewing of initial blood flashback in catheter and reduces additional line contamination*

Action	Rationale

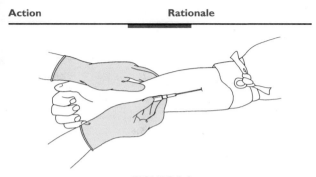

FIGURE 5.4

Butterfly: Pinch "wings" of butterfly together to insert needle.	*Decreases pain during needle insertion*
13. Maintaining sterility, insert catheter into vein with bevel of needle up. Insert needle parallel to straightest section of vein.	*Allows for full insertion of catheter*
Puncture skin at a 30-degree angle, 1 cm below site where the vein will be entered (Fig. 5.5).	*Ensures catheter stability*
14. When needle has entered skin, lower it until it is almost flush with the skin (Fig. 5.6).	*Prevents penetration of both walls of the vein*

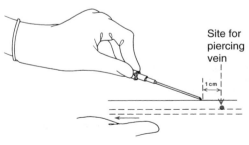

Site for
piercing
vein

1 cm

FIGURE 5.5

Action	Rationale

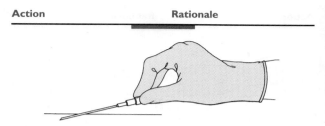

FIGURE 5.6

15. Following path of vein, insert catheter into side of vein wall. (*If using an over-the-needle catheter system, insert needle at a 30-degree angle with bevel and push-off tabs in the up position. Place index finger on the push-off tab and thread the catheter to the desired length.*)

16. Watch for first backflow of blood, then push needle gently into vein.
    Over-the-needle catheter: Push needle into vein about 1/4 inch after blood is noted. Slide catheter over needle and into vein before pulling needle out of vein and skin (Fig. 5.7). IF UNABLE TO INSERT CATHETER FULLY, DO NOT FORCE; WAIT UNTIL FLOW IS INITIATED.

    Indicates that needle has pierced vein wall

    Prevents piercing both walls of vein with needle
    Permits insertion of catheter without needle to prevent puncture of other vein wall

    Fluid infusion facilitates dilatation of vein

17. Holding catheter securely, remove cap from IV tubing and insert into hub of catheter, with IV LOCK twist on infusion plug (Fig. 5.8A).

    Prevents dislodging of catheter

18. Remove tourniquet.

    Prevents vein rupture from infusion of fluid against closed vessel

Action	Rationale

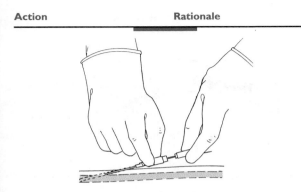

FIGURE 5.7

19. Open roller clamp and allow fluid to flow freely for a few seconds; with **IV lock,** wipe plug with alcohol and flush with saline (Fig. 5.8*B*).

Determines if catheter is in vein or wedged against vessel wall Fluid infusion prevents clot formation

20. Monitor for swelling or pain.

Indicates infiltration

21. Tape catheter in position that allows free flow of the fluid. Tape catheter in one of the following methods:

Eliminates positional flow of IV fluids

   Over-the-needle catheter: Put small piece of tape under hub of catheter and cross over to secure hub to skin. DO NOT PLACE TAPE OVER INSERTION SITE.

Maintains sterility of insertion site by covering with sterile material only

   Butterfly: Put smallest pieces of tape across "wings" of butterfly; put another tape piece across middle to form an H. A second method is to put a small piece of tape under wings and tape over to form a V; then place piece of tape across the V. (See Fig. 5.15 for an example.)

Provides catheter stabilization without tape covering insertion site

Action	Rationale

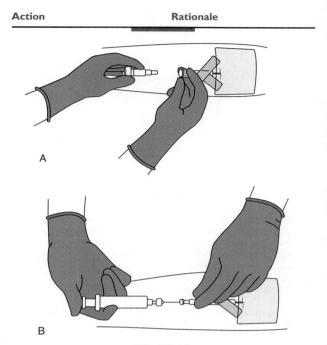

FIGURE 5.8

22. Slow IV fluids to a moderate drip.	*Prevents accidental fluid bolus while completing site care*
23. Place ointment over insertion site, if desired, and cover with adhesive bandage, 2 × 2-inch dressing, or transparent dressing.	*Decreases exposure to and growth of microorganisms*
24. Remove gloves and secure tubing: **Over-the-needle catheter:** Place tape across top of tubing, just below catheter. Loop tubing and tape to dressing. Secure length of tubing to arm with short piece of tape. Tape the tubing/catheter hub junction.	*Prevents disconnection of tubing*

Action	Rationale
Butterfly: Coil needle tubing around and on top of IV site. - Tape across coil and hub of needle.	*Prevents weight of tubing or movement from dislodging needle*
IV lock: Flush with saline or dilute heparin solution (1:100). Tape across infusion plug.	*Prevents clot formation* *Secures needle/catheter*
25. On a piece of tape or label, record: needle size, type, date and time of insertion, and your initials. Place label over top of dressing.	*Provides information needed for follow-up care*
26. Apply armboard if needed.	*Stabilizes sites of frequent movement*
27. Discard gloves and dispose of equipment properly.	*Prevents spread of micro-organisms*
28. Regulate IV flow manually or set infusion device at appropriate rate (see Procedure 5.6).	
29. Review limitations in range of motion with client. Instruct client to notify nurse of problems or discomfort.	*Enlists client's assistance in maintenance of catheter*
30. Remove towel and position client for comfort, with call light within reach.	*Promotes comfort and safety*
31. Check infusion accuracy after 5 min and again after 15 min. Check volume every 1 to 2 hr.	*Determines if rate needs to be adjusted*

Evaluation

Were desired outcomes achieved?

Documentation

The following should be noted on the client's chart:

- Client's tolerance of insertion procedure and fluid infusion
- Status of IV site, dressing, fluids, and tubing
- Size and type of catheter/needle
- Type and rate of infusion (if continuous infusion)
- Client teaching accomplished
- Follow-up assessments of the infusion
- Dilute heparin instillation (if IV lock)

SAMPLE DOCUMENTATION

DATE	TIME	
12/3/02	1200	Client has 20-gauge Jelco inserted in right lower arm. One liter D_5W infusing at 125 ml/hr. Site intact. Client tolerated insertion procedure and fluid infusion without significant changes in vital signs. Teaching done regarding mobility limitations; client voiced understanding.

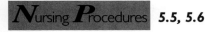

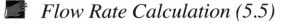 *Flow Rate Calculation (5.5)*

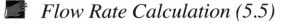 *Intravenous Fluid Regulation (5.6)*

 EQUIPMENT

- IV pole (bed or rolling) or IV pump/controller
- Calculator (or pencil and pad)
- Watch with second hand

Purpose

Ensures delivery of correct amount of IV fluids

Assessment

Assessment should focus on the following:

Orders for type and rate of fluid
Type of infusion control devices available or ordered
Viscosity of ordered fluids

Nursing Diagnoses

The nursing diagnoses may include the following:

Risk of fluid overload related to incorrect fluid rate

Outcome Identification and Planning

Desired Outcome (sample)
Correct volume of fluid is infused within designated time frame

Special Considerations
Viscous solutions may require rate adjustments throughout infusion process based on actual flow due to accumulation in filter or on sides of tubing.

Pediatric and Geriatric

These clients are often volume sensitive and prone to fluid overload, particularly with rapid infusion of large volumes. Infusions must be regulated carefully and checked frequently, and
clients must be watched closely for tolerance.

Delegation

Regulation of IV fluid should remain the responsibility of the
nurse. However, unlicensed personnel can be enlisted to help
monitor the infusion and to report when fluid is nearing completion, so the nurse can discontinue or hang an additional infusion.

IMPLEMENTATION

Action	Rationale

Procedure 5.5 Flow Rate Calculation

1. Check tubing package to
   determine drop factor of
   tubing.

   *Indicates drops per milliliter for
   drip rate calculation*

2. Determine the infusion
   volume in milliliters per hour
   (ml/hr) using the following
   formula:

   *Simplifies calculations by limit-
   ing time to 60 min*
   *Facilitates monitoring of fluid
   and time taping container*

$$\frac{\text{TOTAL VOLUME}}{\text{TOTAL TIME (hours)}} = \boxed{\begin{array}{c}\text{Hourly infusion rate} \\ \text{(volume to infuse each hour)}\end{array}}$$

Example: 1000 ml to be infused over 6 hr

$$1000/6 = 167 \text{ ml/hr}$$

3. Determine *flow rate* by using
   the following formula:

$$\frac{\text{TOTAL FLUID VOLUME}}{\text{TOTAL TIME (minutes)}} \times \begin{array}{c}\text{DROP FACTOR} \\ \text{(drops/ml)}\end{array} = \boxed{\begin{array}{c}\text{INFUSION} \\ \text{RATE} \\ \text{(drops/min)}\end{array}}$$

Example: Volume ordered is 1000 ml of D_5W over 6 hr; tubing
drop factor is 15 drops/ml

$$\frac{1000 \text{ ml}}{6 \ (60) \text{ min}} \times 15 \text{ drops/ml} = \frac{15,000 \text{ drops}}{360 \text{ min}} = \begin{array}{c}41.7 \text{ or } 42 \\ \text{drops/min}\end{array}$$

Or utilize hourly infusion rate (see above):

Action	Rationale

$$\frac{167 \text{ ml} \times 15 \text{ drops}}{60 \text{ min/ml}} = 41.7 \text{ or } 42 \text{ drops/min}$$

Total fluid volume equals the amount of fluid, expressed in milliliters, to infuse over the ordered period of time (if order is 1 L of D_5W over 12 hr, the total volume is 1 L [1000 ml]).

Total time is the number of minutes (hours × 60) over which the fluid should infuse. IF FLUID IS ORDERED PER HOUR OR YOU CALCULATE VOLUME PER HOUR, THE TOTAL TIME WILL EQUAL 60 MINUTES. Total volume will equal hourly infusion rate.

The drop factor is the number of drops from the chosen tubing that will equal 1 ml. This amount is found on the tubing package and is expressed in drops per milliliter.

4. If available, use pre-
   calculated infusion chart by:
   - Looking across chart for   *Indicates drops per minute at*
     drop factor of tubing   *point of intersection*
   - Coming down chart to
     line indicating amount
     of fluid infusing per
     hour (Table 5.1)
5. Regulate fluid or set drop
   rate on fluid regulator (see
   Procedure 5.6).

Procedure 5.6 Intravenous Fluid Regulation

1. Calculate or determine
   appropriate volume per hour
   and drip rate (drops per
   minute; see Procedure 5.5).
2. Prepare time tape for fluid   *Facilitates close monitoring of*
   based on volume of fluid to   *fluid infusion*
   infuse over 1 hr (Fig. 5.9).
   Use felt pen to mark.   *Prevents puncture of container*
   - Tear an 11-inch strip of
     1-inch tape.
   - Place tape on IV fluid
     container beside fluid-
     level indicators.
   - Mark tape at intervals   *Simplifies marking of fluid*
     indicating fluid level after   *amounts (ie, instead of 75*
     each hour of infusion (for   *ml/hr mark 150 ml at 2-hr*
     small hourly volumes,   *intervals)*
     mark the volume for a 2-
     or 3-hr interval instead).

TABLE 5.1 Flow Rates for Intravenous Infusions						
Drop Factor of Tubing (drops/ml)	1000 ml/6 hr (drops/min)	1000 ml/8 hr (drops/min)	1000 ml/10 hr (drops/min)	1000 ml/12 hr (drops/min)	1000 ml/24 hr (drops/min)
10	28	21	17	14	7
15	42	31	25	21	10
20	56	42	34	28	14
60	167	125	100	84	42

Action	Rationale

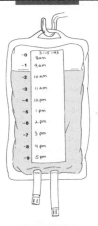

FIGURE 5.9

3. Attach appropriate tubing
   (for infusion pump, with
   chamber, or Dial-A-Flo)
   and clear tubing of air.
   Proceed to appropriate
   section for step 4.

Manual Rate Regulation

4. Open all clamps except
   regulator roller/screw.

   *Limits fluid rate control to
   regulator*

5. Open regulator fully; then
   slowly close regulator while
   observing drip chamber—
   fluid should initially run in
   a stream. (Table 5.2 lists
   troubleshooting tips.)

   Determines catheter patency

6. Close regulator screw until
   fluid is dropping at slow but
   steady pace.

7. Count the number of drops
   falling within 15 sec and
   multiply by 4 (see
   Procedure 5.5).

   *Determines number of drops
   falling per minute*

TABLE 5.2	**Troubleshooting Tips for Intravenous Infusion Management**

Problem	Actions
1. Drip chamber is overfilled.	Close regulator clamp, turn fluid container upside down, and squeeze fluid from drip chamber until half full or slightly below.
2. Air is in tubing.	Check adequacy of fluid level in drip chamber and security of tubing connections. Insert needle and syringe into rubber port distal to air and aspirate to remove air.
3. Blood is backing up into tubing.	Be sure fluid is above the level of the IV catheter site and the level of the heart. Check security of tubing connections. Check that infusing fluid has not run out and that catheter is in a vein, not an artery (note pulsation of blood in tubing).
4. Infusion pump alarms indicate flow problem.	Check drip chamber for excess or inadequate fluid level. Check that clamps and regulators are open, air vent is open (if applicable), and tubing is free of kinks. Check IV catheter site for infiltration, blood clot, kinks, and positional obstruction (open fluid regulator fully and change position of arm to see if fluid flows better in various positions). Insert needle and syringe into medication port and gently flush fluid through catheter. If resistance is met, try to aspirate blood/clot into tubing; if unsuccessful, discontinue IV and restart.
5. IV is positional (ie, runs well only when arm or hand is in a certain position).	Stabilize IV site with armboard or handboard, and monitor fluid infusion every 1 to 2 hr.
6. Fluid is dripping but is also leaking into tissue surrounding puncture site.	Discontinue IV and restart in another site. Place warm soak over infiltrated site. Reassess frequently.

Action	Rationale
8. Open regulator to increase drop flow if drops-per-minute rate is less than calculated drip rate; close regulator if drops-per-minute rate is more than needed.	
9. Count drops again and continue to adjust flow until desired drip rate is obtained.	*Produces correct drip rate*
10. Recheck drip rate after 5 min and again after 15 min. Proceed to finishing steps 11 to 15.	*Detects changes in rate due to expansion/contraction of tubing*

Dial-A-Flo Fluid Regulation
See steps 1 to 3 for initial preparation.

Action	Rationale
4. At end of IV tubing, attach Dial-A-Flo tubing (Fig. 5.10).	
5. Open all clamps and regulator on IV tubing.	
6. Adjust Dial-A-Flo to open position and clear tubing of air (remove cap if needed).	
7. Close fluid regulator roller/screw.	*Prevents fluid flow during connection to IV catheter*
8. Attach Dial-A-Flo to catheter hub (following initial insertion or during tubing change) and open fluid regulator.	
9. Turn Dial-A-Flo regulator until arrow is aligned with desired volume of fluid to infuse over 1 hr.	*Regulates fluid to infuse at desired rate*
10. Check drip rate over 15 sec and multiply by 4 (should coincide with calculated drip rate).	*Verifies fluid infusion rate*
- Adjust height of pole if necessary.	*Gravity facilitates flow*

Action	Rationale

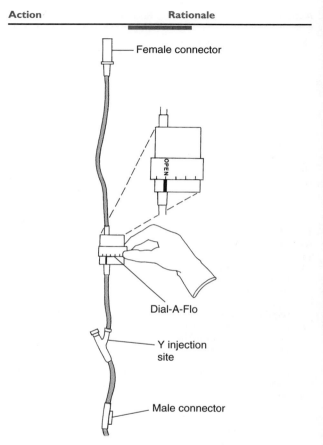

FIGURE 5.10

- Recheck drip rate after 5 min and again after 15 min.
- Proceed to finishing steps 11 to 15.

Detects changes in rate due to expansion/contraction of tubing

Action	Rationale

Infusion Controller or Pump Regulation

See steps 1 to 3 for initial preparation.

4. Insert tubing into infusion pump/regulator according to pump manual.

Ensures proper functioning of infusion regulator

5. Close door to pump/controller and open all tubing clamps and regulator roller/screw.

Allows pump/controller to regulate fluids

6. Set volume dials for appropriate volume per hour or drops per minute (check type of pump *carefully*).

Determines amount of fluid pump/controller will deliver

7. Place electronic eye clamp over drip chamber (optional in some infusion regulators; consult manual; Fig. 5.11).

Allows pump/controller to monitor fluid flow

8. Push ON or START button.

Initiates fluid flow and regulation

9. Check drip rate over 15 sec and multiply by 4 (should coincide with calculated drip rate).

Verifies fluid infusion rate

10. Set volume infusion alarm, if desired (often omitted). If tubing does not contain a regulator cassette, periodically change the sections of tubing placed inside infusion clamp. Proceed to finishing steps 11 to 15.

Notifies nurse when set volume has been infused

Prevents tubing collapse due to constant squeezing by pump

Volume Control Chamber (Buretrol) Regulation

See steps 1 and 2 for initial preparation.

3. Close off regulator 1 (above chamber) and regulator 2 (below chamber). Insert spike into fluid bag.

Controls fluids more precisely

Action   **Rationale**

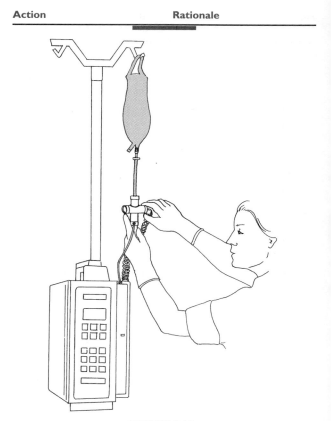

FIGURE 5.11

4. Open regulator 1 and fill   *Facilitates clearing of air from*
   chamber with 10 ml fluid,   *tubing*
   prime drip chamber, and
   close regulator 1. Open
   regulator 2 and clear tubing
   of air (Fig. 5.12 *A*).

5. Fill chamber with volume of   *Allows for close monitoring of*
   fluid to infuse in 1 hr (or 2   *fluid volume (needed for*
   or 3 hr worth if volume is   *volume-sensitive or pediatric*
   small).   *clients)*

Action	Rationale
6. Close regulator 1. Make sure air vent is open (Fig. 5.12*B*).	*Fluid will not flow if regulator 1 and air vent are closed*
7. Open regulator 2 and regulate drops to calculated rate (drip rate should equal volume per hour if minidrip tubing system is used [check drop factor]), *or:* - Attach Dial-A-Flo to	*Sets volume to infuse over an hour*

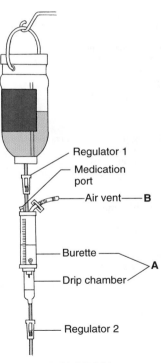

Regulator 1

Medication port

Air vent——**B**

Burette ———

——**A**

Drip chamber

———— Regulator 2

FIGURE 5.12

Action	Rationale
tubing and leave regulator 2 open, *or*	
- Place tubing into infusion pump or controller and leave regulator 2 open.	*Allows infusion pump/controller to regulate fluid*
8. Check drip rate over 15 sec and multiply by 4 (should coincide with calculated drip rate).	*Verifies fluid infusion rate*
9. Put a time tape on the chamber (if pump/ controller is not used).	*Allows for quick, easy check of fluid infusion progress and the need to add fluid to chamber*
10. Check chamber each hour or two and add 1 to 2 hours' more fluid volume as needed. IF CLOSE FLUID MONITORING IS NOT NEEDED, CLAMP AIR VENT AND OPEN REGULATOR 1. Proceed to finishing steps 11 to 15.	*Maintains fluid infusion and catheter patency* *Prevents air entrance into tubing* *Allows fluid to flow directly from bottle/bag into chamber and to client*

Finishing Steps

11. Mark beginning hour of fluid infusion on time tape.	*Sets times for subsequent checks*
12. Check volume every 1 to 2 hr and compare with time tape.	*Determines actual volume infusion*
13. If volume depleted does not coincide with time mark:	
- Check time tape for accuracy.	
- Check settings on pump/ controller or Dial-A-Flo and readjust if indicated.	
- Elevate fluid container on pole.	*Facilitates flow by gravity*
- Check catheter site and position for obstruction (see Table 5.2).	

Action	Rationale
14. Review limitations in range of motion with client. Instruct client to notify nurse of problems or discomfort.	*Facilitates early detection of problems with catheter or fluid flow*
15. Position client for comfort with call light within reach.	*Promotes client comfort and safety*

Evaluation

Were desired outcomes achieved?

Documentation

The following should be noted on the client's chart:

- Time of initiation of fluid infusion
- Type and volume of fluid infusion
- Infusion device used, if applicable
- Status of catheter insertion site
- Problems with infusion procedure and solutions applied (eg, armboard used, catheter repositioned)
- Client tolerance to fluid infusion
- Client teaching and response

SAMPLE DOCUMENTATION

DATE	TIME	
2/9/02	1400	Client receiving D_5W; 1000-ml bag infusing at 125 ml/hr per Dial-A-Flow. Tolerating fluid infusion well. Catheter site clean and dry, without signs of infiltration or infection. Return demonstration noted regarding arm positions to be avoided during IV fluid infusion.

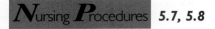

 Intravenous Tubing Change/Conversion to IV Lock (5.7)

 Intravenous Dressing Change (5.8)

EQUIPMENT

- Alcohol pads and Betadine pad (optional)
- Infusion tubing (vented for IV fluid bag, unvented for IV bottles)
- Towel
- Tape 1 inch wide (may cut 2-inch tape)
- Dressing: 2 × 2-inch gauze, adhesive bandage, or transparent dressing (Opsite)
- IV pole (bed or rolling) *or* IV pump/controller
- Ointment (optional)
- Razor and soap (optional)
- Armboard (optional)
- Adhesive labels
- Nonsterile gloves
- IV infusion plug
- Heparin or saline flush

Purpose

Decreases opportunity for growth of microorganisms by removing possible medium for infection

Assessment

Assessment should focus on the following:
Doctor's orders for type and rate of fluid
Status of skin on hand and arms, presence of hair or abrasions
Ability to hold arm and hand without movement or resistance for duration of procedure
Allergy to tape, iodine, antibiotic pads, or ointment

Nursing Diagnoses

The nursing diagnoses may include the following:
Risk of infection related to interruption of skin integrity

Outcome Identification and Planning

Desired Outcomes (sample)

No evidence of infection exists around insertion site over the next 72 hours.
Client verbalizes understanding of movement limitations related to intravenous infusions and of complications to be reported to the nurse.
The client will maintain skin integrity around insertion site, as evidenced by lack of pain, redness, or swelling at site.

Special Considerations

If possible, replace IV fluid and tubing and change dressing at the same time. This reduces risk of introducing microorganisms. Many institutions have specified procedures and times for dressing and tubing change. If unsure, consult policy manual.

Pediatric and Geriatric

If the client is resistant, confused, or frightened, obtain an assistant to immobilize arm to ensure that IV line is not accidentally dislodged during dressing change.

Home Health

In the homebound client, be constantly alert for subtle signs and symptoms of infection associated with long-term IV therapy.

Delegation

Care should be taken when delegating IV dressing changes. Consider the skill level of the personnel to whom you delegate care. Often, special training is needed before an LPN or other personnel performs IV dressing changes.

IMPLEMENTATION

Action	Rationale

Procedure 5.7 Intravenous Tubing
Change/Conversion to IV Lock

Action	Rationale
1. Wash hands and organize equipment.	*Reduces microorganism transfer* *Promotes efficiency*

Action	Rationale
2. Open package and check tubing for cracks or flaws. Be sure that caps are on all ports and that the regulator clamp is closed (rolled down, clamped off, or screwed closed).	*Ensures that no defective materials are used and that tubing remains sterile* *Allows better fluid control, minimizing air in tubing*
3. Check infusing fluid against doctor's orders.	*Validates correct fluid infusion*
4. Tape old tubing to IV pole or pump pole with strip of tape and fill drip chamber full (Fig. 5.13).	*Allows fluid in tubing to infuse into vein while new tubing is being prepared*
5. Remove infusing fluid bag/bottle from IV pole or bottle from IV pole or pump (put pump on hold) and disconnect from old tubing.	*Provides fluid for new tubing*

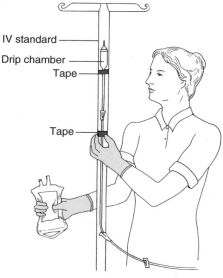

IV standard

Drip chamber

Tape

Tape

FIGURE 5.13

Action	Rationale
6. Attach new tubing to bag/ bottle and prime tubing (remove air):	
- Hang bottle or bag on IV pole (or pole or infusion pump hook).	*Forces air to bottle/bag top and places fluid at entrance to tubing*
- Squeeze and release drip chamber until fluid level reaches ring mark on chamber.	*Fills drip chamber and prevents introduction of air into tubing*
- Remove cap from end of tubing.	
- Open roller clamp and flush tubing until air is removed.	*Allows total removal of air from tubing*
- Hold rubber medication plugs and in-line filter (if present) upside down and tap while fluid is running; close clamp.	*Forces air bubbles from plugs and filters*
7. Loosely cover end of tubing with cap and lay on bed near IV dressing.	*Maintains sterility*
8. Don gloves.	*Prevents exposure to blood*
9. Close off flow from old tubing.	*Prevents wetting of dressing and bed*
10. a. Exchange old tubing for new at IV catheter hub:	*Removes medium for micro-organism growth*
- Place alcohol swab under the catheter hub–tubing junction.	*Decreases blood soiling of dressing or bed*
- Loosen connection at junction of IV catheter and old tubing.	
- Holding catheter firm with one hand, remove old tubing; *and*	*Prevents dislodgment of catheter when changing tubing*
- Quickly insert new tubing into catheter hub (Fig. 5.14*A*), maintaining sterility of catheter and tip of new tubing.	

Action	Rationale

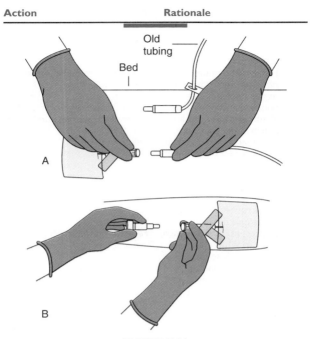

FIGURE 5.14

   b. Begin flow from new tubing.

Prevents clot formation in catheter

   c. Regulate fluid flow or place tubing into pump.

Promotes accurate infusion rate

   d. Tape tubing to dressing and arm unless dressing is to be changed.

Decreases accidental pull on catheter

   e. Tag tubing with date, time hung, and own initials.

Indicates when tubing replacement is due (every 24–48 hr or per agency policy)

11. **Conversion to IV lock**
   a. Perform steps 1 to 9. Remove old tubing, and apply infusion plug/IV lock (Fig. 5.14*B*).
   b. Flush catheter with saline or heparin flush.

Action	Rationale
c. Tape infusion plug and catheter securely in place or perform dressing change, if indicated.	
d. Tag site with date, time, and initials.	
12. Discard old tubing and other trash.	*Promotes clean environment*
13. If performing dressing change, see Procedure 5.8. If not, place tape across junction of tubing and catheter.	*Prevents dislodging of tubing from catheter*
14. Raise side rails and position client for safety and comfort.	*Promotes client comfort and safety*
15. Discard gloves and wash hands.	*Reduces microorganism transfer*

Procedure 5.8 Intravenous Dressing Change

Action	Rationale
1. Wash hands and organize equipment.	*Reduces microorganism transfer* *Promotes efficiency*
2. Explain procedure to client.	*Decreases anxiety*
3. Tear tape strips 3 inches in length, 1 inch wide. Cut one strip down the center. Hang tape pieces from edge of table.	*Secures catheter without covering insertion site* *Places tape in available position without disrupting adhesive*
4. Open alcohol/Betadine pads, dressing and adhesive bandage, and ointment.	*Provides fast access to supplies*
5. Lower side rail and assist client into a supine position.	*Provides easy access to IV site* *Promotes comfort during procedure*
6. Raise bed to high position.	*Decreases strain on nurse's back*
7. Place towel under extremity.	*Prevents soiling of linens*
8. Don gloves.	*Protects against potential contamination*
9. Remove dressing and all tape except tape holding catheter.	*Prevents dislodging of catheter while cleaning site*

Action	Rationale
10. Using alcohol first and then Betadine swabs, clean catheter insertion site beginning at catheter and cleaning outward in a 2-inch diameter circle.	*Removes blood and drainage from site and surrounding area*
11. Holding catheter secure with one hand, remove remaining tape and clean under catheter.	*Prevents catheter dislodgment*
12. Allow area to dry and secure catheter in position:	
- **Over-the-needle catheter:** With tape edges sticking to thumb and fingertip, slide small strip of tape under catheter hub with adhesive side up (Fig. 5.15*A*); cross tape over hub to secure catheter, but DO NOT place tape over insertion site; put other small strip of tape across catheter hub (Fig. 5.15*B*).	*Provides greater control of tape* *Insertion site should be covered with sterile material only* *Adds stability to catheter*
- **Butterfly:** Put smallest pieces of tape across wings of butterfly and another tape piece across middle to form an H; or put small piece of tape under wings, tape over to form a V, and then place piece of tape across the V.	*Eliminates positional flow of IV fluids* *Allows for catheter stabilization without tape covering insertion site*
13. Place ointment over insertion site, if desired, and cover site with adhesive bandage, 2 × 2-inch dressing, or transparent dressing (if client is allergic to iodine, use Neosporin ointment).	

Action	Rationale

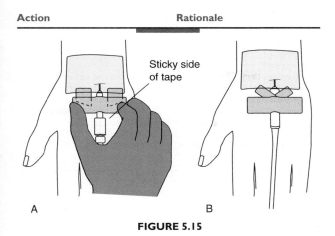

FIGURE 5.15

14. Remove gloves and secure tubing:
    - **Over-the-needle catheter:** Place tape across top of tubing just below catheter, loop tubing and tape to dressing, and secure tubing to arm with short piece of tape (taping the catheter hub–tubing junction is optional). *Prevents disconnection of tubing*
    - **Butterfly:** Coil catheter tubing around on top of IV site; tape across coil and catheter hub. *Prevents weight of tubing or movement from dislodging catheter*
    - **IV lock:** Flush with heparin flush solution and tape across infusion plug. *Prevents clot formation and secures catheter*
15. Apply armboard, if needed. *Stabilizes sites of frequent movement*
16. On a piece of tape or label, record needle size, type, date and time of site care, and your initials; place label over top of dressing. *Provides information needed for follow-up care*

Action	Rationale
17. Raise side rails and position client for comfort.	*Promotes client comfort and safety*
18. Explain limitations of movement to client with return demonstrations, as well as need to report pain or swelling at site.	*Decreases client anxiety regarding proper maintenance of IV needle* *Promotes early detection of infiltration or other complications*
19. Discard or restore supplies; wash hands.	*Decreases the spread of organisms*

Evaluation

Were desired outcomes achieved?

Documentation

The following should be noted on the client's chart:

- Location and status of IV site, dressing, fluids, and tubing
- Size and type of catheter/needle
- Reports of pain at site
- IV site care rendered and client tolerance to care
- Client teaching

SAMPLE DOCUMENTATION

DATE	TIME	
4/9/02	1200	Tubing changed to IV of D_5W infusing at 125 ml/hr in right lower arm. Site care done, #20 Jelco present, site clean without swelling or pain. Client tolerated procedure well. Reinforced teaching regarding mobility limitations; client demonstrated understanding.

Central Line/Peripherally Inserted Central Catheter (PICC) Maintenance

EQUIPMENT

- Sterile gloves
- Sterile gauze pads (2 × 2 inches) and transparent dressing
- Face masks
- 1-inch tape (optional)
- Steri-strips
- Alcohol pads
- Povidone swabs (optional)
- IV fluids and tubing or heparin flush or saline flush
- Prep razor
- Suture with needle holder
- Central line (PICC) insertion kit containing:
  - sterile gloves (multiple sizes)
  - Betadine swabs or solution and gauze
  - sterile towels/drapes
  - 10-ml syringe (slip-tip)
  - 5/8-, 1-, and 1½-inch needles
- Lidocaine/Xylocaine (without epinephrine) 1% or 2%
- Central line with introducer (eg, single-lumen or multilumen catheter, Hickman catheter, angiocath)
- Tape measure (PICC only)
- Dressing change label

Purpose

Permits administration of medications and nutritional support that should not be given via a peripheral route or when peripheral routes cannot be obtained

Assessment

Assessment should focus on the following:

Type of catheter
Location of catheter
Type of infusion(s)
Agency policy regarding central line care

Nursing Diagnoses

The nursing diagnoses may include the following:

Fluid volume deficit related to nausea and vomiting
Altered nutrition: less than body requirements related to anorexia

Outcome Identification and Planning

Desired Outcomes (sample)

Client remains free of embolism, pleural effusion, and infection, both systemic and at catheter site.
Client maintains skin turgor during total parenteral nutrition (TPN) administration.
Central line remains patent.
Client gains 1 to 2 lb per week.

Special Considerations

Delegation

PICCs are often inserted only by physicians or registered nurses specially certified by the hospital. Consult hospital policy for specific PICC insertion and maintenance procedures.
If central line was inserted for infusion of TPN, infuse only $D_{10}W$ or D_5W until TPN is available.
If multilumen catheter is used, select and mark a catheter port for TPN only.
Policy varies greatly regarding use of saline or heparin solution for flushing catheter; consult agency policy manual.

Home Health

In the homebound client, a central line is likely to be in place for a long time. Therefore, be constantly alert for early signs and symptoms of infection.

IMPLEMENTATION

Action	Rationale

Assisting With Central Line or PICC Insertion

1. Wash hands, and organize equipment.	*Reduces microorganism transfer* *Promotes efficiency*
2. Arrange supplies on tray, using appropriate-size gloves for physician.	

Action	Rationale
3. Reinforce explanation of procedure to client. Clarify that his/her face will be covered with towels or drapes but that you will be nearby.	*Reduces client anxiety*

For central line

4. Put bed and client in Trendelenburg's position. If client has respiratory distress, place in supine position with feet elevated 45 to 60 degrees (modified Trendelenburg's).	*Dilates vessels in upper trunk and neck* *Puts less pressure on diaphragm and facilitates breathing*

For PICC insertion

5. Position the arm for ease of access to the upper arm or antecubital vein sites—basilic or cephalic arm extended at 45- to 60-degree angle from the body.	
6. Hold client's hand (obtain assistant and restrain both hands if client is resistant or confused).	*Provides comfort* *Prevents procedure disruption or contamination of field*
7. Don face mask and apply mask to client (optional).	*Decreases contamination of insertion site*
8. Inform client of progression of the procedure, particularly when needle stick is to occur.	*Prepares client for discomfort* *Decreases startle reaction*
9. Monitor client for respiratory distress, complaints of chest pain, dysrhythmias, or other complications.	*Facilitates early detection of pneumothorax, air or catheter embolism, or other complication*
10. After the vein has been punctured, the doctor will remove the syringe from the insertion needle and insert a guidewire through the needle. *In centrally inserted lines, instruct the client to take a deep breath*	*Prevents air from being sucked into the vein by increasing the intrathoracic pressure*

Action	Rationale

and to bear down (Valsalva's maneuver) while the guidewire is inserted.

11. The multilumen central catheter or a PICC is inserted over the guidewire into the vein, and the guidewire is withdrawn. Blood will back up into the catheter lumen(s). Aseptically aspirate air from and then flush saline through each catheter lumen (Fig. 5.16).

Indicates the presence of the catheter in the vein and removes air from the catheter tubing before infusion of fluid

12. Apply IV lock and cap to catheter lumen(s).

Maintains sterility of lumen and prevents blood loss

13. Once the catheter is in place and sutured, apply gel ointment, sterile gauze, or transparent dressing, and, if needed, tape dressing down securely.

Protects IV site from air leak, debris, and organisms while allowing visualization of most of the catheter tubing

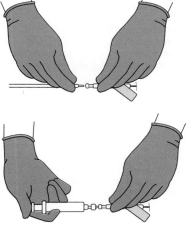

FIGURE 5.16

Action	Rationale
14. Begin regular infusion rate after catheter position has been confirmed.	*Verifies that catheter is in vena cava or right atrium before infusion of large amounts of fluid.*
15. Position client for comfort with call light within reach; instruct client to call nurse if any respiratory distress or pain is experienced.	*Promotes client safety and early detection of complications*

Monitoring and Maintenance

Action	Rationale
1. Mark each lumen of multilumen catheter with name of fluid/medication infusing.	*Prevents mixing of medications*
2. Lumens without continuing infusion of fluids are capped with infusion plug and flushed every 8 hr with heparin solution (usually 1:100 dilution) or normal saline.	*Prevents obstruction of catheter lumen with blood clot*
Depending on length of tubing and size of catheter, 1 to 3 ml is used (use 6 ml or ordered amount of flush for Hickman catheter and short small needle—⅝ inch, 25 gauge). For PICC lines, use a 10-cc syringe or larger for flushing.	*Minimizes leakage of plug or damage to catheter* *Prevents rupture of PICC tubing due to excess syringe pressure*
3. Flush tubings, between infusion of medications and drawing of blood, first using saline, and then heparin.	*Prevents medication interaction or lumen obstruction with blood*
4. ALWAYS ASPIRATE BEFORE INFUSING MEDICATIONS OR FLUSHING TUBINGS.	*Ensures patency of line and validates presence in vessel*
5. Monitor for clot formation in lumen:	

Action	Rationale
If resistance is met when flushing tubing, DO NOT FORCE; aspirate and remove clot, if possible; if not, notify doctor.	*Prevents clot from reaching client and causing emboli*
6. Monitor respirations and breath sounds every 4 hr.	*Promotes early detection of fluid entering chest cavity or of pulmonary embolism*
7. Maintain IV fluids above the level of the heart. Do not allow fluid to run out and air to enter tubing (see Table 5.2 and Procedure 5.6).	*Prevents blood reflux into tubing* *Prevents infusion of air*

Tubing Change

Action	Rationale
1. Review Procedure 5.7. Prepare fluid and tubing (see Procedure 5.3).	*Minimizes exposure to micro-organisms*
2. Don gloves.	*Protects from potential contamination*
3. Expose catheter hub or rubber port of multilumen catheter.	*Precedes connection of tubing*

For centrally inserted lines

Action	Rationale
4. Ask client to take a deep breath and bear down (Valsalva's maneuver).	*Increases intrathoracic pressure* *Prevents air from entering vein*
5. Disconnect old tubing and quickly connect new tubing.	
6. Open fluid and adjust to appropriate infusion rate.	
7. Proceed to dressing change, if needed.	

Dressing Change

Action	Rationale
1. Explain procedure to client.	*Reduces anxiety*
2. Wash hands and gather equipment.	*Reduces microorganism transfer* *Promotes efficiency*
3. Open packages, keeping supplies sterile.	*Prevents contamination of catheter site*
4. Don clean gloves and mask.	
5. Remove tape and previous dressing.	
6. Don sterile gloves.	

Action	Rationale
7. Beginning at catheter and wiping outward to the surrounding skin, clean insertion site with alcohol and povidone.	*Decreases contamination* *Removes microorganisms from site*
8. Place ointment over insertion site (optional) and cover with sterile gauze.	
9. Cover gauze with tape or transparent dressing; wrap tubing on top and cover tubing with tape.	*Secures dressing* *Prevents pull on catheter*
10. Remove gloves and mask.	
11. On a piece of tape or label, record date and time of site care and your initials. Place label over top of dressing.	*Determines next site care* *(required every 48 to 72 hr)*
12. Raise side rails and position client for comfort.	*Promotes client safety and comfort*

Evaluation

Were desired outcomes achieved?

Documentation

The following should be noted on the client's chart:

- Date and time of catheter insertion
- Type and location of catheter
- Care and maintenance procedures performed
- Equipment used with catheter
- Client tolerance to procedures

SAMPLE DOCUMENTATION

DATE	TIME	
1/9/02	0400	Dressing changed at right subclavian triple-lumen catheter site. No redness, edema, or drainage at site. Povidone ointment applied. IV fluid bag and tubing changed. D_5W infusing via IVAC pump at 50 ml/hr.

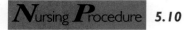

Parenteral Nutrition Management

EQUIPMENT

- IV tubing with filter (for parenteral nutrition [PN])
- IV tubing without filter for lipids, if ordered
- Infusion pumps, if available
- Appropriate labels
- Sterile gloves

Purpose

Permits administration of nutritional support when gastrointestinal tract is traumatized or nonfunctional

Assessment

Assessment should focus on the following:

Doctor's orders for PN type (central or peripheral), contents, and rate
Doctor's orders for lipid infusion frequency and rate
Current nutritional status (weight, height, skin turgor, edema)
Laboratory values, particularly albumin level, glucose, and potassium

Nursing Diagnoses

The nursing diagnoses may include the following:

Altered nutrition: less than body requirements related to anorexia

Outcome Identification and Planning

Desired Outcomes (sample)
Client maintains elastic skin turgor during PN administration.
Client gains 1 to 2 lb per week.
Client has no edema present.
Acceptable laboratory values: albumin and potassium levels within normal range; glucose level within acceptable range.

Special Considerations

High glucose levels in PN provide a good medium for bacterial growth; thus, strict asepsis is needed to prevent septicemia.

Some facilities use 3 in 1 parenteral solution containing lipids; thus, no additional lipids are needed.

Pediatric and Geriatric

Children and the elderly tend to be very sensitive to volume changes; thus, volume should be infused cautiously.

They are also susceptible to infection; therefore, check frequently for temperatures and other signs of infection.

Delegation

DO NOT DELEGATE CENTRAL LINE CARE TO NON-RN PERSONNEL UNLESS HOSPITAL POLICY DICTATES AND YOU HAVE ASSESSED THAT PERSON TO WHOM YOU WILL DELEGATE HAS BEEN PROPERLY INSTRUCTED AND CERTIFIED.

IMPLEMENTATION

Action	Rationale

Central PN

1. Wash hands and organize equipment.

Reduces microorganism transfer
Promotes efficiency

2. Assist in starting central line (see Procedure 5.9) and monitor client appropriately.

Provides venous access for PN

3. Don gloves.

Reduces contamination

4. Mark port intended for PN and close it with infusion plug or prepare infusion of $D_{10}W$ or D_5W to be used until PN solution is available. DO NOT INFUSE MEDICATIONS OR OTHER SOLUTIONS THROUGH PORT.

Preserves sterility of port for PN
Maintains tubing for PN
Minimizes contamination of tubing

5. Compare PN label with doctor's orders.

Verifies correct dosage of nutrients

6. Check client's name band against PN label.

Verifies correct client

7. Prepare PN:
   - If refrigerated, allow bag/bottle to stand at room temperature for 15 to 30 min.

Prevents infusion of cold fluid with resulting discomfort and chilling

Action	Rationale
- Put time tape on bag/bottle.	
- Close drip regulator on filtered tubing.	
- Remove cap from filtered IV tubing to expose spike.	
- Remove tab/cover from PN bag/bottle.	
- Insert tubing spike.	
- Prime drip chamber.	
- Open drip regulator.	
- Clear air from tubing.	
- Close drip regulator.	
- Place tubing at bedside.	
8. Prepare lipids (if lipids and PN are to infuse simultaneously):	
- Put time tape on bottle (mark every 2 hr if small hourly infusion).	*Facilitates correct infusion rate*
- Insert vented, nonfiltered tubing spike into lipid container.	
- Prime drip chamber and clear air from tubing.	*Prevents infusion of air into chest*
- Place needle (21 gauge) on end of tubing and plug into medication plug at distal end of PN tubing (Fig. 5.17).	
9. Attach PN tubing to central line port (see Fig. 5.17).	
10. Discard gloves and disposable materials; position client for comfort with call light within reach.	*Promotes clean environment* *Facilitates communication and client safety*
11. Set pumps to deliver appropriate volumes per hour.	
12. Calculate and check drip rate and monitor infusion every 1 to 2 hr. (If infusion	*Verifies correct infusion rate*

Action	Rationale

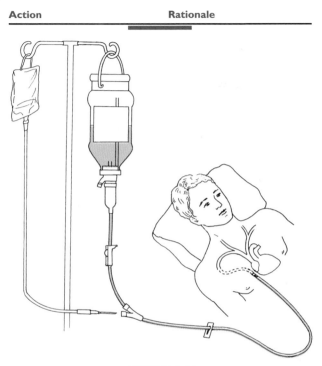

FIGURE 5.17

is behind schedule, DO NOT SPEED UP IN-FUSION RATE. Correct infusion rate and resume proper administration.)	*Prevents volume overload or glucose bolus*
13. Perform client teaching regarding:	
- Need to keep solution higher than chest and avoid manipulating catheter	*Facilitates proper flow of solution*
- Need to report any pain, respiratory distress, warmth, or flushing	*Indicates possible catheter dislodgment or infection*

Action	Rationale
14. Monitor:	
- Vital signs with temperature check every 4 to 8 hr (depending on orders)	*Facilitates early detection of infection or complications*
- Blood glucose level every 12 to 24 hr (more frequently if client is diabetic)	*Detects glucose intolerance*
- Urine glucose and electrolytes in pediatric clients (and watch for signs of hyperglycemia)	
- Central line site every shift; provide care every 72 hr, or per policy. (see Procedure 5.9)	
- For dyspnea (ie, rales in lung bases)	*Indicates possible fluid overload*
15. Weigh client daily and monitor total protein and albumin levels.	*Indicates benefits of nutritional intake*
16. Place PN and lipids on rolling infusion pumps and encourage client ambulation, if allowed.	*Facilitates pulmonary toilet* *Facilitates muscle development* *Promotes sense of well-being*

Evaluation

Were desired outcomes achieved?

Documentation

The following should be noted on the client's chart:

- Time PN bottle/bag is hung, number of bottles/bags, and rate of infusion
- Site of IV catheter and verification of patency
- Status of dressing and site, if visible
- Laboratory results of electrolytes
- Client tolerance to PN

SAMPLE DOCUMENTATION

DATE	TIME	
3/9/02	2400	Bag #3 of PN infusing at 80 ml/hr into middle port of right subclavian triple-lumen catheter. Catheter insertion site intact, with good blood return. Fingerstick blood sugar 110.

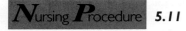

Blood Transfusion Management

 EQUIPMENT

- Blood transfusion tubing (Blood Y set with in-line filter)
- 250- to 500-ml bag/bottle normal saline
- Packed cells or whole blood, as ordered
- Blood warmer or coiled tubing and pan of warm water (optional)
- Order slips for blood
- Flow sheet for vital signs (for frequent checks)
- Nonsterile gloves
- Materials for IV start (see Procedures 5.3 and 5.4)

Purpose

Increases client's hemoglobin and hematocrit for improved circulation and oxygen distribution

Assessment

Assessment should focus on the following:

Baseline vital signs; circulatory and respiratory status
Skin status (eg, rash)
Doctor's orders for type, amount, and rate of blood administration
Size of IV catheter or need for catheter insertion
History of blood transfusions and reactions, if any
Religious or other personal objections to client's receipt of blood
Compatibility of client to blood (matching blood sheet numbers to name band)

Nursing Diagnoses

The nursing diagnoses may include:
Activity intolerance related to weakness (associated with low hemoglobin and hematocrit levels)
Fluid volume deficit related to gastrointestinal hemorrhage

Outcome Identification and Planning

Desired Outcomes (sample)

Blood pressure, pulse, respirations, and temperature are within normal range for client within 48 hrs.

Client's activity tolerance has increased to ambulation in hallway without dyspnea.

Client has adequate circulation, as evidenced by capillary refill time of 2 to 3 sec, pink mucous membranes, and warm, dry skin.

Special Considerations

Some agencies require that two registered nurses perform blood–client identification checks. Refer to agency policy.

Clients with a history of previous transfusions must be watched carefully for a transfusion reaction.

The maximum transfusion time for packed cells or whole blood is 4 hr.

The transfusion must be started within half an hour after getting the blood from the blood bank; otherwise, the blood cannot be reissued.

Geriatric

Fluid-sensitive clients may not tolerate a rapid change in blood volume; they must receive the transfusion as slowly as possible.

Pediatric

Small children and confused or comatose clients must be watched closely for a transfusion reaction because they often cannot communicate discomfort.

Home Health

Remain with the client during the entire transfusion period and for 1 hr afterward.

Because you may be the only licensed caregiver in the home at the time, double-check the date, time, and transfusion information on the blood bag and blood bank slip at two separate points in time or ask the client or relative to verify that the transfusion data are identical.

Have adrenalin on hand in case an anaphylactic reaction occurs.

Delegation

UNLICENSED PERSONNEL MAY BE HELPFUL IN TAKING FREQUENT VITAL SIGNS DURING THE INFUSION, BUT THEY SHOULD PLAY NO PART IN MATCHING OF PATIENT WITH BLOOD OR HANGING OF TRANSFUSION. IT IS THE NURSE'S RESPONSIBILITY TO MONITOR FOR COMPLICATIONS.

IMPLEMENTATION

Action	Rationale
1. Wash hands and organize equipment.	*Reduces microorganism transfer* *Promotes efficiency*
2. Explain procedure to client, particularly the need for frequent vital sign checks.	*Decreases client anxiety*
3. **Prepare tubing:**	
- Open tubing package and close drip regulator (which may be a clamp, roller, or screw). Note red and white caps over tubing spikes.	*Prepares for infusion of saline before and after transfusion*
- Remove white cap to reveal spike on one side of blood tubing (Fig. 5.18*A*).	
- Remove tab from normal saline bag/bottle and insert tubing spike.	
- Remove cap from end of tubing, open saline regulator 1, prime drip chamber with saline, and flush tubing to end.	*Prevents air from entering tubing* *Clears air from tubing*
- Close fluid regulator.	
- Replace cap on tubing end and place on bed near IV catheter.	*Retains sterility*
(If infusing blood rapidly, connect to warming-coil tubing and flush tubing to end. Place coil in warm water bath.)	*Prepares medium for warming blood before infusing* *Prevents infusion of cold blood and lowering of body temperature*
4. Don gloves, and insert IV catheter, if needed (see Procedure 5.4) or if IV catheter is present, verify that it is of adequate size (catheter should be 20 gauge or larger).	*Decreases hemolysis* *Allows free flow of blood*
Remove dressing enough to expose catheter hub.	*Permits access for connection of blood tubing*

Action	Rationale

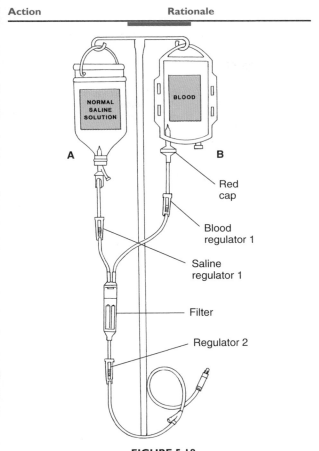

A
B

Red cap

Blood regulator 1

Saline regulator 1

Filter

Regulator 2

FIGURE 5.18

5. Connect blood tubing to catheter hub (discard infusion plug or place needle cap over previous infusion-tubing tip).

Connects blood directly to catheter
Preserves previous infusion for future use

Action	Rationale
6. Open fluid regulator fully and regulate to a rate that will keep vein open (15 to 30 ml/hr) until blood is available.	*Verifies and maintains patency of catheter*
7. **Check for correct identification information.** When blood arrives, check blood and client information with a second nurse; compare blood package with:	*Prevents transfusion of unmatched blood. Failure to identify the blood product or client properly is often linked to severe transfusion reactions*
- *Order slip*, checking client name, hospital number, blood type, expiration date	*Verifies that the patient's name, ABO group, Rh type, and unit number match*
- *Client's name band:* name and hospital number (or emergency department number on name band if typing and cross-matching were done in emergency department). *If discrepancies are noted, notify the blood bank immediately and postpone transfusion until problems are resolved.*	*Ensures transfusion to correct client*
8. Complete blood bank slip with date and time of transfusion initiation and nurses' checking information.	*Provides legal record of blood verification*
9. Check and record pulse, respirations, blood pressure, and temperature.	*Provides baseline vital signs before blood transfusion*
10. Remove red cap to reveal spike on other side of blood tubing and push spike into port on blood bag (Fig. 5.18B).	
11. Close regulator 1 on normal saline side of tubing and open regulator 1 on blood side of tubing.	*Prevents saline from infusing into blood bag* *Allows blood tubing to fill with blood*
12. Regulate drip rate to deliver:	

Action	Rationale
a. A maximum of 30 ml of blood within the first 15 min	*Most reactions occur within the first 15 min*
b. One half to one quarter of the volume of blood each hour (62 to 125 ml/hr—depending on client tolerance of volume change and volume of blood to be infused); if client has poor tolerance of volume change, some blood banks will divide units in half so 8 hr may be used to infuse 1 unit of packed cells.	*Delivers blood volume in 2 to 4 hr* *Allows slower infusion of total unit without violating 4-hr transfusion time limit*
13. Check vital signs and temperature again 15 min after beginning the transfusion, then every half hour or hourly until transfusion is completed (refer to agency policy); check at the completion of delivery of each unit of blood.	*Detects transfusion reaction (Most reactions occur within the first 15 min)*
14. When blood transfusion is complete:	
- Clamp off blood regulator 1.	*Clears bloodline for infusion of other fluids*
- Turn on normal saline.	
- Remove empty blood bag/bottle. Recap spike.	*Maintains sterility for future transfusions*
- Fill in time of completion on blood bank slip, and place copy of slip with empty bag or bottle.	*Complies with agency regulations for confirmation of blood administration*
- Place other copy of slip on chart. (If no further blood is to be given, replace blood transfusion tubing with IV tubing or infusion plug.)	
15. During and after transfusion, monitor client closely for signs of a trans-	*Prevents severe complications from undetected reaction*

Action	Rationale

fusion reaction, which
include the following:
- **Allergic reaction,** | *Indicates incompatibility*
evidenced by rash, chills, | *between transfused red cells*
fever, nausea, or severe | *and host cells*
hypotension (shock)
- **Pyrogenic reaction** | *Indicates sepsis and subsequent*
(usually noted toward | *renal shutdown*
end or after transfusion),
evidenced by nausea,
chilling, fever, and
headache
- **Circulatory overload,** | *Indicates acute pulmonary edema*
evidenced by cough, | *or congestive failure*
dyspnea, distended neck
veins, and rales in lung
bases

16. *If allergic or pyrogenic
reaction is noted:*
- Turn off blood trans- | *Decreases further infusion of*
fusion. | *incompatible or contaminated*
| *blood*
- Remove blood tubing | *Maintains catheter patency*
and replace with tubing
primed with normal
saline.
- Turn on normal saline
at slow rate.
- Contact doctor
immediately.

17. *If fluid overload is noted:*
- Slow blood transfusion | *Decreases workload of the heart*
rate and contact doctor. | *and avoids further overload*
- Take vital signs | *Detects and treats resulting*
frequently (every 10 to | *shock or cardiac insufficiency*
15 min until stable), and
perform emergency
treatment as needed or
ordered.
- Remove and send re-
maining blood and blood
tubing to blood bank
with completed blood
transfusion forms.
- Send first voided urine | *Confirms hemolytic reaction if*
specimen to laboratory. | *red blood cells are present*

Action	Rationale
- Monitor I & O (particularly urinary output).	*Detects renal shutdown secondary to reaction*
- Check vital signs every 4 hr for 24 hr (or per institutional policy).	*Facilitates early detection of complications*
18. Position client for comfort.	
19. Discard supplies, remove gloves, and wash hands.	*Prevents spread of micro-organisms*

Evaluation

Were desired outcomes achieved?

Documentation

The following should be noted on the client's chart:

- Date and initiation and completion times for each unit of blood transfused
- Type of blood infused (packed cells or whole blood)
- Initial and subsequent vital signs
- Presence or absence of transfusion reaction and actions taken
- State of client after transfusion and current IV fluids infusing, if any

SAMPLE DOCUMENTATION

DATE	TIME	
1/9/02	0400	One unit of packed red blood cells (Unit #R46862, O positive) hung at 0345; blood pressure, 120/70; pulse, 80 and regular; respirations, 20 and nonlabored; temperature, 98.4°F after first 15 min of transfusion. Blood regulated at 100 ml/hr to infuse over 3 hr. No signs of transfusion reaction or fluid overload noted.

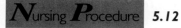 **N**ursing **P**rocedure **5.12**

 Nasogastric/Nasointestinal Tube Insertion

 EQUIPMENT

- Nasogastric (NG) tube (14 to 18 French sump tube) or naso-intestinal (8 to 12 French, small-bore feeding tube)
- Lubricant
- Ice chips or glass of water
- Appropriate-sized syringe:
  - NG: 30- or 60-cc syringe with catheter tip
  - Small bore: 20- to 30-cc luer-lock syringe
- Nonsterile gloves
- Stethoscope
- 1-inch tape (two 3-inch strips and one 1-inch strip)
- Washcloth, gauze, cotton balls, cotton-tipped swab
- Petroleum jelly
- Emesis basin
- Tissues

Purpose

Permits nutritional support through gastrointestinal tract
Allows evacuation of gastric contents
Relieves nausea

Assessment

Assessment should focus on the following:

Doctor's order for type of tube and use of tube
Size of previous tube used, if any
History of nasal or sinus problems

Nursing Diagnoses

The nursing diagnoses may include the following:

Altered nutrition: less than body requirements, related to dysphagia
Nausea and vomiting related to absence of bowel peristalsis

Outcome Identification and Planning

Desired Outcomes (sample)

Client gains 1 to 2 lb per week.
Client has no complaints of nausea or vomiting

Special Considerations

Pediatric

Be prepared to use protective device or enlist family to prevent client pulling on NG tube.
If NG tube is plastic, change every 3 days.
The tube should be taped to side of client's face rather than to nostril to prevent nasal ulceration.

Delegation

Unlicensed personnel are not commonly skilled in NG feeding tube insertion.

IMPLEMENTATION

Action	Rationale
1. Wash hands and organize equipment.	*Reduces microorganism transfer* *Promotes efficiency*
2. Explain procedure to client.	*Reduces anxiety* *Promotes cooperation and participation*
3. Place client in semi-Fowler's position.	*Facilitates passage of tube into esophagus instead of trachea*
4. Check and improve nasal patency:	
- Ask client to breathe through one naris while the other is occluded.	*Determines patency of nasal passage*
- Repeat with other naris.	*Determines patency of nasal passage*
- Have client blow nose with both nares open.	*Clears nasal passage without pushing microorganisms into inner ear*
- Clean mucus and secretions from nares with moist tissues or cotton-tipped swabs	*Clears nasal passage*
5. Measure length of tubing needed by using tube itself as a tape measure:	

Action	Rationale
- Measure distance from tip of nose to earlobe, placing rounded end of tubing at earlobe (Fig. 5.19A).	*Indicates distance from nasal entrance to pharyngeal area*
- Continue measurement from earlobe to sternal notch (Fig. 5.19B).	*Indicates distance from pharyngeal area to stomach*
- Mark location of sternal notch along the tubing with small strip of tape.	*Indicates depth to which tube should be inserted*
- Place tube in ice-water bath (optional).	*Makes tube less pliable*
(If a feeding tube with weighted tip is used [small-bore feeding tube], insert guidewire and prepare the tube as instructed on package insert [usually by flushing with 10–20 cc of irrigation saline]).	*Facilitates insertion of tube*
6. Don gloves and dip feeding tube in water to lubricate tip.	*Reduces contamination* *Promotes smooth insertion of tube*
7. Ask client to tilt head backward; insert tube into clearest naris.	*Facilitates smooth entrance of tube into naris*

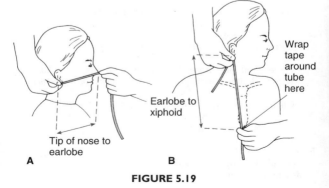

Wrap tape around tube here

Earlobe to xiphoid

Tip of nose to earlobe

A

B

FIGURE 5.19

Action	Rationale
8. As you insert tube deeper into naris, have client hold head and neck straight and open mouth.	*Decreases possibility of insertion into trachea* *Allows nurse to see when tube is in pharynx*
9. When tube is seen and client can feel tube in pharynx, instruct client to swallow (offer ice chips or sips of water).	*Facilitates passage of tube into esophagus*
10. Insert tube further into esophagus as client swallows (if client coughs or tube curls in throat, withdraw tube to pharynx and repeat attempts); between attempts, encourage client to take deep breaths.	*Prevents trauma from forcing tube and prevents tube from entering trachea* *Maintains good oxygenation*
11. When tape mark on tube reaches entrance to naris, stop tube insertion and check placement: - Have client open mouth for tube visualization. - Aspirate with syringe and monitor for gastric drainage (or old tube feeding if reinsertion). - Connect syringe with 10 to 20 cc (10 cc for pediatric clients) air to tube, and push air in while listening to stomach with stethoscope (see Fig. 5.21); if gurgling is heard, secure tube. (If tube is a feeding tube, remove the guidewire and store it.)	*Indicates that tube is in stomach and not curled in mouth or in tracheobronchial tree* *Preserves guidewire for reinsertion of tube, if needed*
12. To secure tube: - Split 2 inches of long tape strip, leaving 1 inch of strip intact. - Apply 1-inch base of tape on bridge of nose.	*Maintains tube placement with client activity*

Action	Rationale
- Wrap first one and then the other side of split tape around tube (Fig. 5.20).	
13. Tape loop of tube to side of client's face (if feeding tube) or pin to client's gown (if sump tube).	*Decreases pull on client's nose and possible dislodgment*
14. Obtain order for chest radiograph; delay tube feeding or flushing with fluid until doctor has read radiograph.	*Confirms placement of tube in stomach or duodenum for type of tube* *Prevents infusion of fluid into lungs*
15. Store stylet from small-bore feeding tube in a plastic bag at the bedside after correct placement is confirmed by x-ray film.	
16. Begin suction or tube feeding as ordered.	

Evaluation

Were desired outcomes achieved?

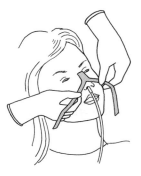 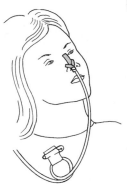

FIGURE 5.20

Documentation

The following should be noted on the client's chart:

- Date and time of tube insertion
- Color and amount of drainage return
- Size and type of tube
- Client tolerance to procedure
- Confirmation of tube placement by radiograph
- Suction applied or tube feeding started and rate

SAMPLE DOCUMENTATION

DATE	TIME	
3/9/02	1230	Sump tube (#18) inserted via left naris, with no obstruction or difficulty, tolerated with no visible clinical problems. Gastric aspirate reveals acidic pH. Gurgling audible with insertion of air; radiograph obtained with placement confirmed by Dr. Wey. Connected to suction at 80 mmHg, with scant green drainage noted.

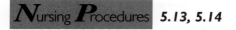

 Nasogastric Tube Maintenance (5.13)

 Nasogastric Tube Discontinuation (5.14)

🔋 EQUIPMENT

- Syringe and container with saline (irrigation kit)
- Tape or tube holder
- Washcloth, gauze, cotton balls, cotton-tipped swabs
- Petroleum jelly or ointment
- Towel or linen saver
- 500- or 1000-ml bottle saline or ordered irrigant
- Stethoscope
- Mouth moistener
- Nonsterile gloves

Purpose

Minimizes damage to naris from tube
Maintains proper tube placement
Promotes proper gastric suctioning or tube feeding
Terminates nasogastric (NG) therapy properly

Assessment

Assessment should focus on the following:

Size and type of tube
Purpose of tube
Doctor's orders regarding type and frequency of tube irrigation
Type and rate of tube feeding

Nursing Diagnoses

The nursing diagnoses may include the following:

Altered nutrition: less than body requirements related to dysphagia

244

Outcome Identification and Planning

Desired Outcomes (sample)

Tubing patency is maintained.
Client will have no episodes of nausea or vomiting.

Special Considerations

General

Aspiration is a primary problem with NG tubes. Clients at risk for aspiration are those with decreased levels of consciousness, those with absent or diminished cough reflex, and those who are noncommunicative and recumbent most of the time (Young & White, 1992).

Home Health

When NG therapy is long term, include in plan of care replacement of tube at specified intervals to avoid complications.
Home caregivers should be taught signs of and ways to avoid aspiration.

 Cost-cutting Tip

Use of 60-cc syringe may be economical because the plastic outer casing that holds the syringe can be used to hold irrigation fluid, thus eliminating the need for an irrigation kit.

Delegation

Unlicensed personnel may administer NG tubefeeding, if skilled in the process. Consult agency policy.

IMPLEMENTATION

Action	Rationale
Procedure 5.13 Nasogastric Tube Maintenance	
1. Question client regarding discomfort from tube and determine need for adjustments.	*Facilitates client comfort*
2. Observe tube insertion site for signs of irritation or pressure.	*Indicates need to adjust or remove tube from current site*
3. Don gloves.	*Reduces contamination*
4. Check tube placement before irrigation or medication administration and every 4 to 8 hr of tube feeding:	

Action	Rationale
- Have client open mouth for tube visualization.	*Indicates that tube is in stomach and not curled in mouth or in tracheobronchial tree*
- Aspirate and monitor for gastric contents (or old tube feeding if reinsertion).	
- Connect syringe with 15 to 20 cc air to NG tube, and push air in while listening to stomach with stethoscope; if gurgling is heard, secure tube (Fig. 5.21).	
5. Cleanse nares with moist gauze or cloth and apply ointment or oil to site.	*Maintains skin integrity and patency of nares*
6. Every 4 hr, perform mouth care: apply moistener to oral cavity and ointment to lips.	*Maintains integrity of oral mucous membranes*

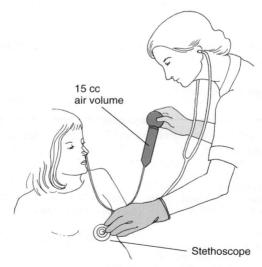

15 cc
air volume

Stethoscope

FIGURE 5.21

Action	Rationale
7. Irrigate tube (if permitted by doctor) with 20 to 30 ml of saline every 3 hr:	*Maintains patency of tube*
- Connect saline-filled syringe to tube.	
- Slowly and gently push fluid into tube.	*Prevents rupture of tube*
- Aspirate fluid gently; note appearance and discard.	*Removes irrigant and detects possible gastric bleeding*
- Repeat irrigation and aspiration.	
- Reconnect tube to suction or tube feeding.	
8. Remove and reapply tape if loose or extremely soiled.	*Prevents dislodgment of tube* *Promotes cleanliness*
9. If entrance to naris is irritated, place tube in other naris, if clear.	*Prevents additional skin break-down*
10. Reconnect to tube feeding (see Procedure 5.15) or suction.	

Gastric Suction

Action	Rationale
11. Every 2 hr, check suction for appropriate suction pressure (usually 80 to 100 mmHg = low suction) and frequency (ie, constant or intermittent).	
12. Monitor drainage in tubing and bag for color, consistency, and odor.	*Indicates presence of bleeding or infection or need for irrigation*
13. Each shift, mark drainage level (if bottle or canister is used) or empty and measure amount of drainage.	*Monitors amounts of drainage*
14. To empty drainage bag (if 75% to 100% full), first turn off suction and wait until suction meter returns to 0. Measure and record drainage.	*Removes suction pressure so canister can be emptied*

Action	Rationale

If Using Canister Suction
(wall or floor suction)
- Loosen seal and remove cap (disconnect tubing leading to NG tube if disposable lining is used).
- Empty contents into graduated container and rinse canister (or discard plastic liner and obtain fresh one).
- Reseal cap and reconnect NG tubing.

If Using Vacuum Suction
- Open door to suction machine (Omnibus).
- Remove bag.
- Remove cap from bag port.
- Pour contents into graduated container.
- Replace cap and place bag into suction machine.
- Reseal door to suction machine.
- Reset and initiate appropriate suction pressure.

15. Every 24 hr (or per institutional policy) replace drainage bag (if used) and clean canister. — *Reduces accumulation of micro-organisms*

16. Discard supplies and wash hands. — *Reduces contamination*

Procedure 5.14 Nasogastric Tube Discontinuation

1. Explain procedure to client. — *Decreases anxiety*
2. Place client in semi-Fowler's position. — *Opens glottis for easy removal*
3. Don gloves. — *Reduces contamination*
4. Remove tape securing tube to cheek or attaching tube to gown and remove or loosen tape across bridge of nose. — *Facilitates smooth removal of tube*

Action	Rationale

5. Remove tube:
  - Place towel under nose and drape over tube.
  - Clamp tube by pinching off or folding over.
  - Slowly withdraw tube until completely removed.
  - Wrap tube in towel and place in trash bag.
	Shields appearance of tube from client during removal
	Prevents aspiration while withdrawing tube (accidental leaking of gastric contents from tube into lungs)

6. Clean nares and apply ointment.	*Promotes skin integrity*
7. Perform mouth care.	
8. Position client with head of bed elevated 45 degrees and call light within reach.	*Facilitates comfort and gastric drainage*
9. Encourage client to call if nausea or discomfort is experienced.	*Facilitates early detection of gastric distention or distress*
10. Monitor bowel sounds and note flatulence.	*Indicates adequate bowel activity*

Evaluation

Were desired outcomes achieved?

Documentation

The following should be noted on the client's chart:

- Type of NG tube and therapy (suction or tube feeding)
- Status of tubing patency and security
- Type and amount of drainage (or of residual if tube feeding)
- Time of NG tube removal
- Client tolerance of continued therapy or tube removal

SAMPLE DOCUMENTATION

DATE	TIME	
2/5/02	1400	NG suction intact per Omnibus suction at 80 mmHg continuous suction pressure. Thick green drainage noted, with scant amounts this shift. Sump tube intact in right naris, with surrounding skin intact. Bilateral nares cleaned with petroleum jelly.
	1800	NG tube removed per orders. Mouth care performed with mouthwash. Active bowel sounds noted. Sips of water provided and tolerated without nausea.

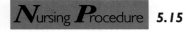

 Tube Feeding Management/Medication by Nasogastric Tube

EQUIPMENT

- Ordered tube feeding
- Syringe
- Tube feeding pump or infusion pump
- Appropriate feeding bag and tubing for pump
- Glass or cup
- Nonsterile gloves

Purpose

Provides nutritional support using the gastrointestinal tract

Assessment

Assessment should focus on the following:

Nutritional status (skin turgor, urine output, weight, caloric intake)
Elimination pattern (diarrhea, constipation, date of last stool)
Response to previous nutritional support

Nursing Diagnoses

The nursing diagnoses may include the following:

Altered nutrition: less than body requirements related to anorexia

Outcome Identification and Planning

Desired Outcomes (sample)

Tube feeding is infused at appropriate volume and rate.
Client has no complaints of nausea or signs of aspiration.
Client gains 1 to 2 lb per week or maintains desired weight.
Client has decreased edema with albumin level within normal
limits.

Special Considerations

If client has endotracheal or tracheostomy tube and is receiving NG tube feedings, check tracheostomy cuff inflation. If cuff is deflated, inflate and maintain for 30 min after feeding to prevent aspiration.

Many tube feeding formulas cause diarrhea; thus, volume and concentration should be increased slowly. If diarrhea persists, report to doctor and administer antidiarrhea medication, if ordered.

Be careful with gastrostomy tube irrigations. Depending on the surgery, irrigation may be contraindicated. Verify this with the doctor.

Pediatric

Feeding time is normally a time for interaction with an infant or child; thus, it is crucial that the nurse or family member administering the tube feeding hold, cuddle, and establish eye contact with the child during feeding (Fig. 5.22). The feeding formula

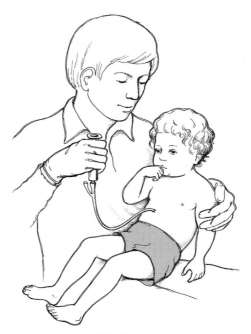

FIGURE 5.22

should be at room temperature. The rate for intermittent feeding should be approximately 10 ml/min.

Delegation

UNLICENSED PERSONNEL MAY BE DELEGATED TO PERFORM TUBE FEEDING IF THEY ARE PROPERLY TRAINED AND AGENCY POLICY PERMITS. THE NURSE MUST MONITOR PATIENT AND RESIDUAL FEEDING LEVELS.

IMPLEMENTATION

Action	Rationale
1. Wash hands and organize supplies.	*Reduces contamination* *Promotes efficiency*
2. Explain procedure to client and insert feeding tube, if needed (see Procedure 5.12).	
3. Verify tube placement:	*Indicates that tube is in stomach*
- Radiograph (chest x-ray), (check last x-ray report if tube has not been newly inserted)	
- Assess the pH level of nasogastric tube aspirant.	*Verifies presence of gastric acid* *Prevents infusion of tube feeding*
- Aspirate and monitor for gastric contents (or old tube feeding if reinsertion).	*into pharynx or pulmonary tree*
- Pinch tube off at the end, connect syringe with 15 to 20 cc air to tube, and push air in while listening with stethoscope over epigastric area for gurgling. Proceed to step 4 for continuous feedings or to step 13 for intermittent feedings.	

Continuous Tube Feeding (steps 4 to 12 only)

4. Prepare tube feeding:	*Prevents muscle cramps from*
- Remove feeding from refrigerator 30 min before hanging (if applicable).	*infusion of cold solution*
- Rinse bag and bag tubing with water.	*Checks for bag or tubing leaks*
- Clamp bag tubing closed.	

Action	Rationale
- Pour 4 hours' volume of feeding in bag (1 hour's volume if medication is added).	*Prevents spoilage of feeding hanging without refrigeration*
- Open bag tubing and allow feeding to flow to end.	*Cleans air from tubing*
- Clamp tubing and insert into pump mechanism, if used (Fig. 5.23).	
- Time tape bag (see Procedure 5.6).	
5. Attach feeding bag tubing to feeding tube.	
6. Set pump to deliver appropriate volume; unclamp bag tubing and start pump or regulate manually after calculating	

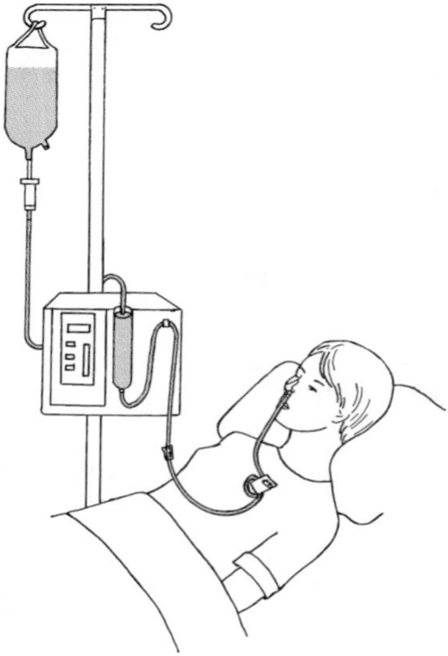

FIGURE 5.23

Action	Rationale

drip rate (see Procedures 5.5 and 5.6).

7. Check infusion hourly or every 2 hr: check time tape and drip rate.

Ensures infusion of proper volume per hour

8. Every 4 hr:
   - Check for residual: stop infusion, slowly aspirate gastric contents, and note amount of residual—may be difficult with small feeding tubes.

Determines degree of absorption of feeding

   (If residual is greater than specified amount per doctor's orders [commonly 100 ml], discard aspirated volume from stomach, cease feedings, and notify doctor.)

Prevents distention of abdomen and possible aspiration

   - Monitor bowel sounds in all abdominal quadrants.

Determines presence of bowel activity (peristalsis)

   - Perform mouth care.

Freshens mouth
Prevents accumulation of micro-organisms

9. Irrigate tube every 3 hr (or after any medication) with 20 to 30 ml saline, or as indicated by doctor's orders or hospital policy.

Maintains patency of tube

10. Once each shift, while irrigating NG tube after completing a supply of tube feeding, rinse bag and tubing with water.

Clears accumulated feeding from bag and tubing

11. Every 24 hr (or 48, if institutional policy), replace old bag and tubing with new.

Removes medium for micro organism growth

12. Elevate head of bed 30 to 45 degrees and maintain throughout feedings.

Decreases aspiration of feeding into lungs

Action	Rationale

Intermittent Tube Feeding

13. Follow steps 1 to 3.
14. Determine amount of water, if any, to be infused and pour into glass or cup.
15. Don gloves.
16. If client previously received feeding, check for and note amount of residual; this may be difficult with small feeding tubes.

    (If residual is greater than specified amount per doctor's orders [commonly 100 ml], discard aspirated volume unless prohibited by doctor's orders or agency policy—delay feeding, and notify doctor.)

    Prevents distention of abdomen and possible aspiration of feeding into lungs

17. Attach syringe to NG tube and aspirate small amount of contents to fill tube and lower portion of syringe.

    Prevents infusion of air into stomach

18. Infuse feeding or medication (see steps 21–24):
    - Hold syringe 6 inches above tube insertion site (nose or abdomen; see Fig. 5.22).
    - Fill syringe with feeding and allow to flow slowly into NG tube; follow with water (30-ml flush if no water is ordered). DO NOT ALLOW SYRINGE TO EMPTY UNTIL FEEDING AND WATER INFUSION ARE COMPLETED.

    Assists flow of feeding by gravity

    Prevents entrance of air into tubing and stomach

19. Clamp NG or gastrostomy tube and place client in semi-Fowler's position.

    Decreases reflux of feeding and possible aspiration into lungs

20. Monitor bowel sounds, stools, and residual continuously.

    Detects loss of or decrease in GI function

Action	Rationale
21. Check NG tube placement and residual before each tube feeding.	*Prevents aspiration of secretions into tracheobronchial tree*

Medication Administration Through NG Tube

22. Check tube placement.	*Prevents obstruction of tube with large medication particles or thick solution*
23. Crush pill (if crushable), and mix with fluid to make a thin solution with small sediment. (*Note:* Be sure guidelines for drug administration are being followed.)	
24. Mix viscous solutions with water or saline (30–60 ml).	*Prevents clogging of tube*
25. Follow medication infusion with 30 ml saline or water.	*Prevents obstruction of tubing*

Evaluation

Were desired outcomes achieved?

Documentation

The following should be noted on the client's chart:

- Type of NG tube and tube feeding
- Status of tubing patency and security
- Type and amount of residual
- Client tolerance of continued therapy or tube removal

SAMPLE DOCUMENTATION

DATE	TIME	
7/8/02	1400	Tube feeding initiated at 0800 with Ensure, 50 ml/hr. Infusing per Dobhoff feeding tube, regulated by infusion pump.
		Active bowel sounds noted; no complaints of nausea. Residual of 30 ml noted after 4 hr of infusion. Tubing flushed with 30 ml water.

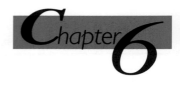

Elimination

OVERVIEW

▶ Adequate elimination of body waste is an essential function
  to sustain life.
▶ Inadequate bladder and bowel elimination ultimately affects
  the body's delicate balance of fluid, electrolyte, and acid–base
  level.
▶ Various means are available clinically to help assess and
  maintain adequate elimination status.
▶ Factors that affect bowel and bladder elimination status
  include food and fluid intake; age; psychological barriers;
  medications; personal hygiene habits; educational level;
  cultural practices; pathology of the renal, urinary, or
  gastrointestinal system; surgery; hormonal variations; muscle

tone of supporting organs and structures; and concurrent medical problems, such as decreased cardiac output or motor disturbances.

▶ Alterations in bowel and bladder elimination mandate careful assessment and monitoring of the upper and lower abdomen, as well as of amounts and appearance of body excretions.

▶ Procedures related to adequate bladder elimination usually require the use of sterile technique to prevent contamination to the highly susceptible urinary tract.

▶ Because clients on peritoneal dialysis or hemodialysis are using final means of adequate renal excretion, it is crucial that the nurse perform these procedures with precision.

▶ Various concentrations of dialysate affect osmolality, rate of fluid removal, electrolyte balance, solute removal, and cardiovascular stability.

▶ Elimination is very personal to the client; therefore, privacy and professionalism should be maintained when assisting clients with elimination needs.

▶ Clients with colostomies frequently experience body-image and self-concept alterations. Psychological support and teaching are crucial in resolving these problems.

▶ All procedures involving elimination of body waste require use of gloves and, occasionally, other protective barriers.

▶ Before planning a procedure, the nurse should determine if same-sex or opposite-sex contact with genitalia is culturally offensive to the client.

▶ Some major nursing diagnostic labels related to elimination are altered urinary elimination, urinary retention, bowel incontinence, constipation, diarrhea, and incontinence (functional, reflex, urge, stress, or total).

▶ For those procedures that can be delegated to unlicensed assistive personnel, emphasis should be placed on procedural accuracy so correct determinations can be made concerning client diagnosis and status of progress.

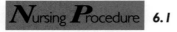

*N*ursing *P*rocedure 6.1

 Midstream Urine Collection

EQUIPMENT

- Basin of warm water
- Soap
- Washcloth
- Towel
- Antiseptic swabs or cotton balls
- Sterile specimen collection container
- Specimen container labels
- Bedpan, urinal, bedside commode, or toilet
- Nonsterile gloves
- Pen

Purpose

Obtains urine specimen by aseptic technique for microbiologic analysis

Assessment

Assessment should focus on the following:

Characteristics of the urine

Symptoms associated with urinary tract infections (eg, pain or discomfort upon voiding, urinary frequency)

Temperature increase

Ability of client to follow instructions for obtaining specimen

Time of day of specimen collection

Fluid intake and output

Nursing Diagnoses

The nursing diagnoses may include the following:

Risk of infection related to poor technique in cleaning perineum

Altered urinary elimination: frequency related to urinary tract infection

Outcome Identification and Planning

Desired Outcomes (sample)

Client shows no signs or symptoms of urinary tract infection.
Client verbalizes relief of discomfort within 3 days.

Special Considerations

Midstream urine collection is frequently performed by the client; however, instructions for the procedure must be clear to obtain reliable laboratory results. Perhaps the most frequent error the client commits is poor cleaning technique. Be certain women understand to cleanse from the front to the back of the perineum, and men from the tip of the penis downward.

If possible, a specimen should be obtained upon first voiding in the morning.

Delegation

This procedure may be delegated. Emphasize importance of procedural accuracy.

IMPLEMENTATION

Action	Rationale
1. Wash hands.	*Reduces microorganism transfer*
2. Explain procedure to client.	*Decreases anxiety*
3. Provide for privacy.	*Decreases embarrassment*
4. Don clean gloves.	*Reduces nurse's exposure to body secretions*
5. Wash perineal area with soap and water, rinse, and pat dry.	*Reduces microorganisms in perineal area*
6. Cleanse meatus with antiseptic solution in same manner as for catheterization in males (see Procedure 6.4, steps 15–17) and females (see Procedure 6.5, steps 23 and 24).	*Reduces microorganisms at urethral opening*
7. Ask client to begin voiding.	*Flushes organisms from urethral opening*
8. After stream of urine begins, place specimen container in place to obtain 30 ml of urine.	*Collects urine at point at which urine is least contaminated*
9. Remove container before client stops voiding.	*Prevents end stream organisms from dripping into container*

Action	Rationale
10. Allow client to complete voiding using urinal, bedpan, or toilet.	
11. Wash perineal area again if stain-producing antiseptic was used.	*Removes antiseptic solution* *Promotes general comfort*
12. Label specimen container with date and time, as well as with client identification information.	
13. Discard equipment and gloves.	*Reduces spread of infection*
14. Wash hands.	*Reduces contamination*

EVALUATION

Were desired outcomes achieved?

DOCUMENTATION

The following should be noted on the client's chart:

- Signs or symptoms of urinary infection
- Amount, color, odor, and consistency of urine obtained
- Specimen collection time
- Total amount voided
- Teaching performed regarding technique for cleaning genitalia

SAMPLE DOCUMENTATION

DATE	TIME	
1/1/02	1100	Clean-catch urine specimen obtained and sent to laboratory—30 ml of cloudy, yellow urine with slightly foul odor noted. Client reports slight perineal burning.

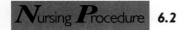

 Urine Specimen Collection From an Indwelling Catheter

EQUIPMENT

- Sterile 3-ml syringe with 23- or 25-gauge needle
- Nonsterile gloves
- Alcohol swab
- Sterile specimen container
- Container labels
- Pen
- Catheter clamp
- Linen saver
- Antiseptic solution

Purpose

Obtains sterile urine specimens for microbiologic analysis

Assessment

Assessment should focus on the following:

Characteristics of the urine
Symptoms associated with urinary tract infections (pain or discomfort)
Temperature increase
Fluid intake and output

Nursing Diagnoses

The nursing diagnoses may include the following:

Risk of infection related to long-term indwelling catheter
Acute pain related to urinary tract infection

Outcome Identification and Planning

Desired Outcomes (sample)
Client shows no signs of urinary tract infection.
Client verbalizes lack of perineal discomfort within 3 days.

Special Considerations

If a specimen is needed and a new catheter is to be inserted, obtain the specimen during catheter insertion procedure. (See Procedure 6.3 or Procedure 6.4.)

Pediatric and Geriatric

If a specimen is needed from a confused or a pediatric client unable to follow directions, obtain assistance to maintain sterility of the specimen and catheter.

Cost-cutting Tip

Rubber band may be used to clamp off catheter.

Delegation

This procedure can be delegated. Emphasize importance of procedural accuracy.

IMPLEMENTATION

Action	Rationale
1. Wash hands.	*Reduces microorganism transfer*
2. Explain procedure to client.	*Decreases anxiety*
3. Provide for privacy.	*Decreases embarrassment*
4. Don clean gloves. Proceed to step 12 for open-system method.	*Reduces nurse's exposure to body secretions*

Closed-System Method

5. Fold or clamp drainage tubing about 4 inches below junction of drainage tubing and catheter.	*Facilitates trapping of urine in tubing at specimen port*
6. Allow urine to pool in drainage tubing; if urine does not pool in tubing immediately, leave it clamped for urine to collect over period of time (usually 10–30 min).	*Allows urine to pool in tubing at specimen port for collection*
7. Cleanse specimen collection port of drainage tubing with alcohol swab or antiseptic solution recommended by agency. (If no collection port is visible, catheter	*Reduces microorganisms at insertion port*

Action	Rationale

tubing is probably designed with a self-sealing material so specimen may be obtained from catheter itself by cleansing and piercing catheter tubing close to junction. However, check package label and instructions. If catheter tubing is self-sealing, cleanse cathether tubing close to junction of drainage tubing.)

8. Carefully insert sterile needle of syringe into specimen-collection port or self-sealing catheter tubing at a 45-degree angle; insert needle slowly, taking care not to puncture other side of catheter tubing (Fig. 6.1).

Prevents accidental puncture of drainage tubing or catheter

9. Pull back on plunger of syringe, and obtain 3 to 10 ml of urine.

Draws urine into syringe

10. Slowly squirt urine into collection container; do not touch inside of specimen container.

Places urine in container, maintaining sterility of container and specimen

11. Complete steps 20 to 24.

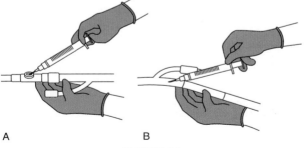

A   B

FIGURE 6.1

Action	Rationale

Open-System Method

12. Place linen saver under tubing at junction of cathether and drainage tubing. — *Prevents soiling of linen*

13. Remove cap from specimen bottle, and place bottle on linen saver.

14. Cleanse junction with antiseptic solution such as Betadine (or antiseptic recommended by agency). — *Reduces microorganisms*

15. Carefully disconnect catheter from drainage tubing at junction. Hold drainage tubing and catheter 1.5 to 2 inches from junction, being careful not to contaminate either end. — *Disconnects catheter to allow for specimen collection* / *Avoids system contamination*

16. Place specimen container under catheter opening, and allow urine to run into container; do not allow catheter tip to touch container. — *Allows urine to run into container* / *Avoids contamination*

17. Place specimen container on bedside table after urine is obtained. — *Prevents contamination of catheter line*

18. Wipe catheter and drainage tubing again with antiseptic solution. — *Reduces microorganism transfer*

19. Firmly reconnect drainage tubing and catheter at junction. — *Reconnects to closed system*

20. Replace top of specimen container. — *Prevents urine waste*

21. Label container with date and time of collection, as well as with client identification information. — *Eliminates errors in client identification*

22. Fill out agency requisition form for specimen. — *Facilitates proper logging and charging in lab*

Action	Rationale
23. Send to laboratory immediately.	*Avoids sending old specimen in which urine constituents may have changed*
24. Discard gloves and wash hands.	*Prevents spread of micro-organisms*

Evaluation

Were desired outcomes achieved?

Documentation

The following should be noted on the client's chart:

- Amount, color, odor, and consistency of urine obtained
- Specimen collection time
- Total amount of urine collected
- Signs or symptoms of urinary infection
- Disposition of specimen to lab

SAMPLE DOCUMENTATION

DATE	TIME	
12/31/02	1000	Sterile urine specimen obtained via indwelling catheter and sent to laboratory. Specimen is 30 ml of cloudy, yellow urine, with slightly foul odor noted. Client reports slight perineal burning.

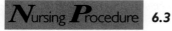

Nursing Procedure 6.3

Condom Catheter Application

EQUIPMENT

- Nonsterile gloves
- Washcloth
- Towel
- Basin of warm, soapy water
- Condom catheter
- Velcro adhesive strip or elastic adhesive strip
- Urine drainage bag with tubing

Purpose

Provides for noninvasive method of urine collection

Assessment

Assessment should focus on the following:

Ability of client to void without incontinent episodes
Appearance of penis (skin intactness, no edema)

Nursing Diagnoses

The nursing diagnoses may include the following:

Urinary incontinence related to neuromuscular disorder
Self-care deficit related to confusion and physical debilitation

Outcome Identification and Planning

Desired Outcomes (sample)
Client voids without spillage of urine.
Client experiences no skin breakdown in area of penile shaft.
Client experiences no constriction of blood flow in area of penile
  shaft.

Special Considerations

Geriatric

Many geriatric clients have condom catheters applied because of confusion coupled with discomfort of soiled skin and linens. Reorient client as necessary to facilitate cooperation with maintaining catheter.

Pediatric

Infant/pediatric boys may receive a condom catheter to facilitate specimen collection or accuracy of output.

Home Health

Clients and caregivers should be taught procedure and importance of reassessment of penis at intervals during the day.

Delegation

This procedure may be delegated to unlicensed assistive personnel. Emphasize the importance of removal during bath and inspection of the penis at intervals. The primary responsbility for inspection, however, lies with the nurse.

IMPLEMENTATION

Action	Rationale
1. Wash hands.	*Reduces microorganism transfer*
2. Explain procedure to client.	*Decreases anxiety*
3. Provide for privacy.	*Decreases embarrassment*
4. Place client in low Fowler's or supine position.	*Facilitates comfort for client and access to full penis length*
5. Place urinary drainage bag on bed so tubing lies on bed, loops off of bed mattress toward bedframe, and hooks onto bedframe (should not be looped through or onto bed rail).	*Facilitates placement of drainage system so it is easily accessible for connection to condom catheter and prevents entanglement in rails to avoid pulling off of penis*
6. Don clean gloves.	*Reduces nurse's exposure to body secretions*
7. Wash and dry penis well.	*Cleans skin, removing debris* *Facilitates adherence of condom appliance*
8. Hold shaft of penis firmly using nondominant hand.	*Positions penis for placement of catheter*

Action	Rationale
9. Obtain condom catheter with dominant hand and roll onto penis from distal tip up shaft, leaving 2.5 to 5 cm (1–2 in) of open space between distal tip of penis at end of catheter to be attached to drainage tubing (Fig. 6.2).	
10. Holding condom catheter in place with nondominant hand, place Velcro or elastic adhesive completely around top end of condom catheter that is on penis. Velcro/elastic adhesive should be on rubber catheter, not penis itself, and should be snug, not tight (Fig. 6.3).	*Positions condom catheter and secures in place with appropriate apparatus and avoids constriction of penile shaft*
11. Connect end of catheter to drainage tubing (Fig 6.4).	*Facilitates drainage into bag rather than urine spillage onto client skin or bed linens*
12. Arrange drainage tubing so it is loose, but not pulling (Fig. 6.5).	*Avoids accidental pulling off of catheter due to weight of tubing*
13. Position client.	*Facilitates comfort*
14. Raise side rails. Place call light within reach.	*Facilitates safety*
15. Discard basin of water and bathing supplies.	*Cleans bedside area*

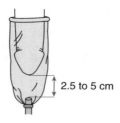

2.5 to 5 cm

FIGURE 6.2

Action	Rationale

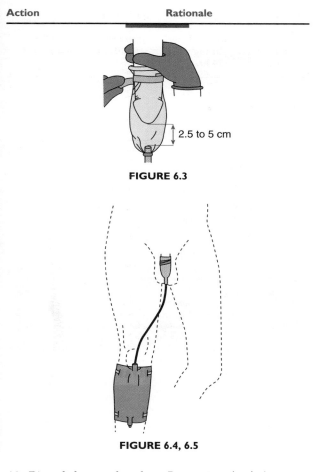

FIGURE 6.3

2.5 to 5 cm

FIGURE 6.4, 6.5

16. Discard gloves and wash hands. — *Prevents transfer of micro-organisms*
17. Document procedure. — *Records prcedure completed*
18. Reassess security of placement, position of catheter on penis, and status of penis and skin every 4 hr. — *Maintains placement and assesses for penile constriction that could cause skin damage or constricted blood flow.*

Action	Rationale
19. Remove condom catheter for half hour during daily bath or every 24 hr.	*Allows for skin care and facilitates full inspection of penis*

Evaluation

Were desired outcomes achieved?

Documentation

The following should be noted on the client's chart:

- Amount, color, odor, and consistency of urine
- Appearance of penis (skin, edema, discharge)
- Status of client comfort

SAMPLE DOCUMENTATION

DATE	TIME	
12/30/02	1000	Condom catheter applied with drainage bag. 300 ml clear yellow urine in bag. No edema of penis noted. Skin at penis area intact. No discharge noted. No c/o pain.

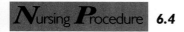

 Male Catheterization

EQUIPMENT

- Urethral catheterization set (includes sterile gloves, specimen-collection container, catheter, two drapes, graduated measurement receptacle, antiseptic solution, cotton balls, forceps, lubricating jelly)
  or
- Indwelling catheterization set (all of the items in urethral catheterization kit except the graduated measurement receptacle, plus a drainage-collection system [tubing and bag that connect to the catheter] and a prefilled saline syringe for inflation)
- Basin of warm soapy water
- Washcloth
- Large towel
- Nonsterile gloves
- Sheet for draping
- Linen saver
- Roll of tape
- Bedpan, urinal, or second collection container
- Specimen container, if specimen is needed
- Goggles (for young boy unable to maintain urinary control during procedure)

Purpose

Facilitates emptying of bladder
Facilitates obtaining sterile urine specimens
Facilitates determining amount of residual urine in bladder
Allows for continuous, accurate monitoring of urinary output
Provides avenue for bladder irrigations

Assessment

Assessment should focus on the following:

Type of catheterization ordered (straight, Foley, residual)
Status of bladder (distention before catheter insertion)
Abnormalities of genitalia or prostate gland
History of conditions that may interfere with smooth insertion
(eg, prostate enlargement, urethral stricture)
Client allergy to iodine-based antiseptics (eg, Betadine)

Nursing Diagnoses

The nursing diagnoses may include the following:

Altered urinary elimination: decreased output related to reduction in total fluid volume

Acute pain related to bladder distention

Urinary retention related to neuromuscular dysfunction

Outcome Identification and Planning

Desired Outcomes (sample)

A urine output of at least 250 ml per shift is attained and maintained during hospital stay.

Client verbalizes relief of lower abdominal pain within 1 hr of catheter insertion.

Special Considerations

Never force a catheter if it does not pass through the urethral canal smoothly. If the catheter still does not pass smoothly after using the suggested troubleshooting methods, discontinue the procedure and notify the physician. Forcing the catheter may result in damage to the urethra and surrounding structures.

Geriatric

A common pathologic feature in elderly men is enlargement of the prostate gland. The enlargement frequently makes inserting a catheter difficult.

Pediatric

In the infant, the bladder is higher and more anterior than in the adult. Common catheter sizes are 8 and 10 French.

Catheterization is a very threatening and anxiety-provoking experience for children. They need explanations, support, and understanding.

Home Health

Because indwelling catheterization is used on a long-term basis for the homebound client, potential is high for infection. Be alert for early signs and symptoms of infection and adhere to a strict schedule for changing catheters.

Explore the possibility of an external catheter as an alternative to the indwelling catheter.

If the client uses intermittent self-catheterization, store sterilized catheters in sterilized jars.

Cost-cutting Tip

If replacing a Foley catheter, note the size of the previous catheter to avoid wastage from insertion of too small a catheter. This occurs frequently with clients on long-term catheterization.

Delegation

In some agencies, catheterization may be delegated to specially trained personnel. Note agency policies concerning delegation of this procedure, and to what level personnel.

IMPLEMENTATION

Action	Rationale
1. Wash hands.	*Reduces microorganism transfer*
2. Explain procedure to client.	*Decreases anxiety*
3. Determine if client is allergic to iodine-based antiseptics.	*Avoids allergic reactions*
4. Provide for privacy.	*Decreases embarrassment*
5. Don nonsterile gloves.	*Reduces nurse's exposure to body secretions*
6. If catheterization is for residual urine, ask client to void in urinal, and measure and record the amount voided; empty urinal.	*Determines amount of urine client is able to void without catheterization* *Determines exact amount*
7. Place linen saver under buttocks.	*Avoids wetting linens*
8. Wash genital area with warm water, rinse, and pat dry with towel.	*Decreases microorganisms around urethral opening*
9. Discard gloves, bath water, wash cloth, and towel; then wash hands.	*Decreases clutter* *Reduces microorganism transfer*
10. Drape client so only penis is exposed.	*Provides privacy* *Reduces embarrassment*
11. Set up work field:	
- Open catheter set and remove from outer plastic package.	*Removes kit without opening inner folds*
- Tape outer package to bedside table with top edge turned inside.	*Provides waste bag*

Action	Rationale
- Place catheter kit beside client's knees and carefully open outer edges.	*Places items within easy reach*
- Ask client to open legs slightly.	*Relaxes pelvic muscles*
- Remove full drape from kit with fingertips and place across thighs, plastic side down, just below penis; keep other side sterile.	*Provides sterile field*
- If catheter and bag are separate, use sterile technique to open package containing bag and place bag on work field.	
12. Don sterile gloves.	*Avoids contaminating other items in kit*
13. Prepare items in kit for use during insertion as follows:	
- Pour iodine solution over cotton balls.	*Prepares cotton balls for cleaning*
- Separate cotton balls with forceps.	*Promotes easy manipulation*
- Lubricate 6 to 7 inches of catheter tip and place carefully on tray so tip is secure in tray.	*Prevents local irritation of meatus on catheter insertion* *Promotes ease of insertion*
- If inserting indwelling catheter, attach prefilled syringe of sterile water to balloon port of catheter.	*Connects to balloon port the syringe needed to inflate balloon*
- Inject 2 to 3 ml of sterile water from prefilled syringe into balloon and observe balloon for leaks as it fills.	*Tests balloon for defects*
- If any leaks are noted, discard and obtain another kit.	*Prevents catheter dislodgment after insertion*
- Deflate balloon, and leave syringe connected.	*Leaves syringe within reach*

Action	Rationale
- Attach catheter to drainage container tubing (or, if drainage tubing is already attached to the catheter, place tubing and bag securely on sterile field, close to the other equipment).	*Facilitates organization while maintaining sterility*
- Check clamp on collection bag to be sure it is closed. Place catheter and collection tray close to perineum.	*Prevents loss of urine before measurement*
- Open specimen collection container and place on sterile field.	*Places container within easy reach for specimen*
14. Remove fenestrated drape from kit and place penis through hole in drape with nondominant hand. KEEP DOMINANT HAND STERILE.	*Expands sterile field*
15. Pull penis up at a 90-degree angle to client's supine body.	*Straightens urethra*
16. With nondominant hand, gently grasp glans (tip) of penis; retract foreskin, if necessary.	*Provides grasp of penis, preventing contamination of sterile field later*
17. With forceps in dominant hand, cleanse meatus and glans with cotton balls, beginning at urethral opening and moving toward shaft of penis; make one complete circle around penis with each cotton ball, discarding cotton ball after each wipe (Fig. 6.6).	*Cleanses meatus without cross-contaminating or contaminating sterile hand*
18. After all cotton balls have been used, discard forceps.	*Prevents contamination of sterile field*

Action	**Rationale**

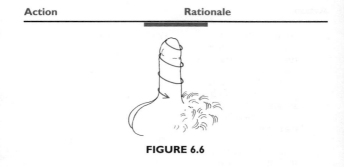

FIGURE 6.6

Action	**Rationale**
19. With thumb and first finger, pick catheter up about 1.5 to 2 inches from tip.	*Gives nurse good control of catheter tip (which easily bends)*
20. Carefully gather additional tubing in hand.	*Gives nurse good control of full catheter length*
21. Ask client to bear down as if voiding and to take slow, deep breaths; encourage him to continue to breathe deeply until catheter is inserted.	*Opens sphincter* *Relaxes sphincter muscles of bladder and urethra*
22. Insert tip of catheter slowly through urethral opening 7 to 9 inches (or until urine returns).	*Inserts catheter*
23. Lower penis to about a 45-degree angle after catheter is inserted about halfway and hold open end of catheter over collection container (if it is not connected to a drainage bag).	*Places penis in position for urine to be released into collection container so accurate amount is measured*
24. If resistance is met: - Stop for a few seconds. - Encourage client to continue taking slow, deep breaths. - Do not force; remove catheter tip and notify doctor if above sequence is unsuccessful.	*Allows sphincters to relax and reduces anxiety* *Prevents injury to prostate, urethra, and surrounding structures*

Action	Rationale
25. After catheter has been advanced an appropriate distance, advance another 1 to 1.5 inches.	*Ensures that catheter advances far enough not to be dislodged*
26. For straight catheterization:	*Obtains sterile specimen*
- Obtain urine specimen in specimen container, if ordered.	
- Allow urine to drain until it stops or UNTIL MAXIMUM NUMBER OF MILLILITERS SPECIFIED BY AGENCY (usually 1000–1500 ml) has drained into container; use second container, bedpan, or urinal, if necessary.	*Empties bladder* *Obtains residual urine amount*
27. For an indwelling catheter, inflate balloon with attached syringe and gently pull back on catheter until it stops (catches).	*Secures catheter placement*
28. Secure catheter loosely with tape to lower abdomen on side from which drainage bag will be hanging (preferably away from door); make certain that tubing is not caught on railing locks or obstructed.	*Stabilizes catheter* *Prevents accidental dislodgment*
29. Clear bed of all equipment.	*Removes waste from bed*
30. Reposition client for comfort, and replace linens for warmth and privacy.	*Promotes general comfort*
31. Raise side rails.	*Prevents falls*
32. Measure amount of urine in collection container or drainage bag and discard.	*Provides assessment data*
33. Gather all additional equipment and discard with gloves.	*Promotes clean environment*
34. Wash hands.	*Reduces microorganism transfer*

Evaluation

Were desired outcomes achieved?

Documentation

The following should be noted on the client's chart:

- Presence of distention before catheterization
- Assessment of genitalia, if abnormalities noted
- Type of catheterization
- Size of catheter
- Amount, color, and consistency of urine returned upon catheterization
- Amount of urine returned before catheterization (if residual urine catheterization)
- Difficulties encountered, if any, in passing the catheter smoothly
- Reports of unusual discomfort during insertion
- Specimen obtained

SAMPLE DOCUMENTATION

DATE	TIME	
4/6/02	1100	Catheter (#16 French Foley) inserted without resistance or report of discomfort. Procedure yielded 700 ml straw-colored urine without sediment or foul odor.

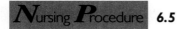

Female Catheterization

🗃 EQUIPMENT

- Urethral catheterization set (includes sterile gloves, specimen-collection container, catheter, two drapes, graduated measurement receptacle, antiseptic solution, cotton balls, forceps, lubricating jelly)
  or
- Indwelling catheterization set (all of the items in urethral catheterization kit except the graduated measurement receptacle, plus a drainage-collection system [tubing and bag that connect to the catheter] and a prefilled saline syringe for balloon inflation)
- Basin of warm soapy water
- Washcloth
- Large towel
- Nonsterile gloves
- One sheet for draping
- Linen saver
- Roll of tape
- Bedpan, urinal, or second collection container
- Specimen container, if specimen is needed
- Extra lighting

Purpose

Facilitates emptying of bladder
Facilitates obtaining sterile urine specimens
Facilitates determining amount of residual urine in bladder
Allows for continuous, accurate monitoring of urinary output
Provides avenue for bladder irrigations

Assessment

Assessment should focus on the following:

Type of catheterization ordered (straight, Foley, residual)
Status of bladder (distention before catheter insertion)
Abnormalities of genitalia
Client allergy to iodine-based antiseptics (eg, Betadine)

Nursing Diagnoses

The nursing diagnoses may include the following:

Altered urinary elimination: decreased output related to reduction in total fluid volume
Acute pain related to bladder distention
Urinary retention related to neuromuscular dysfunction

Outcome Identification and Planning

Desired Outcomes (sample)
A urine output of at least 250 ml per shift is attained and maintained during hospital stay.
Client verbalizes relief of lower abdominal pain within 1 hr of catheter insertion.

Special Considerations
Pediatric

Catheterization is a very threatening and anxiety-producing experience. Children need explanations, support, and understanding.
In the baby girl, the urethra hooks around the symphysis in a C shape. Common catheter size is 8 or 10 French.

Home Health

When indwelling catheterization is used on a long-term basis, there is a high potential for infection. Be alert for early signs and symptoms of infection and adhere to a strict schedule for changing catheters.
If the client uses intermittent self-catheterization, store sterilized catheters in sterilized jars.

Cost-cutting Tip

For female clients, time and money may be saved by using clean gloves to locate the meatus before opening the sterile kit. This minimizes the chance of sterile glove contamination.
If replacing a Foley catheter, note the size of the previous catheter to avoid wastage from insertion of too small a catheter. This occurs frequently with clients on long-term catheterization.

Delegation

In some agencies, catheterization may be delegated to specially trained personnel. Note agency policies concerning delegation of this procedure, and to what level personnel.

IMPLEMENTATION

Action	Rationale

1. Wash hands.

   Reduces microorganism transfer

2. Explain procedure to client, emphasizing need to maintain sterile field.

   Decreases anxiety

3. Determine if client is allergic to iodine-based antiseptics.

   Avoids allergic reactions

4. Provide for privacy.

   Decreases embarrassment

5. Don nonsterile gloves.

   Reduces nurse's exposure to body secretions

6. If catheterization is for residual urine, ask client to void in urinal, and measure and record the amount voided; empty urinal.

   Determines amount of urine client is able to void without catheterization
   Determines exact amount
   Promotes tidiness

7. Place linen saver under buttocks.

   Avoids wetting linens

8. Place light to enhance visualization.

   Promotes clear identification of anatomical parts

9. Separate labia to expose urethral opening:
   - If using dorsal recumbent position (Fig. 6.7*A*), separate labia with thumb and forefinger by gently lifting upward and outward. (Fig. 6.8) illustrates this technique and identifies parts of the female perineum.)

   Allows nurse to identify urethral opening clearly before area is cleansed
   Subtle variations in location of structures of female genitalia often cause a delay that increases chance of contamination of field

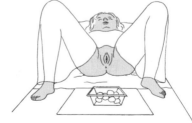

A

FIGURE 6.7A

Action	Rationale

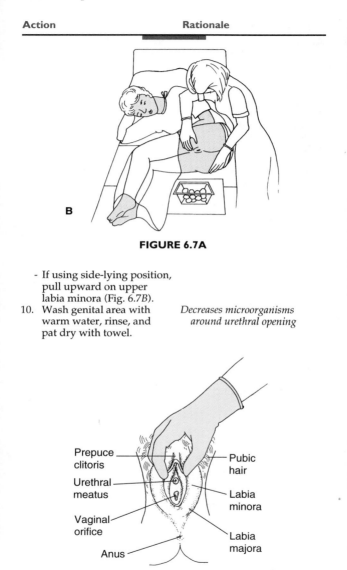

FIGURE 6.7A

- If using side-lying position,
  pull upward on upper
  labia minora (Fig. 6.7B).
10. Wash genital area with   *Decreases microorganisms*
   warm water, rinse, and   *around urethral opening*
   pat dry with towel.

Prepuce
clitoris

Pubic
hair

Urethral
meatus

Labia
minora

Vaginal
orifice

Labia
majora

Anus

FIGURE 6.8

Action	Rationale
11. Discard gloves, bath water, washcloth, and towel; then wash hands.	*Decreases clutter* *Reduces microorganisms*
12. If inserting an indwelling catheter in which the drainage apparatus is separate from the catheter (not preconnected):	
- Check for closed clamp on collection bag.	
- Secure drainage collection bag to bed frame.	*Places drainage tubing within immediate and easy reach, decreasing chance of catheter contamination once inserted*
- Pull tubing up between bed and bed rails to top surface of bed.	
- Check to be sure tubing will not get caught when rails are lowered or raised.	
13. Position client in dorsal recumbent or side-lying position with knees flexed (see Figs. 6.7*A* and *B*); in side-lying position, slide client's hips toward edge of bed.	*Exposes labia*
14. Drape client so only perineum is exposed.	*Provides privacy* *Reduces embarrassment*
15. Remove gloves and wash hands; lift side rails and cover client before leaving bedside.	*Reduces microorganism transfer* *Prevents client from falling* *Reduces embarrassment*
16. Carefully open catheter set and remove it from plastic outer package.	*Removes kit without opening inner folds*
17. Tape outer package to bedside table with top edge turned inside.	*Provides waste bag*
18. Place catheter kit between client's knees and carefully open outer edges (if using side-lying position, place kit about 1 foot from perineal area near thighs).	*Places items within easy reach*

Action	Rationale
19. Remove full drape from kit with fingertips and place, plastic side down, just under buttocks by having client raise hips; keep other side sterile.	*Provides work field*
20. Don sterile gloves.	*Avoids contaminating other items in kit*
21. Prepare items in kit for use during insertion as follows:	
- Pour iodine solution over cotton balls.	*Prepares cotton balls for cleaning*
- Separate cotton balls with forceps.	*Promotes easy manipulation*
- Lubricate 3 to 4 inches of catheter tip and place carefully on tray so that tip is secure in tray.	*Prevents local irritation of meatus on catheter insertion* *Promotes ease of insertion*
- If inserting indwelling catheter, attach prefilled syringe to balloon port of catheter by twisting syringe in clockwise direction.	*Connects syringe needed to inflate balloon to balloon port*
- Push plunger in, inject 2 to 3 ml of sterile water from prefilled syringe into balloon, and observe balloon for leaks as it fills.	*Tests balloon for defects*
- If any leaks are noted, discard and obtain another kit.	*Prevents catheter dislodgment after insertion*
- Deflate balloon, and leave syringe connected.	*Leaves syringe within reach*
- If inserting closed indwelling system with drainage tubing already attached to catheter, move tubing and bag close to other equipment on work field, making certain that drainage system is on the sterile field only.	*Facilitates organization while maintaining sterility*

Action	Rationale
(Check clamp on collection bag to be sure it is closed.)	*Prevents loss of urine before measurement*
- Open specimen collection container and place on sterile field.	*Places container within easy reach for specimen*
22. Remove fenestrated drape from kit and place on perineum such that only labia are exposed (or discard the drape if you prefer).	*Expands sterile field*
23. Separate labia minora with nondominant hand in same manner as in step 9 and hold this position until catheter is inserted (*Note:* Dominant hand is only hand sterile now; contaminated hand continues to separate labia.)	*Exposes urethral opening*
24. Using forceps, cleanse meatus with cotton balls:	
- Making one downward stroke with each cotton ball, begin at labium on side farther from you and move toward labium closer to you.	*Cleanses meatus without cross-contaminating*
- Afterward, wipe once down center of meatus.	
- Wipe once with each cotton ball and discard (Fig. 6.9).	
25. After all cotton balls have been used, remove forceps from field.	*Prevents contamination of sterile field*
26. Move cleaning tray to end of sterile field and move collection container and catheter closer to client.	*Facilitates organization* *Prevents accidental contamination of system*
27. With thumb and first finger, pick catheter up about 1.5 to 2 inches from tip.	*Gives nurse good control of catheter (which easily bends)*

Action	Rationale

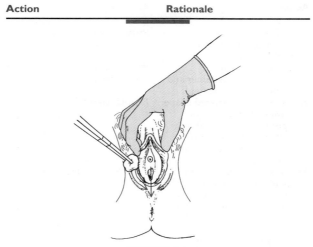

FIGURE 6.9

Action	Rationale
28. Carefully gather additional tubing in hand.	*Gives nurse good control of full catheter length*
29. Ask client to bear down as if voiding and to take slow, deep breaths; encourage her to take deep breaths until catheter is fully inserted.	*Opens sphincter* *Relaxes sphincter muscles of bladder and urethra*
30. Insert tip of catheter slowly through urethral opening 3 to 4 inches (or until urine returns), releasing tubing from hand as insertion continues; direct open end of catheter into collection container.	*Inserts catheter*
31. After catheter has been advanced an appropriate distance (3–4 inches or until urine returns), advance another 1 to 1.5 inches.	*Ensures that catheter advances far enough not to be dislodged*

Action	Rationale
32. Grasp catheter with thumb and first finger of non-dominant hand and hold steady.	*Keeps catheter from being forced out by sphincter muscles* *Avoids contamination*
33. If straight catheterization:	
- Obtain urine specimen in specimen container, if ordered, and replace open end of catheter in collection container.	*Obtains sterile specimen*
- Allow urine to drain until it stops or UNTIL MAXIMUM NUMBER OF MILLILITERS SPECIFIED BY AGENCY (usually 1000–1500 ml) has drained into container; use second container, bedpan, or urinal, if necessary.	*Empties bladder* *Obtains residual urine amount* *Prevents temporary hypovolemic shock state*
- Remove catheter.	
34. If indwelling catheter is being used, inflate balloon with attached syringe and gently pull back on catheter until it stops (catches).	*Secures catheter placement*
35. If the indwelling catheter is separate from bag and tubing, remove protective cap from end of tubing and attach drainage tubing to end of catheter.	*Converts system to closed system*
36. Secure catheter loosely with tape to thigh on side from which drainage bag will be hanging (preferably away from door); make certain that tubing is not caught on railing locks or obstructed.	*Stabilizes catheter* *Prevents accidental dislodgment*
37. Clear bed of all equipment, reposition client for comfort, and replace linens for warmth and privacy; lift side rails.	*Promotes clean environment, comfort, and safety*

Action	Rationale
38. Measure amount of urine in collection container or drainage bag and discard.	*Provides assessment data*
39. Gather up all additional equipment and discard with gloves.	*Promotes clean environment*
40. Wash hands.	*Reduces microorganism transfer*

Evaluation

Were desired outcomes achieved?

Documentation

The following should be noted on the client's chart:

- Assessment of lower abdomen before catheterization
- Assessment of genitalia, if abnormalities noted
- Types of catheterization
- Size of catheter
- Amount, color, and consistency of urine returned upon catheterization
- Amount of urine returned before catheterization (if residual urine was collected)
- Difficulties encountered, if any, in passing catheter smoothly
- Reports of unusual discomfort during insertion
- Specimen obtained

SAMPLE DOCUMENTATION

DATE	TIME	
1/5/02	100	Catheter (#16 French Foley) inserted without resistance or report of discomfort. Procedure yielded 700 ml of straw-colored urine without sediment or foul odor.

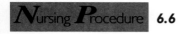 *Bladder/Catheter Irrigation*

EQUIPMENT

- Two-way indwelling catheter set
  or
- Three-way indwelling catheter set
- Solution ordered for irrigation
- Catheter irrigation kit
  - Large catheter-tip syringe with protective cap
  - Sterile linen saver
  - Graduated irrigation container
- Medication additives, as ordered
- Medication labels
- IV tubing
- IV pole
- Two pairs of clean gloves
- Basin of warm water
- Soap
- Washcloth
- Towel
- Linen saver
- Betadine (or recommended antiseptic solution for cleansing irrigation port)
- Catheter clamp or rubber band

Purpose

Maintains bladder and catheter patency by removing or minimizing obstructions such as clots and mucous plugs in bladder
Prevents or treats local bladder inflammation or infection
Instills medications for local bladder treatments

Assessment

Assessment should focus on the following:

Type of irrigation order
Characteristics of urine before irrigation, such as hematuria
Amount of urine output
Distention, pain, or tenderness of the lower abdomen
Signs of inflammation or infection of bladder and perineal structures
Status of catheter (if already inserted) before irrigations

Nursing Diagnoses

The nursing diagnoses may include the following:

Acute pain related to bladder inflammation
Acute urinary retention related to bladder outlet obstruction
  from blood clots

Outcome Identification and Planning

Desired Outcomes (sample)
Client verbalizes decrease in lower abdominal discomfort within
  24 hr.
Client maintains urine output of at least 250 ml per shift.

Special Considerations
When calculating urine output for a client receiving bladder irrigations, subtract the amount of irrigation solution infused
  within a designated period of time from the total amount of
  fluid accumulated within the bag.

Delegation
Unlicensed assistive personnel should help with emptying the
  catheter bag. Irrigation fluid should only be hung by the nurse.

IMPLEMENTATION

Action	Rationale
Bladder Irrigation	
1. Wash hands.	*Reduces microorganism transfer*
2. Explain procedure to client.	*Decreases anxiety*
3. Determine if client is allergic to iodine-based antiseptics or additives to be injected into irrigation fluid.	*Avoids allergic reactions*
4. Prepare irrigation fluid: - Remove fluid and IV tubing from outer packages. - Close roller clamp on tubing. - Insert additives, if ordered, into fluid container additive port. - Insert spike of tubing into insertion port of fluid bag.	*Prepares irrigation solution*

Action	Rationale
- Place on IV pole.	
- Pinch fluid chamber until fluid fills chamber halfway.	*Prevents infusion of air into bladder*
- Remove protective cover from end of tubing line, taking care not to contaminate end of tubing or protective cover.	
- Slowly open roller clamp and fill tubing with fluid.	*Removes air from tubing*
- Close roller clamp and replace protective cover.	*Maintains sterility of tubing*
- Place label on bag of fluid stating type of solution, additives, date, and time solution was opened.	*Identifies contents of irrigant*
5. Provide for privacy.	*Decreases embarrassment*
6. If three-way catheter has not already been inserted, don clean gloves, place linen saver under buttocks, and wash and dry perineal area.	*Reduces microorganisms in local perineal area before catheter insertion*
7. Discard gloves, bath water, washcloth, and towel; then wash hands.	*Decreases bedside clutter* *Reduces microorganism transfer*
8. Insert catheter using Procedure 6.4 for men or Procedure 6.5 for women.	*Inserts catheter for irrigation*
9. Don clean gloves.	*Reduces nurse's exposure to body secretions*
10. Cleanse irrigation port of catheter with antiseptic solution recommended by agency.	*Removes microorganisms from port* *Decreases contamination*
11. Connect tubing of irrigation fluid to irrigation port of three-way catheter (Fig. 6.10).	*Connects tubing to appropriate catheter port for irrigation*
12. Slowly open roller clamp on tubing and adjust drip rate.	*Sets fluid at appropriate infusion rate for type of infusion*

Action   **Rationale**

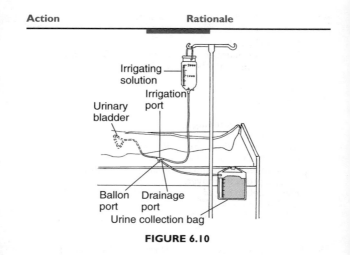

Irrigating — solution

Irrigation port

Urinary bladder

Ballon port   Drainage port

Urine collection bag

FIGURE 6.10

For intermittent irrigation:
- Clamp catheter drainage tubing (or kink tubing and bind with rubber band).
- Open roller clamp so 100 ml of irrigation fluid flows into bladder by gravitational flow; close roller clamp.
- Allow fluid to remain for 15 min (or amount of time specified by physician's order).

Allows proper exchange of electrolytes and fluid

- Unclamp drainage tubing.

Allows fluid to drain from abdomen into drainage bag

- Repeat irrigation at frequency ordered.

For continuous irrigation:
- Leave drainage tubing open.
- Slowly open roller clamp of irrigation fluid tubing.
- Adjust irrigation to ordered drip rate (see Procedure 5.5 to review calculation of drip rates).

Provides continuous flushing of clots and debris from bladder

Action	Rationale
13. Remove linen saver.	*Removes soiled linen saver*
14. Discard gloves and wash hands.	*Prevents spread of micro-organisms*
15. Record urinary output on intake and output flow sheet.	Provides accurate record of urine output

Catheter Irrigation

For catheter irrigation using a two-way catheter:

1. Open catheter irrigation kit.	
2. Remove catheter-tip syringe from sterile container. Remove sterile cap and place syringe back into sterile container. Hold cap between fingers, being careful not to contaminate the open end.	*Ensures continued sterility of syringe tip while allowing use of sterile cap to protect drainage tubing tip*
3. Fill container with saline or ordered irrigant and fill syringe.	*Prepares syringe for irrigation process*
4. Disinfect the drainage tubing–catheter connection using an antimicrobial agent recommended by the institution.	*Decreases microorganisms at the connection site*
5. Open sterile linen saver and spread on bed near catheter.	*Provides sterile field*
6. Disconnect catheter and drainage tubing. Place cap over drainage tube tip, being careful to keep catheter end sterile. Place capped tubing on linen saver.	*Maintains sterility of drainage tubing for reconnection*
7. Remove syringe from container and insert tip securely into catheter, using sterile technique.	*Reestablishes closed sterile system for irrigation*
8. Slowly infuse irrigant into catheter until full amount of ordered fluid has been	*Minimizes discomfort caused by rapid or excessive fluid infusion*

Action	Rationale

    infused or patient com-
plains of inability to
tolerate additional fluid
infusion.

9. Clamp catheter by bending
end above syringe tip and
remove the syringe.
Disinfect the catheter end
with antimicrobial agent.
Remove cap from the
drainage tubing and insert
it into catheter end.

*Prevents leakage of irrigant from
catheter*
*Minimizes microorganisms at
connection site*

10. Repeat irrigation at
frequency ordered.

*Reestablishes closed bladder
drainage system*

11. Proceed to steps 13 to 15
of Bladder Irrigation.

Evaluation

Were desired outcomes achieved?

Documentation

The following should be noted on the client's chart:

- Amount, color, and consistency of fluid obtained
- Type and amount of irrigation solution and medication addi-
tives administered
- Infusion rate
- Abdominal assessment
- Urine output (total fluid volume measured minus irrigation so-
lution instilled)
- Discomfort verbalized by client

SAMPLE DOCUMENTATION

DATE	TIME	
7/6/02	1330	Three-way irrigation catheter inserted and continuous bladder irrigation initiated with 1000 ml sterile normal saline irrigant. Drip rate 50 ml/hr via infusion regulator. Client reports cramping sensation in lower abdomen as if having spasms. Urine and irrigant clear, without sediment or evidence of blood clots.

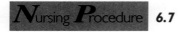

Bladder Scanning

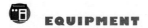 **EQUIPMENT**

- Bladder scanning device
- Ultrasound transmission gel
- Washcloth
- Soap

Purpose

Evaluates bladder volume noninvasively to determine need for catheterization to empty bladder
Assists in evaluating general bladder function

Assessment

Assessment should focus on the following:

Medical diagnosis (urinary retention, urinary incontinence, stroke, spinal cord injury, or other pertinent diagnosis)
Physician order for use of bladder scanning
Bladder palpation for fullness
Patterns of urine amounts upon previous voidings or catheterizations
Previous residual urine volumes, if applicable
Time of last bladder emptying

Nursing Diagnoses

The nursing diagnoses may include the following:

Altered urinary elimination: incomplete bladder emptying related to urinary incontinence
Acute pain related to bladder distention from urinary retention

Outcome Identification and Planning

Desired Outcomes (sample)
Client maintains urine output of at least 250 ml per 8 hr.
Client verbalizes no lower abdominal pain.

Special Considerations

Bladder scanning has been associated with less urinary tract infections in some research studies. BVI 3000 is designed for acute care settings, and BVI 5000 is designed for rehabilitation and home settings.

Geriatric

Urinary incontinence is a significant problem for many elderly clients. Bladder scanning is used in many geriatric rehabilitation settings, because these patients are prone to the development of urinary tract infections.

IMPLEMENTATION

Action	Rationale
1. Wash hands, and gather equipment: BVI 3000 (Fig. 6.11) or BVI 5000 (Fig. 6.12).	*Reduces microorganisms*
2. Explain procedure to client.	*Reduces anxiety*

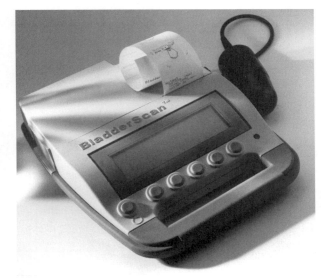

FIGURE 6.11

Action	Rationale

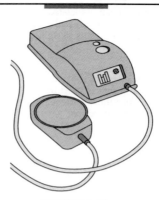

FIGURE 6.12

3. Assist the client into supine position. — *Positions client for obtaining accurate readings*
4. Expose the lower abdomen. — *Determines location of bladder*
5. Palpate the symphysis pubis. — *Identifies starting point for scan*
6. Apply gel pad over bladder area.
7. Place the scanhead device on lower abdomen where symphysis pubis is palpated (Fig. 6.13).
   - Hold the scanhead completely still.
   - Do not raise the dome of the scanhead off the client's body.
8. Press scan button. — *Obtains bladder volume*
9. Check aiming screen. — *Verifies correct position of scanhead*
10. Note the final calculated volume reading on the display screen (Fig. 6.14) in 5 sec (BVI 2500) or in 10 sec (BVI 5000). — *Obtains calculated bladder volume*
11. Press print button (BVI 2500). — *Obtains hard (written) copy of results*

Action	Rationale

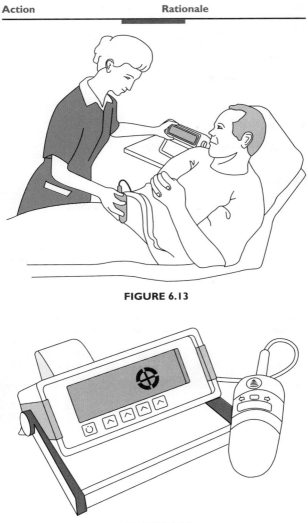

FIGURE 6.13

FIGURE 6.14

Action	Rationale
12. Turn machine off.	
13. Wash gel off client.	*Removes gel*
14. Lower clothing top.	*Reclothes client*
15. Clean and store bladder scanning device.	

Evaluation

Were desired outcomes achieved?

Documentation

The following should be noted on the client's chart:

- Status of bladder on palpation
- Volume amount indicated on bladder scan readings
- Complaints of client discomfort
- Disposition of catheterization as intervention for bladder emptying

SAMPLE DOCUMENTATION

DATE	TIME	
2/20/02	1800	Client has not voided since 1200. Bladder scanning reading volume amount of 450 cc. Straight catheterization done, with 450 ml clear yellow urine return

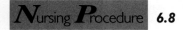

Hemodialysis Shunt, Graft, and Fistula Care

EQUIPMENT

- Nonsterile gloves
- Two pairs of sterile gloves
- Antiseptic cleansing agent or antiseptic swabs
- Topical antiseptic, if ordered
- Sterile 4 × 4-inch gauze pads
- Kerlix/Kling wrap
- Cannula clamps

Purpose

Maintains patency of access for dialysis
Detects complications of a hemodialysis access site related to infection, occlusion, or cannula separation

Assessment

Assessment should focus on the following:

Status of fistula, graft, or cannula site and dressing
Location of shunt, fistula, or graft
Vital signs
Pulses distal to shunt, fistula, or graft
Color and temperature of extremity in which access is located
Presence of pain or numbness in extremity in which access is located
Time of last dressing change

Nursing Diagnoses

The nursing diagnoses may include the following:

Altered tissue perfusion related to shunt/fistula/graft occlusion or infection
Risk of peripheral neurovascular dysfunction related to possible shunt/graft/fistula occlusion

Outcome Identification and Planning

Desired Outcomes (sample)

A bruit is present on auscultation; a thrill is palpable; and there is
no edema, redness, pain, drainage, or bleeding at the hemodialysis access site

Special Considerations

A potential complication related to the presence of the shunt is
cannula separation. Hemorrhage can occur if the shunt is not
clamped off until a new cannula is inserted; therefore, a pair of
cannula clamps should be kept at the client's bedside at all
times.

Home Health

To enable client to change dressings between nursing visits, secure the dressing with a stockinette dressing that the client can
roll down over Kerlix, remove old dressing, and roll up to secure new dressing.

Delegation

This procedure should be performed by the nurse.

IMPLEMENTATION

Action	Rationale
1. Wash hands.	*Reduces microorganism transfer*
2. Explain procedure to client.	*Decreases anxiety*
3. Open several 4 × 4 packages, and soak several gauze pads with antiseptic solution or open antiseptic swabs and position for easy access. Keep one package of gauze 4 × 4s dry.	*Facilitates cleaning process; provides gauze to cover shunt*
4. Don clean gloves.	*Reduces nurse's exposure to body secretions*
5. Remove old dressing, if present, and check access site.	*Exposes access site*
6. Discard dressing and gloves.	*Removes contaminated items*
7. Wash hands and don sterile gloves.	*Avoids site contamination*
8. Cleanse access area with antiseptic agent recom- mended by agency. For	*Reduces contamination*

Action	Rationale

shunt care, begin at exit areas and work outward, discarding antiseptic swab or folded gauze pad after each wipe.

9. Lightly place two or three fingertips over access site and assess for presence of thrill (a palpable vibration should be present); assess site for extreme warmth or coolness. — *Tests for adequate blood flow through shunt*

10. Apply topical ointment, if ordered. — *Prevents infection*

11. Place dry sterile gauze pads over access site. — *Reduces site contamination*

12. For shunt, apply Kerlix or Kling wrap over gauze pads and around extremity (wrap firmly enough that dressing is secure but not so tight as to occlude blood flow) and tape securely; leave small piece of shunt tubing visible. — *Prevents accidental dislodgment of cannula* / *Allows for visualization of continuous blood flow*

13. Discard equipment and gloves; then wash hands. — *Reduces spread of infection*

14. Place call light within reach. — *Enables client to communicate*

15. Assess status of dressing, access site, and pulses in affected extremity every 2 hr. — *Monitors frequently for complications*

16. During immediate post-operative period, inform client, family, and staff of the following care instructions: — *Prevents unnecessary loss of access site due to occlusion, infection, or cannula separation*
    - If shunt is in arm or leg, keep extremity elevated on pillow until instructed otherwise.
    - Keep extremity as still as possible.

Action	Rationale
- Do not apply pressure to or lift heavy objects with extremity. (If shunt is in leg, crutches will be used for a short while when client becomes ambulatory.)	*Prevents rupture and pain*
- Do not allow access area to get wet during showering, bathing, or swimming.	
17. Inform client, family, and staff of the following care instructions:	*Facilitates cooperation with care of site, reduces fear, and prevents undue injury*
- Never perform the following procedures on the affected extremity:	
a. Blood pressure assessment or any procedure that might occlude blood flow.	*Prevents occlusion of blood flow*
b. Venipuncture or any procedure involving a needlestick. PLACE A SIGN OVER BEDSIDE PROHIBITING USE OF AFFECTED EXTREMITY FOR THESE PROCEDURES.	*Prevents injury, clotting, and infection*
- Avoid restricting blood flow in affected extremity with tight-fitting clothes, watches, name bands, knee-high stockings, antiembolytic hose, restraints, etc.	*Prevents restriction of blood flow and injury to graft/shunt/ fistula area*
- Notify nurse immediately if bleeding or cannula disconnection is noted.	*Prevents excessive bleeding*
- Apply cannula clamps if disconnection is noted.	*Prevents hemorrhage*

Evaluation

Were desired outcomes achieved?

Documentation

The following should be noted on the client's chart:

- Location of access site
- Status of site and dressing
- Vital signs
- Status of pulses distal to access area
- Color and temperature of extremity in which access is located
- Presence of pain or numbness in extremity in which access is located

SAMPLE DOCUMENTATION

DATE	TIME	
2/6/02	1115	Left forearm Goretex-graft site care given. Radial pulse normal (3+) in left arm. Left fingers pink with 2-sec capillary refill. Denies pain or numbness of left arm. Thrill palpable at graft site. Site cleaned with Betadine solution and sterile dressing applied.

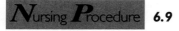

Peritoneal Dialysis Management

 EQUIPMENT

- Dialysate fluid(s) ordered
- Medication additives ordered (usually some combination of potassium chloride, heparin, sodium bicarbonate, and possibly antibiotics)
- Syringes for additives
- Medication labels
- Dialysis flow sheet
- Dialysate tubing
- IV pole
- Peroxide or sterile saline
- Antiseptic recommended by agency
- Masks (for each person in room, including client and visitors)
- Clean gown
- Sterile gloves
- Gauze dressing pads (2 × 2 inches and 4 × 4 inches)
- Tape
- Graduated container

Purpose

Instills solutions into peritoneal cavity to remove metabolic end products, toxins, and excess fluid from body when kidney function is totally or partially ineffective

Treats electrolyte and acid–base imbalances

Assessment

Assessment should focus on the following:

Changes in mental status

Fluid balance indicators (vital signs, weight, skin turgor, condition of mucous membranes, presence or absence of edema, I & O)

Abdominal status, including abdominal girth

Cardiopulmonary status

Status of dressing and catheter site

Status of skin surrounding site

Indicators of peritonitis (sharp abdominal pain, cloudy or pink-tinged dialysate fluid return, increased temperature)

Laboratory data (blood gases, potassium, blood urea nitrogen, creatinine, hemoglobin, hematocrit)
Indicators of electrolyte imbalance

Nursing Diagnoses

The nursing diagnoses may include the following:

Fluid volume excess related to inability of kidneys to remove excess fluids
Risk of infection related to peritoneal catheter

Outcome Identification and Planning

Desired Outcomes (sample)

Cardiopulmonary complications during dialysis, if any, are detected as they occur.
Client verbalizes no acute abdominal pain. Temperature within normal range. Pulse, 88. Dialysate return clear. No redness, edema, or abnormal drainage at catheter insertion site.

Special Considerations

Peritonitis is a frequent complication in clients with peritoneal dialysis; therefore, strict aseptic technique must be maintained to protect the client from peritonitis.

Pediatric

The pediatric client may be anxious, apathetic, or withdrawn: offer understanding and support.

Home Health

Many homebound clients dialyze intermittently at home with use of a cycler. Many also use continuous ambulatory peritoneal dialysis (CAPD) or continuous cycling peritoneal dialysis (CCPD).
Observe return demonstrations until you are certain that the client and family understand the importance of preventing infection.

 Cost-cutting Tip

If not contraindicated by agency's or manufacturer's policy, a blanket warmer may be used to warm dialysate solution and conserve time expenditure in preparation.

Delegation

This procedure cannot be delegated to unlicensed personnel , except in agencies where special training or certification is done (see agency policy). Unlicensed assistive personnel may, however, assist with obtaining weights, emptying draining receptacles/graduated containers, and recording output amounts.

IMPLEMENTATION

Action	Rationale
1. Wash hands.	*Reduces microorganism transfer*
2. Explain procedure to client.	*Decreases anxiety*
3. Weigh client each morning and as ordered for each series of exchanges, and record weight.	*Provides data needed to determine appropriate concentrations of fluids and additives*
4. Place unopened dialysate-fluid bag or bottle in warmer if solution is not at least room temperature.	*Enhances solute and fluid clearance* *Prevents abdominal cramping*
5. Don mask.	*Reduces spread of airborne microorganisms*
6. Prepare dialysate with medication additives as ordered; prepare each bag according to the five rights of drug administration (see Procedure 11.1); place completed medication label on bag.	*Avoids errors that could affect end results of dialysis— concentration affects osmolality, rate of fluid removal, electrolyte balance, solute removal, and cardiovascular stability*
7. Insert dialysate infusion tubing spike into insertion port on dialysate-fluid bag/bottle and prime tubing; place fluid bag/bottle on IV pole. *Note:* Some tubing spikes are designed like a screw cap with a spike in the center of the cap. An antiseptic solution should be placed in the cap before spiking bag.	*Eliminates air that may contribute to client discomfort*

Action	Rationale
8. Adjust position of bed so fluid hangs higher than client's abdomen and drainage bag is lower than abdomen (Fig. 6.15).	*Enhances gravitational flow as fluid infuses and drains*
9. Provide privacy.	*Reduces embarrassment*
10. Open and arrange cleaning supplies (soak 4 × 4 gauze pads, leaving dry pads for covering or other dressing, if ordered).	
11. Don clean gown and sterile gloves; instruct each person in room to don appropriate protective	*Decreases nurse's exposure to microorganisms and client's exposure to airborne microorganisms*

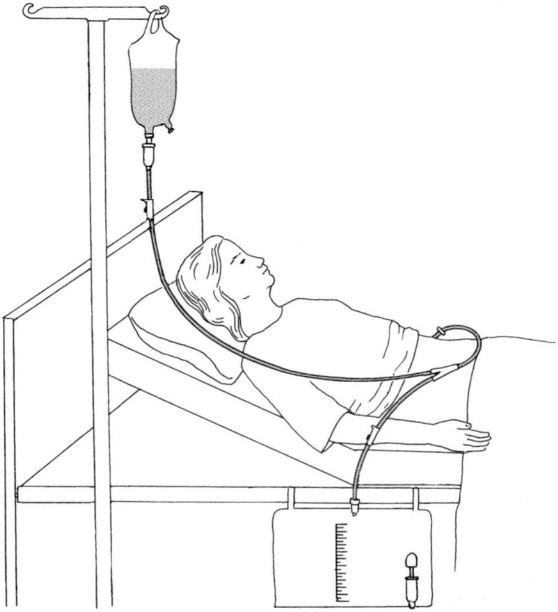

FIGURE 6.15

Action	Rationale
wear (masks for all persons in room, sterile gloves for nurse and assistant handling fluid bags).	*Reduces client's chance of developing peritonitis*
12. Remove old peritoneal catheter dressing and examine catheter site for catheter dislodgment or signs of infection; if leakage or abnormal drainage is noted, culture site.	*Assesses catheter intactness* *Facilitates identification of infectious agent*
13. Discard dressing and gloves; wash hands and don sterile gloves.	*Reduces microorganism transfer*
14. Beginning at catheter insertion site, cleanse site with a circular motion outward, using peroxide or sterile saline on gauze or swab, and allow to dry; apply antiseptic agent recommended by agency or ordered by doctor (discard each gauze or swab after each wipe when cleansing site and applying antiseptic).	*Decreases microorganisms at catheter insertion site* *Reduces risk of peritonitis*
15. Using sterile technique, apply new dressing and secure with tape.	*Protects site from micro-organisms*
16. Discard gloves and wash hands.	*Reduces microorganisms*
17. Label dressing with date and time of change and your initials.	*Provides data needed to determine when next dressing change is due*
18. Don sterile gloves.	*Reduces microorganisms*
19. Connect end of dialysate tubing to abdominal catheter.	*Connects tubing to begin dialysate infusion*
20. Clamp tubing from abdominal catheter to drainage bag (outflow tubing).	*Prevents dialysate from running through*

Action	Rationale

21. Check client's position (abdomen lower than height of fluid, which allows gravity to facilitate flow); check tubing for kinks or bends.

Removes obstructions that could affect infusion rate

22. Open dialysate infusion tubing clamp(s) and allow fluid to drain into peritoneal cavity for 10 to 15 min. Observe respiratory status while fluid infuses and while fluid remains in the abdomen (dwell time).

Infuses dialysate for fluid and electrolyte exchange in peritoneal cavity

23. Allow fluid to dwell in abdomen for 20 min (or amount of time specified by doctor).

Allows time for proper exchange of fluids and electrolytes

24. Open clamp leading to drain bag and allow fluid to drain for specified amount of time or until drainage has decreased to a slow drip (if all the fluid does not return, reposition client and recheck tubing leading to drainage bag). *For CAPD,* client may fold dialysis bag and secure bag and tubing to abdomen or clothing and allow fluid to dwell while performing daily activities. To drain dialysate, client would unfold and lower bag and allow fluid to drain from abdominal cavity (same bag is used for infusion and drainage).
A new bag is then hung, and infusion–dwelling–drainage cycle is repeated continuously.

Allows end products of dialysis to drain

Action	Rationale
25. Record amount of fluid infused and amount drained after each exchange; add balance of fluids infused and drained on appropriate flow sheet (if net output is greater than amount infused by a large margin—200 ml or more—notify doctor).	*Provides accurate record of fluid exchanges for determining fluid balance*
26. Reassess the following client data every 30 to 60 min thereafter throughout exchanges: vital signs, output, respiratory status, mental status, abdominal status, appearance of dialysate return, abdominal dressing (should be kept dry), and signs of lethal electrolyte imbalances.	*Alerts nurse to impending complications or need to change fluid and additive concentrations*
27. Weigh client at end of appropriate number of fluid exchanges.	*Provides data regarding efficiency of exchanges in removing excess fluid*
28. Obtain laboratory data, as ordered and as needed (check doctor's orders and agency policy regarding p.r.n. laboratory data).	*Provides data about clearance of metabolic wastes as well as electrolyte status*
29. When the total series of exchanges is completed, empty drainage bag into graduated container, discard bag and tubing, and cap peritoneal catheter.	*Removes fluid waste so other fluid may drain*
30. Discard or restore equipment appropriately.	*Promotes clean environment*
31. Wash hands.	*Reduces microorganisms*

Evaluation

Were desired outcomes achieved?

Documentation

The following should be noted on the client's chart:

- Fluid balance indicators (vital signs, weight, skin turgor, condition of mucous membranes, presence or absence of edema, I & O) before and after dialysis
- Mental status before and after dialysis
- Cardiopulmonary assessment
- Abdominal assessment, including abdominal girth
- Status of dressing and catheter site
- Status of skin surrounding site
- Indicators of peritonitis (sharp abdominal pain, cloudy or pink-tinged dialysate-fluid return, increased temperature)
- Changes in laboratory data (blood gases, potassium, blood urea nitrogen, creatinine, hemoglobin, hematocrit)
- Acute indicators of electrolyte imbalance
- Type and amount of dialysate infused
- Medication additives in dialysate

SAMPLE DOCUMENTATION

DATE	TIME	
5/9/02	1400	First series of dialysis exchanges begun. Twelve bags of 1.5% dialysate fluid hung to infuse via dialysis cycler. Abdominal dressing clean, dry, and intact. Client denies abdominal pain. Dialysate return clear. Predialysis weight, 88 lb. Postdialysis weight, 87 lb.

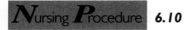

Fecal Impaction Removal

EQUIPMENT

- Three pairs of nonsterile gloves
- Packet of water-soluble lubricant
- Bedpan
- Linen saver
- Basin of warm water
- Soap
- Washcloth
- Towel
- Air freshener

Purpose

Manually removes hardened stool blocking normal evacuation
    passage in lower part of colon
Relieves pain and discomfort
Facilitates normal peristalsis
Prevents rectal and anal injury

Assessment

Assessment should focus on the following:

Agency policy and physician's order regarding performance of
    procedure
Status of anus and skin surrounding buttocks (ie, presence of ul-
    cerations, tears, hemorrhoids, and excoriation)
Indicators of impaction (ie, lower abdominal and rectal pain,
    seepage of liquid stools, inability to pass stool, general malaise,
    urge to defecate without being able to do so, nausea and vom-
    iting, shortness of breath)
Abdominal status
Vital signs before, during, and after removal
Time of last bowel movement and usual bowel evacuation pattern
History of factors that may contraindicate or present complica-
    tions during impaction removal (such as cardiac instability or
    spinal cord injury)
Client history regarding dietary habits (ie, intake of bulk and liq-
    uids), changes in activity pattern, frequency of use of laxatives
    or enemas

Client knowledge regarding promotion of normal bowel elimination

Medications that decrease peristalsis, such as narcotics

Nursing Diagnoses

The nursing diagnoses may include the following:

Constipation related to decreased activity
Acute abdominal pain related to bowel distention from impaction

Outcome Identification and Planning

Desired Outcomes (sample)

Client has normal bowel movement within 24 hr.
Client verbalizes pain relief within 1 hr.

Special Considerations

Digital removal of impacted stool stretches the anal sphincter, causing vagal stimulation. As a result, electrical impulses may be inhibited at the SA node of the heart, causing a decrease in pulse rate as well as dysrhythmias. Therefore, this procedure is contraindicated in cardiac clients.

Consult agency policy and physician's orders regarding the performance of this procedure on any client.

Certain tube feeding formulas (hypertonic) promote constipation and fecal impaction. Check medication record and nutritional supplement list if impaction occurs.

Geriatric

Many elderly clients are especially prone to dysrhythmias and palpitations related to vagal stimulation because of chronic cardiac problems. Observe such clients closely during procedure.

Many elderly clients are especially prone to fecal impaction because of decreased metabolic rate, decreased activity levels, inadequate dietary intake, and tendency to overuse laxatives and enemas as a routine means of promoting bowel evacuation. A thorough history related to these factors should be obtained.

Pediatric

Use little finger when removing impaction in small children.

Delegation

Procedure may be delegated to unlicensed assistive personnel; however, reinforce observation for Valsalva response.

IMPLEMENTATION

Action	Rationale
1. Wash hands.	*Reduces microorganism transfer*
2. Explain procedure to client, admitting that the procedure will cause some discomfort.	*Reduces anxiety*
3. Assess blood pressure and rate and rhythm of pulse.	*Provides baseline data in case of complications*
4. Provide privacy; drape client so only buttocks are exposed.	*Reduces embarrassment*
5. Don gloves, placing one on nondominant hand and two gloves on dominant hand.	*Decreases nurse's exposure to body secretions in case hardened fecal mass tears glove*
6. Position client in side-lying position with knees flexed.	*Allows good exposure of anal opening*
7. Place linen saver under buttocks.	*Prevents soiling of linens*
8. Place bedpan on bed within easy reach.	*Facilitates disposal of fecal mass*
9. Raise side rail on side facing client.	*Prevents injury due to fall*
10. Generously lubricate first two gloved fingers of dominant hand.	*Prevents injury to anus and rectum*
11. Gently spread buttocks with nondominant hand.	*Exposes anal opening*
12. Instruct client to take slow, deep breaths through mouth.	*Relaxes sphincter muscles, facilitating entry*
13. Insert index finger into rectum (directed toward umbilicus) until fecal mass is palpable (Fig. 6.16).	*Prevents rectal trauma*
14. Gently break up hardened stool and remove one piece at a time, until all stool is removed; place stool in bedpan as it is removed.	*Manually removes impacted stool*
15. Observe client for untoward reactions or unusual discomfort during stool removal; obtain pulse and blood pressure if unusual reaction is suspected.	*Prevents complications from vagal stimulation*

Action	Rationale

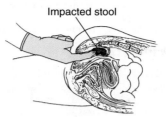

Impacted stool

FIGURE 6.16

Action	Rationale
16. Remove finger, wipe excess lubricant from perineal area, and release buttocks.	*Promotes comfort*
17. Empty bedpan and discard gloves.	*Promotes clean environment*
18. Wash hands.	*Reduces microorganism transfer*
19. Don new pair of gloves.	
20. Wash, rinse, and dry buttocks.	
21. Reposition client and raise side rails.	*Promotes comfort and safety*
22. Leave bedpan within easy reach.	*Impaction removal may have stimulated defecation reflex*
23. Discard bathwater and gloves.	*Promotes clean environment*
24. Spray air freshener at bedside.	*Eliminates odor*
25. Wash hands.	*Reduces microorganism transfer*

Evaluation

Were desired outcomes achieved?

Documentation

The following should be noted on the client's chart:

- Color, consistency, and amount of stool removed
- Condition of anus and surrounding area

- Status of vital signs before and after removal
- Description of adverse reactions during removal
- Abdominal assessment before and after removal
- Presence of discomfort after removal
- Client teaching regarding prevention of fecal impaction

SAMPLE DOCUMENTATION

DATE	TIME	
6/6/02	1100	Large, dark brown, impacted stool removed manually, with no signs of adverse effects. Pulse, 75 and regular before removal and 68 and regular afterward. Bowel sounds auscultated in four quadrants after removal. Abdomen soft and nondistended. Discussed with client factors preventing constipation and impaction. Factors verbalized by client.

Enema Administration

EQUIPMENT

- Two pairs of nonsterile gloves
- Enema setup (administration bag or bucket with rectal tubing, Castile soap, protective plastic linen saver, packet water-soluble lubricant)
- Solution for enema (for adults, 750–1000 ml; for children, up to 350 ml; for infants, up to 250 ml)
- Bath thermometer
- Bedpan
- Linen saver
- Basin of warm water
- Soap
- Washcloth
- Towel
- Air freshener

Purpose

Relieves abdominal distention and discomfort
Stimulates peristalsis
Resumes normal bowel evacuation
Cleanses and evacuates colon

Assessment

Assessment should focus on the following:

Physician's order for type of enema
Agency policy and physician's order regarding performance of procedure
Status of anus and skin surrounding buttocks (ie, presence of ulcerations, tears, hemorrhoids, and excoriation)
Indicators of constipation (ie, lower abdominal pain or hard, small stools)
Abdominal status
Vital signs before, during, and after enema
Time of last bowel movement and usual bowel evacuation pattern
History of factors that may contraindicate enema or present complications during enema administration (such as cardiac instability)

Client history regarding dietary habits (eg, intake of bulk and liquids), changes in activity pattern, frequency of use of laxatives
or enemas
Client knowledge regarding promotion of normal bowel evacuation
Client medications that decrease peristalsis, such as narcotics

Nursing Diagnoses

The nursing diagnoses may include the following:

Constipation related to decreased activity
Chronic pain related to bowel distention from constipation

Outcome Identification and Planning

Desired Outcomes (sample)
Client evacuates moderate to large stool.
Client verbalizes pain relief within 1 hour.

Special Considerations
Geriatric

Many elderly clients are especially prone to dysrhythmias and
palpitations related to vagal stimulation because of chronic cardiac problems. Observe such clients closely during procedure.
Many elderly clients are especially prone to constipation and impaction because of decreased metabolic rate, decreased activity
levels, inadequate dietary intake, and tendency to overuse laxatives and enemas as a routine means of promoting bowel evacuation. A thorough history related to these factors should be
obtained.

Pediatric

Minimal elevation of fluid above the anus (4–18 inches) is needed
to achieve adequate influx of solution.

    Cost-cutting Tip

If bath thermometer is not available to test solution temperature,
use the inner aspect of your forearm.

Delegation

This procedure may be delegated to unlicensed assistive personnel. Emphasize the importance of monitoring client comfort and
monitoring closely for Valsalva response.

IMPLEMENTATION

Action	Rationale
1. Wash hands.	*Reduces microorganism transfer*
2. Explain procedure to client, admitting that the procedure may cause some mild discomfort.	*Reduces anxiety*
3. Prepare solution, making certain that temperature of solution is lukewarm (about 105°F–110°F).	*Reduces abdominal cramping during procedure*
4. Prime tubing with fluid and close tubing clamp; place container on bedside IV pole.	*Prevents distention of colon and abdominal discomfort from air*
5. Lower pole so enema solution hangs no more than 18 to 24 inches above buttocks (Fig. 6.17; for infants and children, solution hangs no more than 4 to 18 inches above the anus).	*Slows rate of fluid infusion and prevents cramping*
6. Provide privacy by draping client so only buttocks are exposed.	*Reduces embarrassment*
7. Don gloves.	*Decreases nurse's exposure to body secretions*

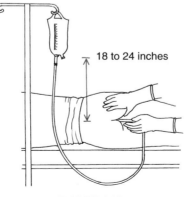

18 to 24 inches

FIGURE 6.17

Action	Rationale
8. Place linen saver under buttocks.	*Prevents soiling of linens*
9. Position client in side-lying position with knees flexed, if not contraindicated.	*Allows good exposure of anal opening*
10. Lubricate 4 to 5 inches of catheter tip.	*Reduces anorectal trauma*
11. Place bedpan on bed within easy reach.	*Facilitates disposal of enema solution*
12. Raise side rail on side facing client.	*Prevents injury due to fall*
13. Gently spread buttocks with nondominant hand.	*Exposes anal opening*
14. Instruct client to take slow, deep breaths through mouth.	*Relaxes sphincter muscles, facilitating entry*
15. With dominant hand, insert rectal tube into rectum (directed toward umbilicus) about 3 to 4 inches and hold in place with dominant hand (1–1½ inches for infants; 2–3 inches for a child).	*Prevents rectal trauma* *Places tube in far enough to cleanse colon*
16. Release tubing clamp.	*Allows solution to flow*
17. Allow solution to flow into colon slowly, observing client closely.	*Avoids cramping*
18. If cramping, extreme anxiety, or complaint of inability to retain solution occurs: - Lower solution container. - Clamp or pinch tubing off for a few minutes. - Resume instillation of solution.	*Decreases or stops solution flow, allowing client to readjust and gain composure*
19. Administer all of solution or as much as client can tolerate; be sure to clamp tubing just before all of solution clears tubing.	*Delivers enough solution for proper effect* *Prevents infusion of air*
20. Slowly remove rectal tubing while gently holding buttocks together.	*Prevents accidental evacuation of solution*

Action	Rationale
21. Remind client to hold solution for amount of time appropriate for type of enema.	*Ensures optimal effect*
22. Reposition client.	*Facilitates comfort*
23. Place call light and bedpan or bedside commode within easy reach.	*Provides means of contacting nurse* *Provides receptacle for enema solution*
24. Discard or restore equipment appropriately.	*Promotes clean environment*
25. Wash hands.	*Reduces microorganism transfer*
26. Check client every 5 to 10 min.	*Reassesses client's condition and results of enema*
27. Assist client on bedpan or toilet after retention time has expired.	*Facilitates evacuation of solution*
28. Spray air freshener after evacuation.	*Eliminates odor*
29. Wash hands.	*Reduces microorganism transfer*

Evaluation

Were desired outcomes achieved?

Documentation

The following should be noted on the client's chart:

- Type and amount of solution used
- Color, consistency, and amount of stool return
- Condition of anus and surrounding area
- Status of vital signs before and after enema
- Description of adverse reactions during enema
- Abdominal assessment before and after enema
- Presence of discomfort after enema
- Client teaching regarding prevention of constipation

SAMPLE DOCUMENTATION

DATE	TIME	
2/6/02	2200	Soap suds enema (750 ml) given. Large, dark brown stool returned from enema. No signs of adverse effects. Bowel sounds auscultated in four quadrants. Abdomen soft and nondistended. Discussed factors for promoting normal bowel evacuation with client. Factors verbalized by client.

Colostomy Stoma Care

EQUIPMENT

- Two pairs of nonsterile gloves (add pair for client, if desired)
- Graduated container
- Two linen savers
- Basin of warm water
- Mild soap (without oils, perfumes, or creams)
- Washcloth
- Towel
- Air freshener
- New pouch appliance
- Scissors
- Pen or pencil
- Mirror
- Peristomal skin paste or powder
- Ostomy pouch deodorizer
- Toilet paper

Purpose

Maintains integrity of stoma and peristomal skin (skin surrounding stoma)

Prevents lesions, ulcerations, excoriation, and other skin breakdown caused by fecal contaminants

Prevents infection

Promotes general comfort

Promotes positive self-concept

Assessment

Assessment should focus on the following:

Appearance of stoma (should be pink and moist) and peristomal skin (should be intact)

Characteristics of fecal waste

Abdominal status

Teaching needs, ability, and preference of client for self-care

Nursing Diagnoses

The nursing diagnoses may include the following:

Risk of impaired skin integrity related to fecal diversion
Knowledge deficit related to lack of information regarding stoma care

Outcome Identification and Planning

Desired Outcomes (sample)

No redness, edema, swelling, tears, breaks, ulceration, or fistulas appear at stoma area.
Client performs procedure with 100% accuracy.

Special Considerations

Once client (or family member) shows readiness to begin learning how to perform ostomy care, supervise client's performance of procedure until it is accomplished accurately and comfortably.
Ostomy care alters a person's self-concept significantly; perform care unhurriedly, and discuss care in a positive manner with the client.

Home Health

Homebound clients may dry the skin after cleaning the stoma by using a hair dryer on a low setting.

Pediatric

Minimal pressure should be used when providing stomal care to prevent prolapse of the small stoma.

Delegation

This procedure may be delegated to unlicensed assistive personnel. Emphasize importance of observations of stoma for irritation or other problems.

IMPLEMENTATION

Action	Rationale
1. Wash hands.	*Reduces microorganism transfer*
2. Explain general procedure to client.	*Reduces anxiety*
3. Explain each step as it is performed, allowing client to ask questions or perform any part of the procedure.	*Reinforces detailed instructions client will need to perform self-care*

Action	Rationale
4. Provide privacy.	*Reduces embarrassment*
5. Position mirror.	*Permits client to observe and learn procedure*
6. Don gloves.	*Avoids nurse's exposure to body secretions*
7. Place linen saver on abdomen around and below stoma opening.	*Prevents seepage of feces onto skin*
8. Carefully remove pouch appliance (bag and skin barrier) and place in plastic waste bag (save tail closure for reuse); remove pouch and skin barrier by gently lifting corner with fingers of dominant hand while pressing skin downward with fingers of non-dominant hand; remove small sections at a time until entire barrier wafer is removed.	*Avoids tearing skin*
9. Empty pouch; measure, discard, and record amount of fecal contents (see Procedure 6.14).	*Maintains records*
10. Wash hands and re-glove.	*Reduces contamination*
11. Gently clean entire stoma and peristomal skin with gauze or washcloth soaked in warm, soapy water (if some of fecal matter is difficult to remove, leave wet gauze or cloth on area for a few minutes before gently removing fecal matter); rinse and pat dry.	*Removes fecal matter from skin and stoma opening*
12. Dry skin thoroughly and apply new pouch device (see Procedure 6.13).	*Provides skin protection from fecal contaminants*
13. Remove gloves and restore or discard all equipment appropriately.	*Promotes clean environment*

Action	Rationale
14. Spray room deodorizer, if needed.	*Eliminates unpleasant odor*
15. Wash hands.	*Reduces microorganism transfer*

Evaluation

Were desired outcomes achieved?

Documentation

The following should be noted on the client's chart:

- Color, consistency, and amount of feces in pouch
- Condition of stoma and peristomal skin
- Abdominal assessment
- Emotional status of client
- Verbal and nonverbal indicators of altered self-concept during procedure
- Verbal and nonverbal indicators of readiness to perform self-care
- Teaching and client participation in performance of procedure
- Additional teaching needs of client

SAMPLE DOCUMENTATION

DATE	TIME	
2/3/02	1600	Stoma care performed by client with 100% accuracy. Discarded large amount of semiformed brown stool. Stoma pink and moist, peristomal skin intact without erythema, excoriation or abnormal discharge. New pouch applied.

Colostomy Pouch Application

EQUIPMENT

- Three pairs of nonsterile gloves
- Graduated container
- Two linen savers
- Basin of warm water
- Mild soap (without oils, perfumes, or creams)
- Washcloth
- Towel
- Air freshener
- New pouch appliance
- Scissors
- Pen or pencil
- Mirror
- Peristomal skin paste
- Ostomy pouch deodorizer

Purpose

Provides clean ostomy pouch for fecal evacuation
Reduces odor from overuse of old pouch
Promotes positive self-image

Assessment

Assessment should focus on the following:

Appearance of stoma and peristomal skin
Characteristics of fecal waste
Type of appliance needed for type of colostomy, nature of
drainage, and client preference
Teaching needs, ability, and preference of client for self-care

Nursing Diagnoses

The nursing diagnoses may include the following:

Risk of impaired skin integrity related to incorrect application of
pouch
Knowledge deficit related to lack of information regarding application of ostomy pouch

331

Outcome Identification and Planning

Desired Outcomes (sample)

No seepage of fecal material from pouch occurs.

Pouch is secured without dislodgment.

Client demonstrates application of new pouch appliance with 100% accuracy.

Special Considerations

A wide variety of ostomy appliances is available to meet clients' personal preferences and needs. Minor variations in techniques of application may be needed to ensure adequate skin protection and pouch security. Some ostomy appliances are permanent and should be discarded only every few months.

Consult appliance manuals for complete information regarding application and recommended usage time for the pouch.

Once client (or family member) shows readiness to learn how to perform ostomy care, supervise client's performance of the procedure until it is accomplished accurately and comfortably.

Ostomy care alters a person's self-concept significantly. Perform care unhurriedly, and discuss care in a positive manner with the client.

Delegation

This procedure may be delegated to unlicensed assistive personnel. Emphasize importance of observations of stoma for irritation or other problems.

IMPLEMENTATION

Action	Rationale
1. Wash hands.	*Reduces microorganism transfer*
2. Explain general procedure to client.	*Reduces anxiety*
3. Explain each step as it is performed, allowing client to ask questions or perform any part of the procedure.	*Reinforces detailed instructions client will need to perform self-care*
4. Provide privacy.	*Reduces embarrassment*
5. Don gloves and offer client gloves.	*Avoids nurse's exposure to body secretions*
6. Place towel or linen saver around stoma pouch close to stoma, remove old pouch, and discard contents; discard gloves.	*Removes old pouch for new pouch application* *Maintains clean environment*

Action	Rationale
7. Wash hands and don fresh gloves.	*Reduces microorganism transfer*
8. Assess stoma and peristomal skin.	*Provides assessment data*
9. Perform stoma care (see Procedure 6.12).	
10. Wash hands.	*Reduces microorganism transfer*
11. Position mirror.	*Allows client to observe and learn procedure*
12. Reglove.	
13. Place linen saver in client's lap or on bed under client's side where colostomy opening is located.	*Protects skin and linens during pouch change*
14. Measure stoma with measuring guide.	*Provides for accurate fit of pouch appliances*
15. Leaving intact adhesive covering of skin-barrier wafer (a flat, platelike piece, without pouch attached, that fits on skin around stoma), use measuring guide to trace a circle on adhesive liner the same size as stoma; cut out circle.	*Cuts barrier to size appropriate for stoma*
16. Cut circular adhesive back of ostomy pouch so it measures about ⅛ inch larger than actual stoma size.	*Allows pouch to be placed over and around stoma without adhering to stoma membrane*
17. Open bottom of pouch and apply a small amount of pouch deodorizer, if client prefers; reclose pouch securely.	*Reduces odor and embarrassment* *Avoids leakage of feces*
18. Apply stomal paste around stoma or apply stomal paste to edges of opening in wafer.	*Prevents skin irritation of uncovered peristomal skin*
19. Remove adhesive covering of skin-barrier wafer, and place wafer on skin with hole centered over stoma; HOLD IN PLACE FOR ABOUT 30 SECONDS.	*Adheres barrier wafer to skin* *Warmth of skin and fingers enhances adhesiveness once wafer makes contact with skin*

Action	Rationale
20. Center pouch over stoma, and place on skin-barrier wafer. (If applying a two-piece appliance, snap pouch on the flange of the skin-barrier wafer (Fig. 6.18).	*Secures pouch for collection of feces*
21. Remove gloves; restore or discard all equipment appropriately.	*Promotes clean environment*
22. Spray room freshener, if needed.	*Eliminates unpleasant odor*
23. Wash hands.	*Reduces microorganism transfer*

Evaluation

Were desired outcomes achieved?

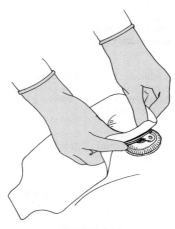

FIGURE 6.18

Documentation

The following should be noted on the client's chart:

- Color, consistency, and amount of feces in pouch
- Condition of stoma and peristomal skin
- Abdominal assessment
- Emotional status of client
- Verbal and nonverbal indicators of altered self-concept during procedure
- Verbal and nonverbal indicators of readiness to perform self-care
- Teaching and client participation in performance of procedure
- Additional teaching needs of client
- Type of appliance client prefers

SAMPLE DOCUMENTATION

DATE	TIME	
2/3/02	1100	New colostomy pouch applied by client with 100% accuracy. Discarded large amount of semiformed brown stool. Stoma pink, without excoriation or abnormal discharge. Client verbalized anxiety about how wife will accept assisting with his care and stated preference for pouch appliance with flange rings.

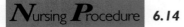

Nursing Procedure 6.14

Colostomy Pouch Evacuation and Cleaning

EQUIPMENT

- Three pairs of nonsterile gloves
- Bedpan and/or graduated container
- Two linen savers
- Air freshener
- Two washcloths
- Mirror
- Ostomy pouch deodorizer
- Toilet paper
- Paper towels

Purpose

Removes fecal material from ostomy pouch
Cleans pouch for reuse
Maintains integrity of stoma and peristomal skin
Promotes general comfort
Promotes positive self-concept

Assessment

Assessment should focus on the following:

Appearance of stoma and peristomal skin (should be pink and moist) and peristomal skin (should be intact with no erythema)
Characteristics of fecal waste
Abdominal status
Type of ostomy appliance (reusable or disposable)
Teaching needs, ability, and preference of client for self-care

Nursing Diagnoses

The nursing diagnoses may include the following:

Risk of impaired skin integrity related to fecal diversion
Knowledge deficit related to lack of information regarding evacuation and cleaning of pouch

Situational low self-esteem related to perceived loss of independent functioning

Outcome Identification and Planning

Desired Outcomes (sample)

No redness, edema, swelling, tears, breaks, ulceration, or fistulas are present in stoma area.
Client performs procedure with 100% accuracy within 2 weeks.
Client verbalizes feelings about fecal diversion.

Special Considerations

Once client (or family member) show readiness to learn how to perform ostomy care, supervise client's performance of the procedure until it is accomplished accurately and comfortably.
Ostomy care alters a person's self-concept significantly. Perform care unhurriedly, and discuss care in a positive manner with the client.

 Cost-cutting Tip

If pouch *clamp* is not available, use sturdy rubber bands.

Delegation

This procedure may be delegated to unlicensed assistive personnel. Emphasize importance of observations of stoma for irritation or other problems.

IMPLEMENTATION

Action	Rationale
1. Wash hands.	*Reduces microorganism transfer*
2. Explain general procedure to client.	*Reduces anxiety*
3. Explain each step as it is performed, allowing client to ask questions or perform any part of the procedure.	*Reinforces detailed instructions client will need to perform self-care*
4. Provide privacy.	*Reduces embarrassment*
5. Position mirror.	*Allows client to observe and learn procedure*
6. Don gloves.	*Avoids nurse's exposure to body secretions*
7. Place linen saver on abdomen around and below pouch.	*Prevents seepage of feces onto skin*

Action	Rationale
8. If using toilet, seat client on toilet or in a chair facing toilet, with pouch over toilet; if using bedpan, place pouch over bedpan.	*Positions client so feces drain into receptacle*
9. Remove clamp on bottom of pouch and place within easy reach. (Fold bottom of pouch up to form a cuff before emptying.)	*Promotes efficiency* *Cuff keeps bottom of pouch clean, which helps to prevent odor and helps keep hands clean during procedure*
10. Slowly unfold end of pouch and allow feces to drain into bedpan or toilet (Fig. 6.19).	*Removes feces from pouch*

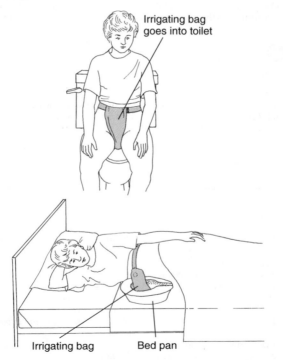

Irrigating bag goes into toilet

Irrigating bag   Bed pan

FIGURE 6.19

Action	Rationale
11. Press sides of lower end of pouch together (Fig. 6.20).	*Expels additional feces from pouch*
12. Open lower end of pouch and wipe out with toilet paper.	*Removes excess feces from lower end of pouch*
13. Flush toilet or, if using bedpan, take time to resecure end of pouch with rubber band and then empty bedpan.	*Reduces client embarrassment and room odor*
14. Wash hands and reglove.	*Reduces microorganism transfer*
15. Wash clamp while in bathroom and dry with paper towel.	*Cleans exterior clamp*
16. Apply pouch deodorizer to lower end of pouch.	*Reduces unpleasant odor*
17. Reclamp pouch with cleaned clamp.	*Prevents leakage of feces*
18. Wipe outside of pouch with clean, wet washcloth; be sure to wipe around clamp at bottom of pouch.	*Completes cleaning of pouch*
19. Remove gloves and restore or discard all equipment appropriately.	*Promotes clean environment*

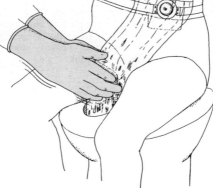

FIGURE 6.20

Action	Rationale
20. Spray room freshener, if needed.	*Eliminates unpleasant odor*
21. Wash hands.	*Reduces microorganism transfer*

Evaluation

Were desired outcomes achieved?

Documentation

The following should be noted on the client's chart:

- Color, consistency, and amount of feces in pouch
- Condition of stoma and peristomal skin
- Abdominal assessment
- Emotional status of client
- Verbal and nonverbal indicators of altered self-concept during procedure
- Verbal and nonverbal indicators of readiness to perform self-care
- Teaching and client participation in performance of procedure
- Additional teaching needs of client

SAMPLE DOCUMENTATION

DATE	TIME	
8/31/02	1430	Ostomy pouch cleaning and evacuation performed by client with 100% accuracy. Discarded large amount of semiformed brown stool. Stoma moist and pink.

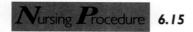

Colostomy Irrigation

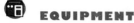

EQUIPMENT

- IV pole or wall hook
- Irrigation bag and tubing
- Irrigation cone
- Water-soluble lubricant
- Commode or commode chair
- Warm saline or tap water
- Bath thermometer
- Two towels
- Two washcloths
- Linen savers
- Bath basin or sink
- Fresh pouch
- Nonsterile gloves

Purpose

Facilitates emptying of colon

Assessment

Assessment should focus on the following:

Doctor's order for frequency of irrigation and type and amount of
    solution
Type of colostomy and nature of drainage
Client's ability and preference to perform colostomy care
Client teaching needs

Nursing Diagnoses

The nursing diagnoses may include the following:

Constipation related to decreased roughage and activity
Acute pain related to constipation
Knowledge deficit regarding irrigation related to information
    misinterpretation

Outcome Identification and Planning

Desired Outcomes (sample)

Stool passes freely through stomal opening.

Client demonstrates correct procedure.

Client experiences no excessive cramping or pain during irrigation.

Special Considerations

If no stool returns and irrigant is retained, reposition client and apply drainable pouch, if needed. You may have client ambulate, if permissible. Notify doctor if there is no return or if abdominal distention is noted. Distention of the colon with irrigation fluid can cause a vasovagal reaction (bradycardia, hypotension, and possible loss of consciousness). Therefore, it is recommended that the initial irrigation be performed with the client in bed.

Pediatric

Routine irrigations are seldom done for the purpose of bowel regulation.

Caution should be exercised because of the small size of the stoma.

Home Health

If homebound client plans to irrigate colostomy while sitting on commode, teach client the proper procedure and have the client demonstrate it to you. Correct client's technique, if necessary.

Delegation

This procedure may be delegated to unlicensed assistive personnel in most agencies. Check agency policies.

Implementation

Action	Rationale
1. Explain procedure to client.	*Reduces anxiety*
2. Wash hands and organize equipment.	*Reduces microorganism transfer and promotes efficiency*
3. Obtain extra lighting, if needed.	
4. Provide for warmth and privacy.	*Promotes comfort and reduces embarrassment*
5. Prepare irrigating solution as follows:	*Ensures proper preparation of solution and tubing*

Action	Rationale
- Obtain irrigation bag and solution (usually tepid water); use 250 to 500 ml for initial irrigation, 500 to 1000 ml for subsequent irrigations (minimal amounts are recommended).	*Allows bowel to adjust to fluid pressure*
- Check temperature of solution (should feel warm to touch but not hot).	*Prevents injury from hot solution or cramping from cold solution*
- Close tubing clamp.	*Allows better fluid control*
- Fill bag with tap water or ordered solution at appropriate temperature.	
- Open clamp and expel air from tubing.	*Prevents air infusion into bowel*
- Close off clamp.	
- Hang bag and tubing on pole or hook.	*Permits drainage by gravity*
- Lubricate the cone tip with water-soluble gel.	*Prevents irritation of stomal tissue*
6. Don gloves.	*Prevents nurse's contact with body secretions*
7. Place client comfortably in any of the following positions (place linen saver under client if performing procedure in bed): - On commode - Sitting on chair facing toilet - In side-lying position, turned toward side of stomal opening, with head of bed elevated 30 to 45 degrees - In supine position	*Provides for effective irrigation*
8. Gently remove existing pouch from stomal area.	*Avoids skin irritation or injury*
9. Assess site for redness, swelling, tenderness, and excoriation.	*Determines need for other skin care measures*
10. Gently wash stomal area with warm, soapy water.	*Removes secretions*

Action	Rationale
11. Rinse with clear water and dry thoroughly.	
12. Apply irrigation sleeve and belt: - Round opening of irrigation sleeve fits over stoma. - Belt fits around waist.	*Holds irrigation bag in place to prevent spillage*
13. Position irrigation bag (with tubing attached) at a height of 18 inches above stoma (approximately shoulder level).	*Avoids undue pressure on mucosal tissues from rushing of fluid*
14. Place lower end of sleeve into toilet or large bedpan and unclamp.	*Provides receptacle for drainage and begins flow of irrigant*
15. Expose stoma through upper opening of sleeve.	
16. Lubricate tip of cone and gently ease into stomal opening (Fig. 6.21). Hold tip securely in place to prevent backflow.	*Prevents escape of bowel content onto skin*
17. Release irrigation tubing clamp and allow solution to infuse over 10 to 15 min. (Fig. 6.22)	*Slow infusion prevents cramping from over-distention*

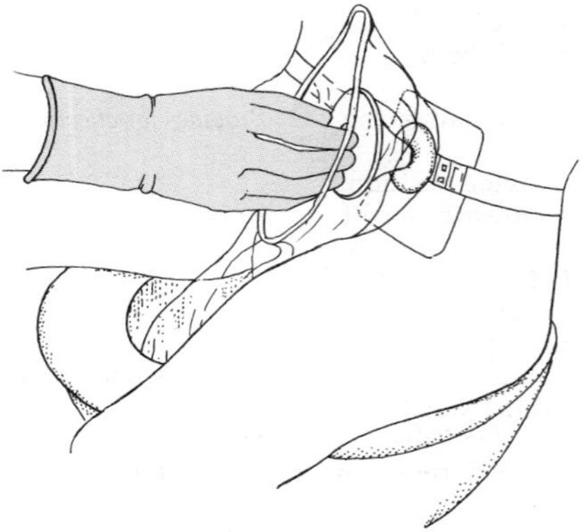

FIGURE 6.21

Action	Rationale
18. Encourage client to take slow, deep breaths as solution is infusing.	*Relaxes client and decreases cramping of bowel*
19. If client complains of cramping, stop infusion for several minutes; then resume infusion slowly.	*Allows bowel time to adjust to fluid*
20. Observe for return of fecal material and solution and assess drainage.	*Indicates effectiveness of irrigation*
21. Remove bottom of sleeve from drainage receptacle and flush toilet or empty bedpan.	*Restores room cleanliness*
22. Dry bottom of sleeve and clamp.	*Prevents soiling and collects further drainage*

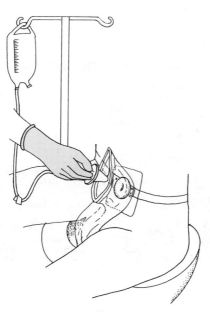

FIGURE 6.22

Action	Rationale
23. Remove irrigation sleeve and belt.	*Concludes irrigation procedure*
24. Clean bedpan.	*Restores room cleanliness and order*
25. Discard or restore equipment.	*Promotes clean, organized environment*
26. Discard old gloves and don new pair.	*Reduces contamination*
27. Wash, rinse, and dry stoma area.	*Cleanses peristomial area*
28. Apply new dressing or ostomy pouch, if needed.	
29. Wash hands.	*Reduces microorganism transfer*

Evaluation

Were desired outcomes achieved?

Documentation

The following should be noted on the client's chart:

- Condition of stoma site
- Amount of irrigant infused
- Amount and nature of drainage
- Client tolerance for procedure
- Client teaching accomplished and/or needed

SAMPLE DOCUMENTATION

DATE	TIME	
3/23/02	1250	Colostomy irrigation done with 600 ml tap water infused. Approximately 800 ml soft and liquid brown drainage noted. Client tolerated procedure without cramping or pain. Client demonstrated correct technique.

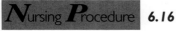

Stool Testing for Occult Blood With Hemoccult Slide

EQUIPMENT

- Stool specimen
- Hemoccult specimen collection card
- Chemical reagent (developer)
- Tongue blade
- Nonsterile gloves
- Stop watch or watch with second hand
- Specimen container labels
- Pen

Purpose

Obtains stool specimen to detect occult blood related to gastrointestinal bleeding and anemia

Serves as a preliminary screening test for colorectal cancer

Assessment

Assessment should focus on the following:

Specific orders regarding specimen collection
Characteristics of stool
Manifestations associated with gastrointestinal bleeding or anemia
History of gastrointestinal bleeding or anemia
Dietary intake of foods or drugs that could alter test reliability
Intake of medications that cause occult bleeding

Nursing Diagnoses

The nursing diagnoses may include the following:
Risk of fluid volume deficit related to gastrointestinal bleeding

Outcome Identification and Planning

Desired Outcome (sample)

Signs and symptoms of gastrointestinal bleeding (bloody or dark black stools, fatigue, decreased bowel sounds, abdominal discomfort) are detected early.

Special Considerations

Some vitamins and minerals (such as vitamin C and iron) can cause erratic test results. Consult a pharmacy reference for a complete listing of such preparations and the amounts necessary to alter results.

Many clients are placed on special diagnostic diets 2 to 3 days before hemoccult testing. Emphasize to client the importance of adhering to diet restrictions.

IMPLEMENTATION

Action	Rationale
1. Wash hands.	*Reduces microorganism transfer*
2. Explain procedure to client.	*Decreases anxiety*
3. Provide for privacy.	*Decreases embarrassment*
4. Don clean gloves.	*Reduces nurse's exposure to body secretions*
5. Obtain stool specimen with tongue blade and smear thin specimen onto guaiac test paper: - Smear specimen onto slot A on front of card. - Smear a second specimen from another part of stool onto slot B. - Close card.	*Prepares specimen for test*
6. Turn card over and open back window; apply two drops of reagent to slot over each specimen and wait 60 sec.	*Activates chemical components necessary for results*
7. Read results (consult product instructions for visual comparison): - If either slot has bluish discoloration, test is positive.	*Determines if results are posiive or negative*

Action	Rationale
- If there is no bluish discoloration, test is negative.	
8. Restore or discard equipment appropriately (test card may be discarded).	*Promotes clean environment*
9. Wash hands.	*Reduces microorganism transfer*

Evaluation

Were desired outcomes achieved?

Documentation

The following should be noted on the client's chart:

- Amount, color, odor, and consistency of stool obtained
- Specimen collection time
- Signs and symptoms consistent with gastrointestinal bleeding

SAMPLE DOCUMENTATION

DATE	TIME	
3/2/02	1100	Second stool tested for occult blood with hemoccult slide. Results negative. Stool is dark brown, large, and formed. Client reports no discomfort during defecation.

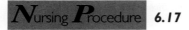

Care of Nephrostomy Tubes

EQUIPMENT

- Clean drainage bag and connecting tube
- Disposable gloves
- Alcohol swabs
- Sterile gauze pads
- Adhesive tape
- Paper bag for disposal of soiled dressing

Purpose

Allows urine to drain from the kidney to a drainage bag in cases of ureters obstructed by tumors, calculi, strictures, or fistulae

Assessment

Assessment should focus on the following:

Continuous flow of urine
Doctor's order for dressing change
Client's knowledge of the procedure
Rise in temperature, purulent discharge at insertion site, odorous urine, flank pain, integrity of skin around the insertion site
Appearance of urine
Client's cognitive status, vision, and manual dexterity
Family member's or significant other's reliability to care for the tube successfully

Outcome Identification and Planning

Desired Outcomes (sample)

Maintenance of adequate urine output
Maintenance of nephrostomy tube without infection or skin breakdown
Resumption of a high level of independent functioning
Verbalize when to call for assistance

Special Considerations

Instruct the patient to notify the health care provider immediately if the tube comes out. The tract closes quickly in 2 to 3 hr.

Keep the drainage bag lower than the nephrostomy tube to en-
hance gravitational flow.
NEVER IRRIGATE THE NEPHROSTOMY TUBE UNLESS OR-
DERED.

IMPLEMENTATION

Action	Rationale
1. Explain procedure to client.	*Decreases anxiety*
2. Wash hands.	*Avoids transfer of micro-organisms*
3. Organize equipment within reach.	*Promotes efficiency*
4. Put on disposable gloves.	*Minimizes exposure to body secretions*
5. Disconnect the nephrostomy tube from the used tubing and drainage bag. Clean end of the nephrostomy tube with an alcohol swab.	*Reduces microorganism transfer*
6. Attach the ends of the nephrostomy tube and the connecting tube securely. Don't touch the ends of the tubes.	*Maintains the sterility of system*
7. Check the tubing for kinks.	*Maintains patency of system*
8. Change the dressing daily according to doctor's order. Put soiled dressing in paper bag for disposal.	*Removes medium for micro-organism growth*
9. Gently wash around the nephrostomy tube.	*Decreases microorganisms around the nephrostomy tube*
10. Inspect the skin around the tube. Note color and character of any drainage.	*Redness, or white, yellow, or green drainage may indicate infection* *Drainage that smells like urine may indicate tube displacement* *Either condition should be reported to the doctor immediately*
11. Fold several gauze pads in half and place them around the base of the nephrostomy tube. Secure the pads with tape. Cover the nephrostomy tube entry site with a dry sterile 4 × 4 and tape securely.	*Protects the skin and is more comfortable for the client*

Action	Rationale
12. Bring all the tubing forward, and tape securely to the body.	*Allows the client to turn without obstructing urine flow or dislodging the tube from the kidney*
13. Keep separate output records for each kidney, if both have tubes.	*Promotes more accurate assessment of kidney function*
14. Irrigate the tube gently with 5 ml of sterile warm saline solution, if ordered. ALERT DOCTOR IMMEDIATELY IF TUBE IS NOT PATENT	*To determine patency*
15. Wash the used bag and connecting tube with a weak detergent daily. Rinse with plain water and hang on clothes hanger to air dry.	*A biodegradable or chlorine product may erode the bag*
16. Twice weekly wash the bag and tubing with a solution of one part white vinegar to three parts water.	*Avoids crystalline buildup*

Evaluation

Were desired outcomes achieved?

Documentation

The following will be noted on the client's chart:

- Teaching done
- Functional limitations that interfere with performance of procedure
- Client toleration of procedure
- Condition of the insertion site
- Quality and quantity of urinary output
- Plans for future visits
- Discharge planning

SAMPLE DOCUMENTATION

DATE	TIME	
9/26/02	0900	Left flank nephrostomy tube site care given and sterile dressing applied. Observed continuous clear amber urine flow. Denies flank pain. Temperature 98.8° F. No redness or drainage noted at insertion site.

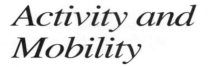

Chapter 7

Activity and Mobility

OVERVIEW

▶ The ability to remain physically active and mobile is essential in maintaining health and well-being. Immobility may pose psychological as well as physiologic hazards. Nurses should be alert for such physical complications of immobility as the following:
  - Hypostatic pneumonia
  - Pulmonary embolism
  - Thrombophlebitis
  - Orthostatic hypotension
  - Pressure ulcers or pressure areas
  - Decreased peristalsis with constipation and fecal impaction
  - Urinary stasis with renal calculi formation
  - Contractures and muscle atrophy
  - Altered fluid and electrolyte status

▶ Proper positioning and correct support surfaces are important factors in managing tissue loads for clients in bed.

► Psychological hazards of immobility may range from mild anxiety to psychosis.

► Improper use of body mechanics when moving a client could result in injury to client and nurse. Knowledge of principles of body mechanics and proper body alignment is essential to injury prevention.

► The occupational group documented as most frequently absent from work with back injury for more than 3 days is nurses.

► Proper body mechanics, with prevention of injury, conserves time and energy expenditure, as well as preventing financial expense resulting from injury.

► Some major nursing diagnostic labels related to activity and mobility are impaired physical mobility, risk of physical injury, activity intolerance, risk of peripheral neurovascular dysfunction, and risk of disuse syndrome.

► Unlicensed assistive personnel should receive training on how to correctly move or transfer clients and monitor for signs of complications; however, routine monitoring remains the responsibility of the nurse.

► Some techniques should only be delegated to assistive personnel specifically trained or certified in physical rehabilitation maneuvers.

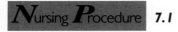

Using Principles of Body Mechanics

🔲 EQUIPMENT

- Equipment needed to move client or lift object (eg, Hoyer lift, sling scales, trapeze bar)
- Turn sheets
- Chair, stretcher, or bed for client
- Adequate lighting
- Positioning equipment (eg, trochanter rolls, pillows, footboards)
- Nonsterile gloves
- Visual and hearing aids needed by client

Purpose

Prevents physical injury of caregiver and client
Promotes correct body alignment
Facilitates coordinated, efficient muscle use when moving clients
Conserves energy of caregiver for accomplishment of other tasks

Assessment

Assessment should focus on the following:

Presence of deformities or abnormalities of vertebrae
Physical characteristics of client and caregiver that will influence techniques used (eg, weight, size, height, age, physical limitations and abilities, condition of target muscles to be used in moving client, problems related to equilibrium)
Characteristics of object to be moved during client care (eg, weight, height, shape)
Immediate environment (amount of space available to work in; distance to be traveled; presence of obstructions in pathway; condition of floor; placement of chairs, stretchers, and other equipment being used; lighting)
Adequacy of function and stability of all equipment to be used
Extent of knowledge of assistive personnel, client, and family regarding proper use of body mechanics and body alignment
Status of equipment attached to client that must be moved (eg, IV machines, tubes, drains)

Nursing Diagnoses

The nursing diagnoses may include the following:

Risk of physical injury related to improper use of body mechanics
Knowledge deficit related to inadequate information on proper
   use of body mechanics

Outcome Identification and Planning

Desired Outcomes (sample)

Client displays no evidence of physical injury, such as new
   bruises, tears, or skeletal trauma after moving.
Before discharge, client demonstrates proper use of body mechanics to be used in performing major lifting and moving tasks
   at home.

Special Considerations

Secure as much additional assistance as is needed for safe moves.
   NEVER BECOME SO IMPATIENT THAT UNSAFE RISK IS
   TAKEN WITH ANY TYPE OF MOVE. As a general rule, if
   equipment is available that will make lifting, turning, pulling,
   or positioning easier, use it.
Check all equipment to be used, including chairs, for adequate
   function and stability.
If physical injury of personnel is sustained because of performance of any work-related activity, follow agency policies regarding follow-up medical attention and completion of incident
   report forms. This provides for proper care and ensures financial assistance as needed.
Avoid excessive pressure and shearing on skin when moving the
   client.

Pediatric and Geriatric

If client is restless, agitated, confused, or has a condition that
   causes loss of muscle control, secure assistance to prevent injury
   during the moving process.

Home Health

The home environment should be assessed to determine the need
   to rearrange furniture and other items and to secure mechanical equipment to ensure the safety of client and family as they
   perform care.

Delegation

If special precautions are to be used with moving a client, be sure to reinforce to assistive personnel to ascertain verbal understanding of care needs. If physical injury of personnel is sustained because of performance of any work-related activity, follow agency policies regarding follow-up medical attention and completion of incident report forms.

IMPLEMENTATION

Action	Rationale
1. Wash hands.	*Reduces microorganism transfer*
2. Determine factors indicating need for additional personnel such as:	*Promotes efficiency and enhances safety of patient and caregiver*
- Equipment attached to client	
- Does move require persons of approximately the same height?	
3. Apply client's glasses and hearing aids if client is able to assist.	*Enables client to assist in making a safe move*
4. Explain required movement techniques to assistive personnel, family, and client; instruct and allow client to do as much as possible.	*Facilitates coordinated movement and prevents physical injury* *Promotes independence*
5. Don gloves if contact with body fluids is likely.	*Prevents exposure to body secretions*
6. Organize equipment so it is within easy reach, stabilized, and in proper position:	*Avoids risks once movement begins*
- If moving client to chair, place chair so back of chair is in same direction as head of bed.	*Keeps number of actions needed for the move to a minimum*
- If placing client on stretcher, align stretcher with side of bed.	
7. Raise or lower bed and other equipment to comfortable and suitable height.	*Prevents unnecessary use of back muscles in performing tasks*

Action	Rationale

8. Maintain proper body alignment by using the following principles when handling equipment and when moving, lifting, turning, and positioning client:

- Stand with back, neck, shoulders, pelvis, and feet in as straight a line as possible; knees should be slightly flexed and toes pointed forward (Fig. 7.1).

Maintains proper body alignment

- Keep feet apart to establish broad support base; keep feet flat on floor (Fig. 7.2).

Provides greater stability

- Flex knees and hips to lower center of gravity (heaviest area of body) close to object to be moved (Fig. 7.3).

Establishes more stable position
Prevents pulling on spine

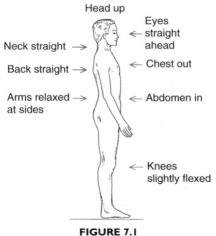

Head up

Eyes ← straight ahead

Neck straight →

← Chest out

Back straight →

Arms relaxed → at sides

← Abdomen in

← Knees slightly flexed

FIGURE 7.1

Action	Rationale

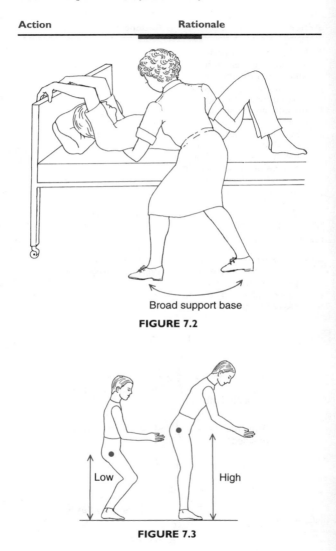

Broad support base

FIGURE 7.2

Low   High

FIGURE 7.3

Action	Rationale
- Move close to object to be moved or adjusted; do not lean or bend at waist.	*Promotes use of muscles of extremities rather than of spine*
- Use smooth, rhythmic motions when using bedcranks or any equipment requiring a pumping motion.	*Prevents improper alignment and inefficient muscle use*
- Use arm muscles for cranking or pumping and arm and leg muscles for lifting.	*Avoids use of spine and back muscles*
9. Secure tubes, drains, traction, and other equipment by whatever means are needed for proper functioning during moving, lifting, turning, and positioning.	*Prevents dislodgment of tubes and reflux of contaminants into body*
10. Move client close to edge of bed in one unit or move client to side of bed at any time during procedure, moving one unit of the body at a time from top to bottom or vice versa (ie, head and shoulders first, trunk and hips second, and legs last). Coordinate move so everyone exerts greatest effort on count of three; the person carrying the heaviest load should direct the count.	*Maintains correct alignment Facilitates comfort* *Prevents physical injury*
11. Use the following principles to move a heavy object or client:	
a. Review each move again before move is made.	*Reinforces original plan*
b. Face client or object to be moved.	*Allows full use of arm and leg muscles*

Action	Rationale
c. Place hands or arms fully under client or object; lock hands with assistant on opposite side, if necessary.	*Provides extra leverage*
d. Prepare for move by taking in a deep breath, tightening abdominal and gluteal muscles, and tucking chin toward chest. (If client is unable to provide assistance, instruct client to cross arms on chest.)	*Facilitates use of large muscle groups*
e. Allow adequate rest periods, if needed.	*Prevents fatigue and subsequent physical injury*
f. When performing move, keep heaviest part of body within base of support.	*Promotes stability*
g. Perform pulling motions by leaning backward and pushing motions by leaning forward, maintaining wide base of support with feet, keeping knees flexed and one foot behind the other; pushing and pulling (use instead of lifting, whenever possible) should be done with muscles of the arms and legs, not back.	*Prevents injury to vertebrae and back muscles*
h. Always lower head of bed as much as permissible.	*Avoids pulling against gravity*
i. When moving from a bending to a standing position, stop momentarily once in standing position before completing next move.	*Allows time to straighten spine and reestablish stability*

Action	Rationale
When getting client into a chair, stop to allow client and self to stand to establish stability before pivoting into chair.	
j. Move in as straight and direct a path as possible, avoiding twisting and turning of spine.	*Avoids vertebral and back injury related to rotating and twisting spine*
k. When turning is unavoidable, use a pivoting turn; when positioning client in chair or carrying client to a stretcher, pivot toward chair or stretcher together.	
12. Position props and body parts for appropriate body alignment of client after move is completed:	
- When client is sitting, hips, shoulders, and neck should be in line with trunk; knees, hips, and ankles should be flexed at a 90-degree angle, and toes should be pointed forward.	
- When client is in bed, neck, shoulders, pelvis, and ankles should be in line with trunk, and knees and elbows should be slightly flexed.	
13. After move is completed, provide for comfort and safety of client with the following actions, if applicable:	
- Raise protective rails.	*Prevents falls*
- Apply safety belts on stretchers and wheelchairs.	*Promotes safety*

Action	Rationale
- Lower height of bed.	*Promotes safety*
- Elevate head properly.	*Supports airway clearance*
- Restore all tubes, drains, and equipment being used by client to proper functioning and placement.	*Reestablishes proper functioning of equipment*
- Place pillows and position equipment properly.	*Promotes proper body alignment and supports airway*
- Replace covers.	*Provides warmth and privacy*
- Place call light within reach.	*Provides means of communication*
- Place items of frequent use within client reach.	*Enhances comfort and general satisfaction*
14. Discard gloves and wash hands.	*Reduces microorganism transfer*

Evaluation

Were desired outcomes achieved?

Documentation

The following should be noted on the client's chart:

- Amount of assistance given by client
- Position in which client was placed (eg, in chair, returned to bed, placed on stretcher)
- Reports of discomfort, dizziness, or faintness during or after move
- Reestablishment of proper functioning of equipment
- Safety belts applied
- Status of side rails
- Auxiliary equipment used
- Status of equipment being used to maintain alignment

SAMPLE DOCUMENTATION

DATE	TIME	
10/19/02	1030	Assisted client into chair. Able to provide partial assistance; reported slight dizziness when standing. IV remains intact and infusing correctly. Posey vest reapplied. Call light within reach.

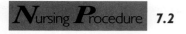

Nursing Procedure 7.2

Body Positioning

EQUIPMENT

- Support devices required by client (eg, trochanter roll, foot-board, heel protectors, sandbags, hand rolls, restraints)
- Pillow for head and extra pillows needed for support

Purpose

Positions client for comfort, body alignment, and tissue load management (pressure distribution, friction, and shear on the tissue)

Positions client for a variety of clinical procedures

Assessment

Assessment should focus on the following:

Client's age and medical diagnosis
Physical ability of client to maintain position
Integumentary and musculoskeletal assessment
Risk of development of pressure ulcers
Length of time client has maintained present body positioning
Doctor's orders for specific restrictions in positioning client or for special position required by impending procedure

Nursing Diagnoses

The nursing diagnoses may include the following:

Risk of impaired skin integrity related to prolonged pressure on bony prominences
Impaired physical mobility related to decreased muscle strength

Outcome Identification and Planning

Desired Outcome (sample)

Client's skin is warm, dry, intact, and without discoloration over pressure points.

Special Considerations

To avoid injury when positioning clients, it is important that body alignment of the client and nurse or assistant be supported and that appropriate body mechanics be used. (Nursing Procedure 7.1 presents the principles of body mechanics.) Secure additional assistance as needed for the safe repositioning of the client and for protection of your back. NEVER BECOME SO IMPATIENT THAT RISKS ARE TAKEN.

Foot drop, pressure ulcers, shoulder subluxation, and internal and external rotation of large joint areas are preventable complications if the client is positioned and supported correctly. Be sure that pillows, trochanter rolls, footboards, and other supportive equipment are positioned to maintain body alignment; that joint and ligament pulling is prevented; that head, feet, and hands do not droop; that large joint areas do not rotate internally or externally; and that excess pressure on any body area is avoided.

Immobile clients with existing pressure ulcers who are at risk of new pressure ulcers and are immobile should not be positioned directly on their trochanters.

Geriatric

Bedridden elderly clients are particularly susceptible to impaired skin integrity when they are not repositioned frequently; this is due to a decreased amount of subcutaneous fat and to skin that is less elastic, thinner, drier, and, thus, more fragile than that of a younger person.

Home Health

In the home, pillows, sofa cushions, or rolled linen may be used for positioning. A recliner may be used to maintain a Fowler's or semi-Fowler's position.

IMPLEMENTATION

Action	Rationale
1. Wash hands.	*Reduces microorganism transfer*
2. Explain procedure to client, emphasizing importance of maintaining proper position.	*Decreases anxiety* *Increases compliance*
3. Provide for privacy.	*Decreases embarrassment*
4. Adjust bed to comfortable working height.	*Prevents back and muscle strain in nurse*
5. Place or assist client into appropriate position. Avoid	*Avoids shearing of skin tissue*

Action	Rationale

dragging client on sheet or bed. (Various positions are illustrated in Fig. 7.4 and described in Table 7.1.)

6. Use the following guidelines in repositioning client:

- Place all equipment, lines, and drains attached to client so dislodgment will not occur.

  Prevents accidental dislodgment and client injury

- Close off drains, if necessary, and remember to reopen them after positioning client.

  Prevents reflux of drainage

- Be sure an assistant is designated to handle extremities bound by heavy stabilizers (such as casts and traction) and heavy equipment that must be moved with client (such as traction apparatus).

  Maintains stability of body part to prevent injury and pain

- Maintain head elevation for clients prone to dyspnea when flat; allow brief rest periods, as needed, during procedure.

  Facilitates breathing and reduces anxiety
  Prevents exertion

- When moving client to side of bed, move major portions of the body sequentially, from top to bottom or vice versa (eg, head and shoulders first, trunk and hips second, legs last).

  Maintains body alignment
  Facilitates comfort

- Use pillows, trochanter rolls, and special positioning supports as needed to maintain body alignment, normal position of extremities, and undue pressure on vulnerable skin surfaces.

  Prevents injury and promotes comfort
  Balances weight to manage tissue load

Action	Rationale

A. Fowler's

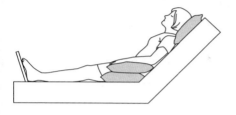

B. Supine

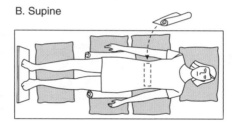

C. Prone

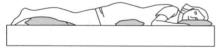

D. Side-lying

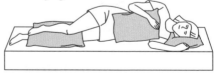

FIGURE 7.4

Action	Rationale

E. Sim's

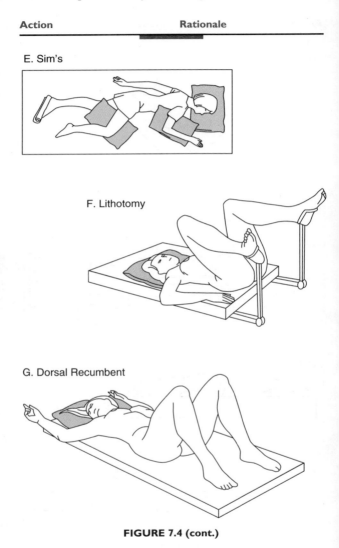

F. Lithotomy

G. Dorsal Recumbent

FIGURE 7.4 (cont.)

TABLE 7.1 Body Positioning

Position	Purpose	Description
Fowler's (low to high)	Improves breathing capacity Prevents aspiration Promotes comfort	Head of bed up 30 to 90 degrees Client in a semisitting position Knees slightly flexed
Supine	Prevents bending at crucial areas, such as groin or spine, after diagnostic procedures	Client flat on back in bed Body straight and in alignment Feet protected with footboard to support 90-degree flexion
Prone	Serves as positioning alternative in turning procedure for immobilized clients	Client flat on abdomen with knees slightly flexed Head turned to side Arms flexed at sides, hands near head Feet over end of mattress or protected with foot-board to support normal flexion
Side-lying (lateral)	Serves as position for some procedures and alternative position for turning procedure	Client lying on side with upper leg flexed at hip and knee Top arm flexed Lower arm flexed and shoulder positioned to avoid pulling and excessive weight of body or shoulder
Sim's	Serves as position for some procedures and alternative position for turning procedure	Client halfway between side-lying and prone positions with bottom knee slightly flexed Knee and hip of top leg flexed (about 90 degrees) Lower arm behind back Upper arm flexed, hand near head

TABLE 7.1 Body Positioning (cont.)

Position	Purpose	Description
Lithotomy	Places client in position for vaginal or anorectal exams	Client on back with legs flexed 90 degrees at hips and knees Feet up in stirrups
Dorsal recumbent	Places client in position for vaginal exams and insertion of catheters	Client on back with legs flexed at hips and knees Feet flat on mattress
Modified Trendelenburg's	Places client in "shock" position to increase blood flow to heart and cerebral tissue	Client flat on back with legs straight and elevated at hips Head and shoulders slightly raised

Pillows and other support equipment are placed to support alignment and normal flexion points, and to prevent pressure on any body area.

Action	Rationale
- Be certain that client's face is not pressed into bed or pillows while turning and that body position does not prevent full expansion of diaphragm.	*Maintains adequate respirations*
- Use appropriate body mechanics (see Nursing Procedure 7.1).	*Prevents injury*
7. Assess status of client's comfort and character of respirations; recheck client periodically.	*Determines if position adjustment is needed.*
8. Lift side rails and place bed in low position. If traction apparatus is being used, be certain that weights are not dragging on floor or touching bed.	*Prevents falls*
9. Place call light within reach.	*Facilitates communication*
10. Move overbed table close to bed and place items of frequent use on table.	*Places items used frequently within easy reach*
11. Wash hands.	*Decreases microorganism transfer*

Evaluation

Were desired outcomes achieved?

Documentation

The following should be noted on the client's chart:
- Client's position
- Client reports of pain, dyspnea, discomfort
- Exertion or dyspnea observed during repositioning
- Abnormal findings on integumentary assessment
- Status of equipment needed for stabilization of body parts (eg, traction, casts)
- Teaching regarding importance of maintaining position

SAMPLE DOCUMENTATION

DATE	TIME	
10/5/02	1430	Client repositioned into right side-lying position. Slight shortness of breath reported during repositioning. Given a brief rest period and no further shortness of breath reported. No redness, breaks, or discoloration noted over bony prominences

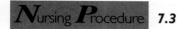

Hoyer Lift Usage

EQUIPMENT

- Hoyer lift (should include base, canvas mat, and two pairs of canvas straps)
- Large chair with arm support for client to sit in

Purpose

Helps move and transfer heavy clients who are unable to assist mover

Prevents undue strain on mover's body

Assessment

Assessment should focus on the following:

Medical diagnosis

Doctor's activity orders (positions contraindicated and number and amount of time client may be up)

Client's ability to keep head erect

Chart to determine client's previous tolerance of sitting position (eg, orthostatic hypotension, amount of time client tolerated sitting up)

Client's need for restraints while sitting up

Room environment (eg, adequate lighting, presence of clutter and furniture in pathway between chair and bed)

Condition of Hoyer device, hooks, and canvas mats

Nursing Diagnoses

The nursing diagnoses may include the following:

Impaired physical mobility related to activity intolerance and decreased coordination.

Outcome Identification and Planning

Desired Outcome (sample)

Client is moved from and returned to bed by Hoyer lift without injury.

375

Special Considerations

It is important for the nurse to be familiar with the Hoyer lift in order to operate it correctly (parts of the lift are labeled in Fig. 7.5). Practice using the lift without a client on the mat if you are unfamiliar with this device.

Organization is crucial when performing numerous moving procedures on heavy clients to avoid client exertion and physical injury to the movers. Plan activities such as changing bed linens while client is out of bed; encourage client to use bedside toilet once out of bed.

Geriatric

Chronic conditions in elderly clients require extra caution when moving them using the Hoyer lift. Clients with chronic cardiopulmonary conditions should be observed closely while sitting up and during transfer for exertion, respiratory difficulty, chest pain, and general discomfort.

Pediatric

Using the Hoyer lift can be frightening to a child. Demonstrate the procedure, using a puppet or game, and allow the child to participate in some way.

Home Health

Help family obtain the equipment, if needed. Educate the family on the use of the equipment and on proper body mechanics.

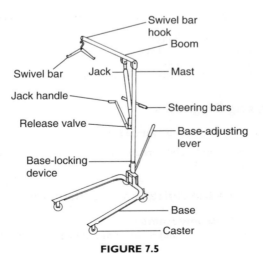

FIGURE 7.5

Delegation

Ascertain that assistive personnel have been trained in use of the Hoyer lift before use with clients. Reinforce the importance of monitoring cardiopulmonary status of clients vulnerable to experiencing breathing difficulty, chest pain, or general discomfort.

IMPLEMENTATION

Action	Rationale
1. Wash hands.	*Reduces microorganism transfer*
2. Explain procedure and assure client that precaution will be taken to prevent falls.	*Decreases anxiety*
3. Provide for and maintain privacy throughout procedure.	*Decreases embarrassment*
4. Place chair on side of bed client will be sitting on (lock wheels, if wheelchair).	*Places chair at close distance*
5. Adjust bed to comfortable working height.	*Prevents back and muscle strain in nurse*
6. Lock bed.	*Prevents bed movement*
7. Place client on mat as follows:	*Centers heaviest parts of body on mat*
- Roll client to one side and place half of mat under client from shoulders to midthigh.	*Positions client on mat with minimal movement*
- Roll client to other side and finish pulling mat under client.	
- Be sure one or both side rails are up as you move from one side of bed to the other.	*Prevents accidental falls*
8. Roll base of Hoyer lift under side of bed nearest to chair with boom in center of client's trunk; lock wheels of lift.	*Moves mechanical part of lift to bedside* *Prevents lift from rolling*
9. Using base-adjustment lever, widen stance of base.	*Provides greater stability to lift*
10. Raise and then push jack handle in toward mast, lowering boom (this is	*Lowers booms close enough to attach hooks*

Action	Rationale
accomplished with appropriate button or control device in the electric Hoyer).	
11. Place the strap or chain hooks through the holes of the mat (hooks of short straps go into holes behind back and hooks of long straps into holes at other end), making certain that hooks are not indenting client's skin.	*Secures hook placement into mat holes* *Attaches rest of device to mat*
12. Place all equipment, lines, and drains attached to client so dislodgment will not occur and close off drains, if necessary (remember to reopen them after moving client).	*Prevents accidental dislodgment and client injury* *Prevents reflux of drainage*
13. Instruct client to fold arms across chest.	*Prevents accidental injury*
14. Using jack handle, pump jack enough for mat to clear bed about 6 inches and tighten release valve.	*Safely assesses client stability and centering on mat*
15. Determine if client is fully supported and can maintain head support. Provide head support as needed throughout the procedure.	*Assesses stability in relation to weight and placement*
16. Unlock wheels and pull Hoyer lift straight back and away from bed; instruct assistant to provide support for equipment and client's legs throughout procedure.	*Promotes stability*
17. Move toward chair, with open end of lift's base straddling chair; continue until client's back is almost flush with back of chair.	*Moves and guides client into chair*
18. Lock wheels of lift.	*Provides Hoyer stability*

Action	Rationale
19. Slowly lift up jack handle and lower client into chair until hooks are slightly loosened from mat; guide client into chair with your hands as mat lowers. Avoid lowering client onto chair handles.	*Lowers client fully into chair*
20. Remove mat (unless difficult to replace or client's first time out of bed).	*Facilitates comfort*
21. Place tubes, drains, and support equipment for proper functioning, comfort, and safety:	*Prevents accidental dislodgment of tubes and drains and maintains necessary functions*
- Pillow behind head	*Ensures client's stability in chair*
- Sheet over knees and thighs	
- Restraints, if needed (eg, Posey vest, sheet, arm restraints)	*Facilitates adequate support of other body parts*
- Phone and items of frequent use within close range	*Places items desired or needed by client within reach*
- Catheter hooked to lower portion of chair	
- IV pole close enough to avoid pulling	
- Call light	*Facilitates communication*
22. Assess client tolerance to sitting up.	*Reduces risk of falling*
23. Leave door to client's room open when leaving room unless someone else will be with client.	*Allows visual observation of unattended client*
24. Monitor client at 15- to 60-min intervals.	*Reduces risk of falling*
25. Return client to bed using above steps.	*Prevents injury and discomfort during transfer*
26. Wash hands and restore equipment.	*Reduces microorganism transfer* *Promotes clean environment*

Evaluation

Were desired outcomes achieved?

Documentation

The following should be noted on the client's chart:

- Status update with indication for continued use of mobility-assist device
- Time of client transfer and type of lift used
- Client tolerance of procedure
- Duration of time in chair

SAMPLE DOCUMENTATION

DATE	TIME	
7/15/02	1400	Client lifted out of bed using Hoyer lift. Placed in bedside chair. Tolerated procedure well, with respirations regular and nonlabored. Call light within reach. Door left partially open.

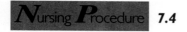

Range-of-Motion Exercises

EQUIPMENT

No equipment needed except gloves if contact with body fluids is likely

Purpose

Maintains present level of functioning and mobility of extremity involved
Prevents contractures and shortening of musculoskeletal structures
Prevents vascular complications of immobility
Facilitates comfort

Assessment

Assessment should focus on the following:

Medical diagnosis
Doctor's orders for indications of specific restrictions
Present range of motion of each extremity
Physical and mental ability of client to perform the activity, including normal age-related changes
History of factors that contraindicate or limit the type or amount of exercise

Nursing Diagnoses

The nursing diagnoses may include the following:

Impaired physical mobility related to unhealed fracture and decreased range of motion
Risk of impaired skin integrity related to prolonged bed rest
Risk of disuse syndrome related to neuromuscular dysfunction

Outcome Identification and Planning

Desired Outcomes (sample)

Client's present range of motion is maintained.
Range of motion of left elbow increased from 30- to 40-degree flexion.

No signs or symptoms of complications of immobility are present (such as pressure ulcers or pressure areas, contractures, decreased peristalsis, constipation and fecal impaction, orthostatic hypotension, pulmonary embolism, thrombophlebitis).

Special Considerations

A client able to perform all or part of a range-of-motion exercise program should be allowed to do so and should be properly instructed. Observe the client performing activities of daily living to determine the limitations of movement and the need, if any, for passive range-of-motion exercise to various joints.

When performing a range-of-motion exercise, a joint should be moved only to the point of resistance, pain, or spasm, whichever comes first.

Consult doctor's orders before performing a range-of-motion exercise on a client with acute cardiac, vascular, or pulmonary problems or a client with musculoskeletal trauma and acute flare-ups of arthritis.

Geriatric

The presence of various chronic conditions in elderly clients requires the use of extra caution when performing range-of-motion exercises. Clients with chronic cardiopulmonary conditions should be observed closely during range-of-motion activity for respiratory difficulty, chest pain, and general discomfort.

Decreased muscle mass, degenerative changes of joints, and degenerative connective tissue changes result in limited range of motion.

Pediatric

Demonstrate the procedure using a doll; instruct the child to perform simple techniques on the doll.

Home Health

Instruct family members in performance of range-of-motion techniques to be used during periods between nurse visits.

Delegation

Ascertain that assistive personnel have been trained in performance of range-of-motion exercises. Reinforce the importance of monitoring cardiopulmonary status of clients vulnerable to experiencing breathing difficulty, chest pain, or general discomfort.

IMPLEMENTATION

Action	Rationale
1. Wash hands.	*Reduces microorganism transfer*
2. Explain procedure to client.	*Decreases anxiety*
3. Provide for privacy.	*Decreases embarrassment*
4. Adjust bed to comfortable working height.	*Prevents back and muscle strain in nurse*
5. Move client to side of bed closest to you.	*Facilitates use of proper body mechanics*
6. Beginning at top and moving downward on one side of body at a time, perform passive (or instruct client through active) range-of-motion exercises of joints in each of the following areas, as applicable for client (Fig. 7.6): - Head and neck (Fig 7.6 *A, B*) - Spine (Fig. 7.6*C*) - Shoulder (Fig. 7.6*D–F*)	*Exercises all joint areas*

HEAD-NECK

A   Flexion   Extension

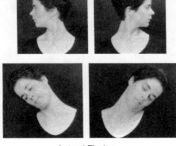

B   Lateral Flexion

FIGURE 7.6

Action	Rationale

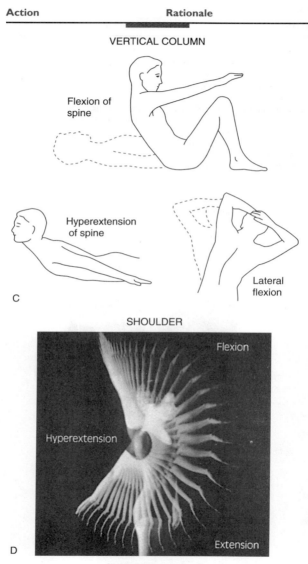

VERTICAL COLUMN

Flexion of spine

Hyperextension of spine

Lateral flexion

C

SHOULDER

Flexion

Hyperextension

Extension

D

FIGURE 7.6 (cont.)

Action	Rationale

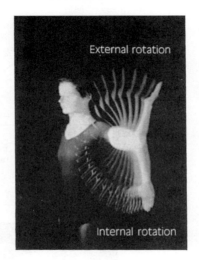

E

SHOULDER *(continued)*

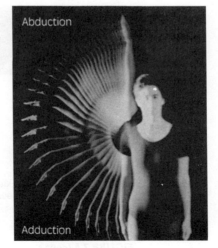

F

FIGURE 7.6 (cont.)

Action	Rationale

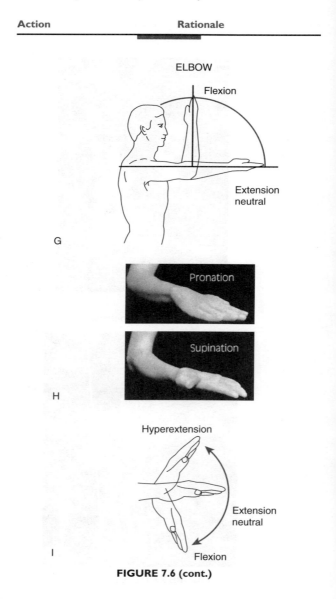

ELBOW

Flexion

Extension neutral

G

Pronation

Supination

H

Hyperextension

Extension neutral

Flexion

I

FIGURE 7.6 (cont.)

Action	Rationale

FINGERS

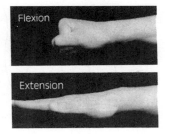

J

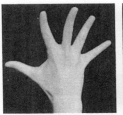 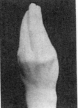

K

Abduction   Adduction

HIPS

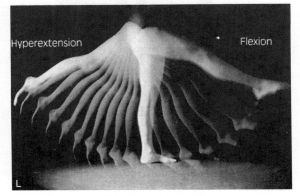

FIGURE 7.6 (cont.)

Action	Rationale

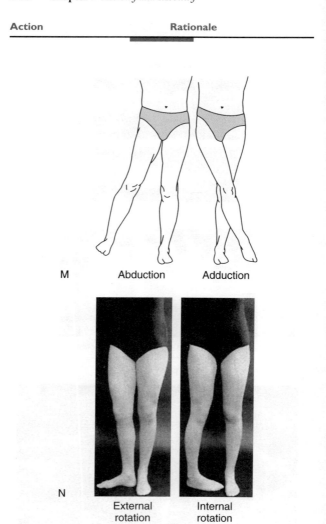

M   Abduction   Adduction

N   External rotation   Internal rotation

FIGURE 7.6 (cont.)

Action	Rationale

KNEE

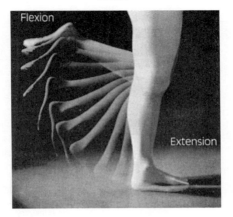

O

KNEE *(continued)*

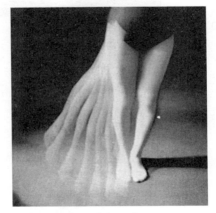

P

FIGURE 7.6 (cont.)

Action	Rationale

TOES

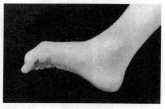

Flexion

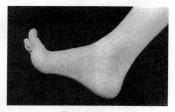

Q

Extension

FIGURE 7.6 (cont.)

Action	Rationale

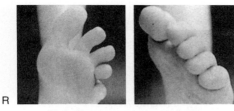

Abduction   Adduction

ANKLES

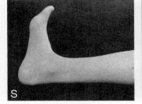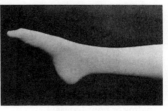

Dorsiflexion   Plantar flexion

FIGURE 7.6 (cont.)

Action	Rationale

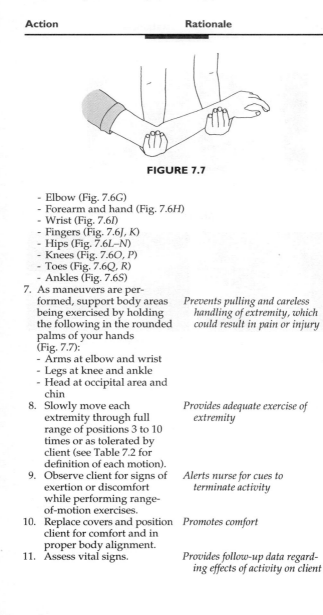

FIGURE 7.7

- Elbow (Fig. 7.6*G*)
- Forearm and hand (Fig. 7.6*H*)
- Wrist (Fig. 7.6*I*)
- Fingers (Fig. 7.6*J, K*)
- Hips (Fig. 7.6*L–N*)
- Knees (Fig. 7.6*O, P*)
- Toes (Fig. 7.6*Q, R*)
- Ankles (Fig. 7.6*S*)

7. As maneuvers are performed, support body areas being exercised by holding the following in the rounded palms of your hands (Fig. 7.7):
   - Arms at elbow and wrist
   - Legs at knee and ankle
   - Head at occipital area and chin

   Prevents pulling and careless handling of extremity, which could result in pain or injury

8. Slowly move each extremity through full range of positions 3 to 10 times or as tolerated by client (see Table 7.2 for definition of each motion).

   Provides adequate exercise of extremity

9. Observe client for signs of exertion or discomfort while performing range-of-motion exercises.

   Alerts nurse for cues to terminate activity

10. Replace covers and position client for comfort and in proper body alignment.

    Promotes comfort

11. Assess vital signs.

    Provides follow-up data regarding effects of activity on client

TABLE 7.2	Descriptions of Range-of-Motion Maneuvers	
Maneuver	Description	Applicable Areas
Flexion	Bending joint at point of normal anatomical fold	All areas
Extension	Straightening joint into as straight a line as possible	All areas
Hyperextension	Straightening joint into extension, then moving past that point	Neck, fingers, wrists, toes, spine
Abduction	Moving extremity away from midline of body	Arms, legs, fingers, toes
Adduction	Moving extremity toward midline of body	Arms, legs, fingers, toes
Internal rotation	Rotating extremity toward midline of body	Hips, ankles, shoulders
External rotation	Rotating extremity away from midline	Hips, ankles, shoulders
Supination	Turning palm upward	Hands
Pronation	Turning palm downward	Hands
Circumduction	Rotating extremity in a complete circle	Shoulders, hips

Action	Rationale
12. Lift side rails, and place bed in position.	*Prevents falls*
13. Place call light within reach.	*Facilitates communication*
14. Wash hands.	*Reduces microorganism transfer*

Evaluation

Were desired outcomes achieved?

Documentation

The following should be noted on the client's chart:

- Areas on which range-of-motion exercises are performed
- Areas of limited range of motion and the degree of limitation
- Areas of passive versus active range of motion
- Reports of pain or discomfort
- Observations of physiologic intolerance to activity

SAMPLE DOCUMENTATION

DATE	TIME	
11/12/02	1400	Passive range-of-motion exercises performed on all extremities. Client has full range of motion of all joints and reports no pain or discomfort during exercises. No signs of activity intolerance.

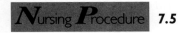
Crutch Walking

EQUIPMENT

- Appropriate-size crutches
- Safety belt (gait belt)
- Shoes
- Housecoat
- Eyeglasses or contacts, if worn

Purpose

Facilitates mobility and activity for client

Increases self-esteem by decreasing dependence

Decreases physical stress on weight-bearing joints and unhealed skeletal injuries

Assessment

Assessment should focus on the following:

Medical diagnosis

Doctor's orders for activity restrictions

Type of crutch–gait movement indicated

Neuromuscular status (muscle tone, strength, and range of motion of arms, legs, and trunk; gait pattern; body alignment when walking; ability to maintain balance)

Focal point of injury and reason for crutches

Measurement parameters of crutches

Ability of client to comprehend instructions regarding use of crutches

Additional learning needs of client

Nature of walking area (ie, presence of clutter, scatter rugs, adequacy of floor for good traction, proximity of adequate rest area)

General environment for safety hazards that could cause falls

Nursing Diagnoses

The nursing diagnoses may include the following:

Risk of physical injury related to unsteady gait pattern

Knowledge deficit related to lack of instruction regarding crutch-walking principles and techniques

Outcome Identification and Planning

Desired Outcomes (sample)

Client does not fall while on crutches.
Client demonstrates correct techniques for crutch-walking maneuvers.

Special Considerations

Crutch walking on slippery, cluttered surfaces and on stairs can be hazardous. Clients should use railing of staircase (or walk close to walls) during crutch walking.
Clients with visual deficits should wear visual aids when crutch walking.

Pediatric and Geriatric

Pediatric and geriatric clients are especially prone to injuries from falls because of brittle or underdeveloped bones. Safety belts should always be used when assisting these clients with crutch walking.
In elderly clients, extra time should be allotted because of decreased muscle strength, decreased coordination, and functional changes in vision.

Home Health

The client's home environment should be assessed carefully for hazards and adequate space. Assist client with arrangement of furniture and decorative items to eliminate hazards in the home while client is on crutches.

Delegation

Crutch walking should only be delegated to assistive personnel trained in physical rehabilitation assistive techniques. Instruct on monitoring for undue fatigue and discomfort.

IMPLEMENTATION

Action	Rationale
1. Wash hands.	*Reduces microorganism transfer*
2. Explain procedure to client, emphasizing that it will take time to learn techniques; stress safety and the importance of moving slowly initially; when providing explanations, include demonstrations.	*Decreases anxiety and frustration* *Increases compliance* *Prevents injury*

Action	Rationale
3. Assist client into shoes that are comfortable, non-skid, hard soled, and low heeled.	*Prevents falls*
4. Assist client into housecoat or loose, comfortable clothes.	*Facilitates comfort*
5. Measure client for correct crutch fit:	*Prevents damage to brachial and radial nerves*
- Have client lie flat in bed with proper shoes on.	*Prevents fall by measuring crutch height using shoes person usually wears*
- Measure from axillary pit outward 6 to 8 inches and from axillary pit to side of heel (Fig. 7.8).	*Promotes correct body alignment*
- Have client stand with elbows slightly flexed; measure distance between axillary pit and top of crutch to be sure that a space at least the width of two or three fingers exists.	*Avoids damage to brachial plexus, which can result in paralysis of extremity*
6. Lower height of bed; then lock wheels.	*Prevents falls*
7. Slowly help client into sitting position; assess for dizziness, faintness, or decrease in orientation.	*Prevents injury from sudden change in blood pressure when sitting up*
8. Apply safety belt.	*Prevents client injury*
9. Assist client with maneuvers appropriate	*Provides assistance and ensures client safety*

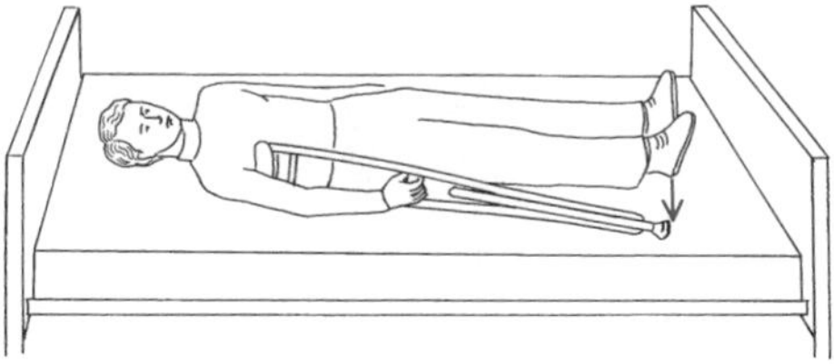

FIGURE 7.8

Action	Rationale
for type of gait and with other general crutch-walking techniques (steps 10 and 11). Initially, always have someone with client but allow greater independence as techniques are performed more proficiently and client demonstrates ability to crutch walk in all areas safely (encourage client to use rails and walk close to walls when climbing stairs).	
10. In general, demonstrate correct technique for type of gait to be used before client gets out of bed; have client demonstrate these techniques to you; reinforce instructions and make corrections as client performs crutch walking.	*Permits concentration on maneuvers before client attempts them.*
11. Begin demonstrating gait technique from tripod position with crutches 6 inches to side and 6 inches to front (Fig. 7.9).	*Promotes stability and balance*

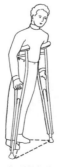

FIGURE 7.9

Action	Rationale
a. *Four-point gait:* Advance right crutch, then left foot, then left crutch, then right foot (Fig. 7.10).	*Places weight on legs while crutches provide stability*
b. *Three-point gait:* Advance both crutches and affected extremity at same time; advance unaffected extremity (Fig. 7.11).	*Places weight on unaffected leg and crutches, with light weight on affected leg*
c. *Two-point gait:* Advance right crutch and left foot together, then left crutch and right foot together (Fig. 7.12).	*Places partial weight on both legs*
d. Swing-to or swing-through gait: Advance both crutches at same time and swing body forward to crutches or past them (Fig. 7.13).	*Provides additional stability for clients with bilateral leg disability*

12. Demonstrate correct techniques for sitting, standing, and stair

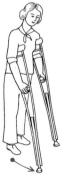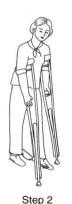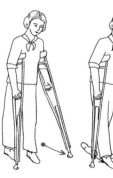

Step 1   Step 2   Step 3   Step 4

FIGURE 7.10

Action	Rationale

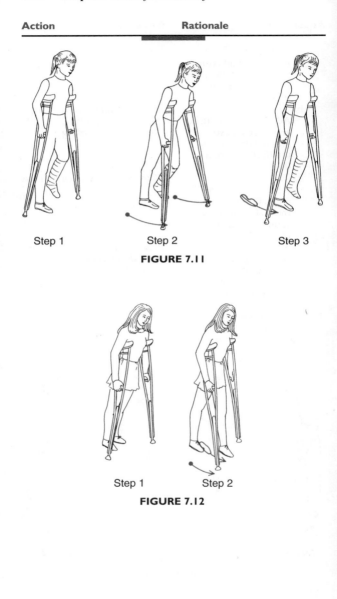

Step 1   Step 2   Step 3

FIGURE 7.11

Step 1   Step 2

FIGURE 7.12

Action	Rationale

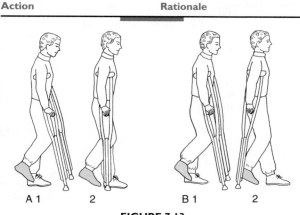

FIGURE 7.13

walking with crutches
(Display 7.1).
Figures 7.14 and 7.15
illustrate stair walking
with crutches.

13. Observe return
demonstrations and help
client practice until
proficiency in crutch
walking is attained
(provide intermittent
praise and encourage-
ment); encourage rest
between activity periods,
assisting client, as needed,
to a comfortable position.

Ensures procedure has been learned

Provides avenue for feedback

14. Wash hands and properly
store equipment.

Reduces microorganism transfer
Maintains order

Evaluation

Were desired outcomes achieved?

DISPLAY 7.1	Techniques for General Crutch-Walking Maneuvers

Moving From Sitting to Standing	**Moving From Standing to Sitting**
- Place both crutches in hand on affected side (holding crutches together and even). - Push down on stable support base (locked bed, arm, or seat of chair) with free hand, put weight on stronger leg, and lift body. - Stand with a straight back, bearing weight on stronger leg and crutches. - Place both crutches on same level as feet. - Advance unaffected leg to next step while bearing down on crutch handles. - Pull affected leg and crutches up to step while bearing weight on stronger leg.	- Inch back until backs of lower legs touch bed or center of chair. - Hold crutches together in hand on unaffected side. - Begin easing down onto chair or bed with back straight, using crutches and stronger leg as support. - When close enough, gently hold on to arm of chair and complete the move.

Walking Up Stairs (see Fig. 7.14)	**Walking Down Stairs (see Fig. 7.15)**
- Place both crutches on same level as feet. - Advance unaffected leg to next step while bearing down on crutch handles. - Pull affected leg and crutches up to step while bearing weight on stronger leg.	- Place both crutches on same level as feet. - Shift weight to stronger leg. - Lower affected leg and crutches to next step while bearing down on crutch handles. - Advance unaffected leg last.

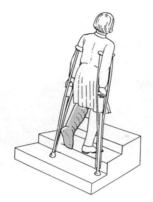

FIGURE 7.14

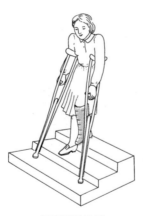

FIGURE 7.15

Documentation

The following should be noted on the client's chart:
- Gait pattern used
- Crutch height
- Steadiness of gait and amount of assistance needed
- Distance walked by client

- Client tolerance of procedure
- Teaching done and additional learning needs of client

SAMPLE DOCUMENTATION

DATE	TIME	
4/28/02	1200	Client completed first week of crutch walking. Efficient with use of four-point gait pattern. Steady with good body alignment while on crutches. Walking entire hall length three times per day without fatigue or reports of discomfort. Has not begun stair walking.

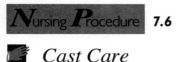

*N*ursing *P*rocedure 7.6

Cast Care

EQUIPMENT

- Washcloth
- Towel
- Soap
- Basin of warm water
- Linen savers for bed
- Pen
- Roll of 1- or 2-inch tape
- Pillows wrapped in linen saver or plastic bag
- Bed linens with pull/turn sheet
- Sterile gloves

Purpose

Prevents neurovascular impairment of areas encircled by cast
Maintains cast for immobilization of treatment area
Prevents infection

Assessment

Assessment should focus on the following:

Medical diagnosis
Doctor's orders for special care of treatment area
Client's report of pain or discomfort
Integumentary status
Neurovascular indicators of health of extremities, particularly of
  areas distal to cast: color, temperature, capillary refill, sensation,
  pulse quality, ability to move toes or fingers
Indicators of infection (foul odor from cast, pain, fever, edema,
  extreme warmth over a particular area of cast)
Indicators of complications of immobility: pressure ulcers or
  pressure areas; reduced joint movement; decreased peristalsis,
  constipation, and fecal impaction; signs of pulmonary embolism (chest pain, dyspnea, wheezing, increased heart rate);
  signs of thrombophlebitis (redness, heat, swelling, or pain in local area)

Nursing Diagnoses

The nursing diagnoses may include the following:

Risk of peripheral neurovascular dysfunction related to edema, bleeding, nerve compression, or vascular compression

Knowledge deficit related to lack of information regarding general cast care

Outcome Identification and Planning

Desired Outcomes (sample)

Signs of neurovascular deficits are detected early.

Client verbalizes actions necessary for cast maintenance by discharge.

Special Consideration

If client experienced traumatic injury to the extremity in the cast, watch for a sudden decrease in capillary refill and loss of pulse during first 24 to 48 hr due to development of compartment syndrome.

Geriatric

Watch client closely during initial gait retraining; additional weight of cast could cause lack of balance and result in stress and fracture of fragile bones.

Home Health

Inform the homebound client that a wet cast may be dried with a hair dryer on the LOW setting.

Delegation

Instruct assistive personnel on transfer or moving of clients with casts. ROUTINE MONITORING OF NEUROVASCULAR STATUS REMAINS THE RESPONSIBILITY OF LICENSED PERSONNEL.

IMPLEMENTATION

Action	Rationale
1. Wash hands.	*Reduces microorganism transfer*
2. Place pull/turn sheet and linen savers on bed before client returns from casting area (place these items on bed with each linen change).	*Promotes ease of positioning client* *Prevents unnecessary pain when moving client*

Action	Rationale
3. Explain procedure to client, emphasizing importance of maintaining elevation of extremity, of not handling wet cast, and of frequent assessment; instruct client not to insert anything between cast and extremity.	*Decreases anxiety* *Increases compliance* *Prevents injury and infection*
4. Don gloves.	*Avoids contact with body fluids*
5. Provide for privacy.	*Decreases embarrassment*
6. Handle casted extremity or body area with palms of hands for first 24 to 36 hr until cast is fully dry.	*Avoids dents that could ultimately result in edema and pressure areas*
7. If cast is slow to dry, place small fan directly facing cast (about 24 inches away). DO NOT PLACE LINEN OVER CAST UNTIL CAST IS DRY.	*Enhances speed of drying* *Allows air to circulate and assist in drying cast*
8. If cast is on extremity, elevate on pillows (cover pillow with linen savers or plastic bags) so normal curvatures created with casting are maintained.	*Prevents edema* *Enhances venous return* *Prevents soiling of pillows* *Prevents flattened areas on cast as it dries and prevents pressure areas*
9. Wash excess antimicrobial agents (such as povidone) from skin. Rinse and pat dry.	*Allows for clear skin and vascular assessment*
10. Perform skin and neurovascular assessment (every ½ to 1 hr for first 24 hr, every 2 hr for next 24 hr, then every 4 hr thereafter); if cast is on extremity, compare to opposite extremity.	*Detects signs of abnormal neurovascular function, such as vascular or nerve compression* *Suggests possible nature of neurovascular deficit*
11. If breakthrough bleeding is noted on cast, circle area, then write date and time on cast; if moderate to	*Provides baseline data for amount of bleeding* *Facilitates early intervention and prevention of complications*

Action	Rationale
large amount of bleeding, notify doctor (otherwise, follow orders as written for bleeding).	
12. Assess for signs of infection under cast; obtain temperature.	*Detects infectious process at early stage*
13. Reposition client every 2 hr; if client has body or spica cast, secure three assistants to help turn client.	*Prevents client discomfort* *Makes turning quick, efficient, and safe*
14. Provide back and skin care frequently.	*Prevents skin breakdown*
15. If flaking of cast around edges is noted, remove flakes, pull stockinette over cast edges, and tape down.	*Prevents accumulation of particles inside cast, which cause infection*
16. Place client with leg or body cast on fracture pan for elimination: for clients with good bowel and bladder control, temporarily line edge of cast close to perineal area with plastic; if client has little or no elimination control (eg, some pediatric and elderly clients), maintain plastic lining on cast edges and change once a shift.	*Provides for elimination needs* *Prevents soiling of cast*
17. Perform range-of-motion exercises on all joint areas every 4 hr (except where contraindicated).	
18. Instruct client to cough and deep breathe and reposition client (within guidelines for orders) every 2 hr.	*Prevents pneumonia, decubitus ulcers, and other complications of immobility*
19. Lift side rails and lower height of bed.	*Prevents falls*
20. Place call light within reach.	*Facilitates communication*

Action	Rationale
21. Restore or discard equipment properly.	*Removes waste and clutter*
22. Wash hands.	*Removes microorganisms*

Evaluation

Were desired outcomes achieved?

Documentation

The following should be noted on the client's chart:

- Data from neurovascular assessment
- Abnormal data indicating inflammation or infection
- Indicators of complications of immobility
- Frequency of body alignment and repositioning and positions into which client is placed
- Frequency and nature of skin care given
- Frequency of coughing and deep breathing exercises performed
- Frequency and nature of range-of-motion exercises performed
- Teaching completed and additional teaching needs of client

SAMPLE DOCUMENTATION

DATE	TIME	
12/19/02	1030	Fourth hour since return of client from casting room. Left leg full-length cast remains cold and wet. Toes of both left and right feet are pink, warm, and dry. Able to wiggle toes and identify which toe is being touched. Cough and deep breathing done. Repositioned every 2 hours. Active range-of-motion exercise performed to all extremities except left leg.

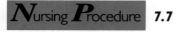

 Traction Maintenance

EQUIPMENT

- Alcohol wipes
- Antimicrobial agent for cleaning pins (skeletal tractions)
- One sterile gauze pad (2 × 2 or 4 × 3) for each traction pin
- Sterile gloves
- Sterile dressings, if needed
- Equipment for supporting body positioning (eg, trochanter roll, pillows, sandbag, footboard)
- Traction setup

Purpose

Maintains traction apparatus with appropriate counterbalance
Prevents infection at site of insertion of traction pins

Assessment

Assessment should focus on the following:

Medical diagnosis
Doctor's orders for traction weight, line of pull maintained, and pin care
Type of skin traction or skeletal traction
Status of weights, ropes, and pulleys
Reports of pain or discomfort
Integumentary status
Neurovascular indicators distal to pin sites (skin color and temperature, capillary refill, sensation, presence of pulse, ability to move toes or fingers)
Indicators of complications of immobility: pressure ulcers or pressure areas; contractures; decreased peristalsis, constipation, and fecal impaction; signs of pulmonary embolism (chest pain, dyspnea, wheezing, increased heart rate); signs of thrombophlebitis (redness, heat, swelling, or pain in local area)

Nursing Diagnoses

The nursing diagnoses may include the following:

Risk of infection related to disrupted skin integrity at insertion site of metal pin of skeletal traction

Risk of physical injury related to immobility from bed rest associated with spinal fracture

Outcome Identification and Planning

Desired Outcomes (sample)
No redness, swelling, pain, discharge, or odor occurs at pin site. There is no evidence of complications of immobility.

Special Considerations
If weights do not swing freely, traction can be counterproductive. Assess status of weights every 1 to 2 hr and after moving client.

Geriatric
Elderly clients are particularly prone to the development of broken skin integrity when they are bedridden and not repositioned frequently; this tendency is due to a decreased amount of subcutaneous fat and to skin that is less elastic, thinner, drier, and more fragile than that of a younger person.

Pediatric
Arrange for quiet play activities, of appropriate developmental level, to occupy child during confinement. Include child in moving procedure (eg, by letting child count aloud to time movement).

Home Health
When the homebound client is mobile, with intermittent traction on an extremity, install traction setup over a door with a measured source of weight (eg, flour bag with sand, rocks, bricks).

Delegation
Instruct assistive personnnel on moving and assisting with bathing of clients with specific types of traction.
Routine monitoring of neurovascular and skin status remains the responsibility of licensed personnel.

IMPLEMENTATION

Action	Rationale
1. Wash hands.	*Reduces microorganism transfer*
2. Explain procedure to client, emphasizing importance of maintaining counterbalance and position.	*Decreases anxiety*

Action	Rationale
3. Provide for privacy.	*Decreases embarrassment*
4. Assess traction setup (Fig. 7.16):	*Ensures accurate counterbalance and function of traction*
- Weights hanging freely and not touching bed or floor	
- Ordered amount of weight applied	
- Ropes moving freely through pulleys	
- All knots tight in ropes and away from pulleys	
- Pulleys free of linens	
5. Check client's position (client's head should be near head of bed and properly aligned).	*Maintains proper counterbalance*
6. Assess skin for signs of pressure areas or friction under skin traction belts.	*Detects early signs of skin breakdown*
7. Assess neurovascular status of extremity distal to traction.	*Detects neurovascular complications*
8. Assess site at and around pin for redness, edema, discharge, or odor.	*Determines presence of infection*

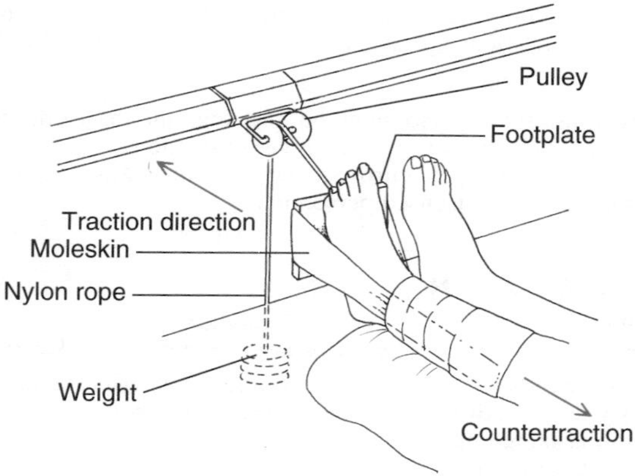

FIGURE 7.16

Action	Rationale
9. Wash hands.	*Reduces microorganism transfer*
10. Don gloves.	*Prevents exposure to body fluids*
11. Wash, rinse, and dry skin thoroughly; if permissible, remove skin traction periodically to wash under skin (check doctor's order and agency policy).	*Promotes circulation to skin*
12. Discard gloves, wash hands, and don sterile gloves.	*Prevents contamination*
13. Cleanse pin site and complete site care using sterile technique.	*Prevents infection*
14. Discard gloves and wash hands.	*Removes microorganisms*
15. Perform range-of-motion exercises on all joint areas, except those contra-indicated, every 4 hr.	*Prevents pneumonia, decubitus ulcers, and complications of immobility*
16. Instruct client to cough and deep breathe, and reposition client (within guidelines for orders) every 2 hr; use trochanter rolls and foot-board to prevent internal and external hip rotation and footdrop.	*Prevents complications related to improper positioning*
17. Lift side rails.	*Prevents falls*
18. Place call light within reach.	*Facilitates communication*
19. Wash hands.	*Reduces microorganism transfer*

Evaluation

Were desired outcomes achieved?

Documentation

The following should be noted on the client's chart:

• Type of traction and amount of weight used

- Status of ropes, pulleys, and weights
- Body alignment of client
- Repositioning (frequency and last position)
- Pin care given
- Skin care given
- Coughing and deep breathing exercises performed
- Range-of-motion exercises performed
- Client teaching completed and additional teaching needs of client

SAMPLE DOCUMENTATION

DATE	TIME	
10/19/02	1030	Maintains intermittent pelvic traction with 20 lb of weight. Traction removed twice this shift for client to go to restroom. Skin in pelvic area clean, warm, pink, and dry. Range-of-motion exercises of upper and lower extremities performed by client every 4 hr. Doing own coughing and deep breathing every 2 hr; breath sounds clear bilaterally.

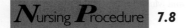

Nursing Procedure 7.8

Antiembolism Hose/Pneumatic Compression Device Application

EQUIPMENT

- Pneumatic compression equipment with comfort stockings or hose

or

- Antiembolic hose
- Washcloth
- Towel
- Soap
- Basin of warm water
- Tape measure (if not included in package)

Purpose

Promotes venous blood return to heart by maintaining pressure on capillaries and veins

Prevents development of venous thrombosis secondary to stagnant circulation

Assessment

Assessment should focus on the following:

Medical diagnosis

Doctor's orders for hose length and frequency of application

Reports of pain or discomfort of lower extremities

Skin status of legs and feet

Neurovascular indicators of lower extremities (skin color and temperature, capillary refill, sensation, pulse presence and quality)

Indicators of venous disorders of lower extremities (redness, heat, swelling, or pain in local area)

Nursing Diagnoses

The nursing diagnoses may include the following:

Risk of peripheral neurovascular dysfunction related to prolonged immobility

415

Risk of peripheral neurovascular dysfunction related to lack of
knowledge regarding application of hose

Outcome Identification and Planning

Desired Outcomes (sample)

By end of day
Client states two ways to reduce risk of developing venous
thrombosis.
Client remains free of signs of venous thrombosis throughout
confinement.

Special Considerations

Clients with known or suspected peripheral vascular disorders
should not wear hose because thrombus dislodgment may occur.
Poor maintenance of hose could result in circulatory restriction;
hose must remain free of wrinkles, rolls, or kinks.

Geriatric

Elderly clients are particularly prone to development of venous
disorders of lower extremities because of age-related physiologic changes that occur in the tissue of veins. In addition,
chronic cardiac and peripheral vascular dysfunctions reduce
venous return.

Delegation

Assistive personnel may apply these devices, after proper training, and should be instructed to report pain, skin abnormalities,
or discoloration of extremities.

IMPLEMENTATION

Action	Rationale
1. Wash hands.	*Reduces microorganism transfer*
2. Explain procedure to client, emphasizing importance of maintaining hose on extremity for specified amount of time and of wearing hose properly.	*Decreases anxiety* *Increases compliance*
3. Provide for privacy.	*Decreases embarrassment*
4. Measure for appropriate-size hose according to package directions (large, medium, or small)	*Promotes proper functioning of hose* *Prevents reduced circulation to legs*

Action	Rationale

or
obtain vinyl sleeves and
comfort stockings/hose.

5. Wash, rinse, and dry legs;　　*Promotes comfort*
   apply light talcum　　　　　　*Promotes clean, dry skin*
   powder, if desired.

6. Turn hose (except foot　　　　*Promotes proper application of*
   portion) inside out.　　　　　　　*hose*

7. Place foot of hose over　　　　*Applies hose, making certain that*
   client's toes and foot.　　　　　*kinks and wrinkles are*
   Using both hands, slide　　　　*smoothed out*
   hose up leg until　　　　　　　*Prevents tourniquet effect*
   completely on (smooth
   and straighten hose as it
   is pulled up); do not turn
   top of hose down.

8. Apply second hose in same
   manner.

Pneumatic Compression Device

9. Slide vinyl surgical sleeve
   over each calf (Fig. 7.17)
   or　　　　　　　　　　　　　*Places source of intermittent*
   apply Velcro-secured　　　　*compression over the veins of*
   vinyl compression hose　　　*the extremities*
   by placing open hose
   under thigh and leg with
   knee-opening site under
   the popliteal area.

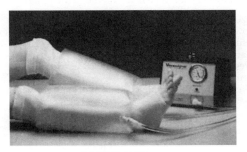

FIGURE 7.17

Action	Rationale
10. Establish the vinyl hose by overlapping the edges and securing the Velcro connectors.	*Establishes air pump source; prepares unit for function*
11. Turn the power on to the unit.	
12. Monitor several inflation/ deflation compression cycles.	*Permits early detection of excessive compression*
13. Replace covers.	*Provides privacy and warmth*
14. Observe extremities every 2 to 3 hr to assess circulation and hose placement.	*Prevents complications*
15. Remove hose twice a day for 20 min or per agency policy (ideally during morning and evening care).	*Allows for skin aeration and reassessment*
16. Wash hands and restore equipment.	*Reduces microorganism transfer Maintains organized environment*

Evaluation

Were desired outcomes achieved?

Documentation

The following should be noted on the client's chart:

- Size and length of hose applied
- Lower extremity skin color, temperature, sensation, capillary refill
- Status of pulses in lower extremities
- Presence of pain or discomfort in lower extremities
- Removal of hose twice daily
- Client teaching completed and additional teaching needs of client

SAMPLE DOCUMENTATION

DATE	TIME	
4/29/02	0830	Full-length embolic hose applied to lower legs—size, large/long. Skin of both lower extremities warm. No tears or abrasions noted. Toes pink, with 2-second capillary refill. Bilateral pedal pulses 2+. Client stated purpose of hose correctly and related care measures.

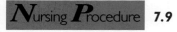

Continuous Passive Motion (CPM) Device

📠 EQUIPMENT

- CPM device
- Softgoods kit (single-patient use)
- Tape measure
- Goniometer

Purpose

Increases range of motion
Decreases effects of immobility
Stimulates healing of the articular cartilage
Reduces adhesions and swelling

Assessment

Assessment should focus on the following:

Doctor's orders for degrees of flexion and extension
Neurovascular status of extremity before start of CPM
Presence of pulses and capillary refill in affected extremity
Skin color and temperature, sensation, and movement of extremity
Reports of pain or discomfort

Nursing Diagnoses

The nursing diagnoses may include the following:

Impaired physical mobility related to surgical intervention
Risk of peripheral neurovascular dysfunction related to surgical
    intervention and immobility

Outcome Identification and Planning

Desired Outcomes (sample)
Client tolerates progressive increase in flexion and extension with
    CPM device.

Client demonstrates increasing mobility of affected extremity.

Special Considerations

Geriatric

Elderly clients are particularly prone to the development of broken skin when they are immobilized.

Pediatric

Explain the CPM device clearly, demonstrating with a doll or stuffed animal.

Arrange for quiet play activities that are developmentally appropriate.

Delegation

Instruct assistive personnel in techniques of moving clients with CPM machines in bed.

IMPLEMENTATION

Action	Rationale
1. Wash hands.	*Reduces microorganism transfer*
Organize equipment.	*Promotes efficiency*
Apply softgoods to CPM device (Fig. 7.18).	*Prevents friction to extremity during motion*
2. Check doctor's order for degrees of flexion and extension. Speed will be determined by patient comfort. Begin with a midpoint setting.	*May change on a daily or per-shift basis as the patient progresses*

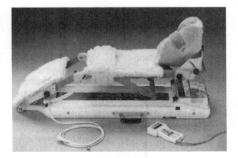

FIGURE 7.18

Action	Rationale
3. Explain procedure to client.	*Decreases anxiety and facilitates cooperation*
4. Using the tape measure, determine the distance between the gluteal crease and the popliteal space.	*Determines the distance to adjust the Thigh Length Adjustment knobs on the CPM device*
5. Measure the length of client's leg from the knee to ¼ inch beyond the bottom of the foot.	*Determines the distance to adjust the position of the footplate*
6. Position the client in the middle of the bed, with the extremity in a slightly abducted position.	*Promotes proper body alignment* *Prevents CPM device from exerting pressure on opposite extremity*
7. Elevate client's leg and place in padded CPM device (Fig. 7.19).	*Prepares client for therapy*
8. Note proper anatomical placement of device: Client's knee should be at the hinged joint of the machine.	*Improper positioning of the device may cause injury*
9. Adjust the footplate to maintain the client's foot in a neutral position. Make certain that the leg is neither internally nor externally rotated.	*Improper positioning of the device may cause injury*
10. Apply the soft restraining straps under CPM device and around extremity	*The soft restraints maintain the extremity in position.* *Allowing several fingers to fit*

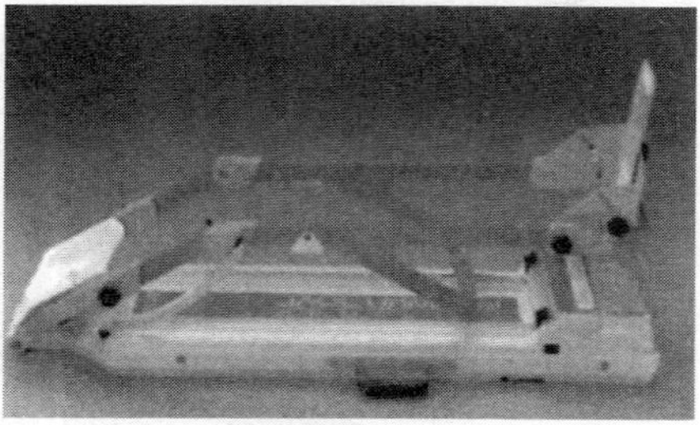

FIGURE 7.19

Action	**Rationale**
loosely enough to fit several fingers under it.	*under the restraint prevents pressure from restraint strap on affected extremity*
11. Turn unit on at mainpower switch. Set controls to levels prescribed by physician.	*Cannot adjust controls and setting unless power is on; prepares client for onset of therapeutic intervention*
12. Instruct the client in the use of the GO/STOP button.	*Client participates in care, thus decreasing anxiety*
13. Set CPM device in the ON stage and press GO button (Fig. 7.20).	*Initiates therapeutic intervention*
14. Determine angle of flexion when device has reached its greatest height using the goniometer. *Note:* If unit is not anatomical, there might be a slight difference between reading on the device and the actual angle of the patient's knee.	

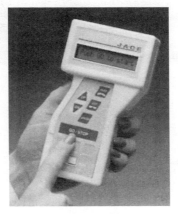

FIGURE 7.20

Evaluation

Were desired outcomes achieved?

Documentation

The following should be noted on the client's chart:

- Onset of therapy
- Tolerance of procedure
- Degree of extension and flexion and speed of machine
- Amount of time client used device
- Neurovascular status of extremity
- Successive therapeutic aids, immobilizer, etc.

SAMPLE DOCUMENTATION

DATE	TIME	
8/4/02	1100	CPM device applied to left leg at 0 degrees of extension and 35 degrees of flexion started at slow speed. Verified by goniometer. Client instructed in use of go/stop button. Denies need for pain medication at this time. Padding to all soft tissue near CPM device. Call bell within reach.
	1400	CPM device removed from left leg. Left lower extremity warm and dry to touch. Distal pulses are present; client denies numbness or tingling; no edema noted. Immobilizer applied.

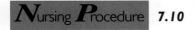

General Muscle-Strengthening Exercises (Home/Home Transition)

EQUIPMENT

- Unopened cans of food, of different sizes
- Well-fitted, rubber-soled shoes; socks

Purpose

Promotes general increase in strength and activity

Assessment

Assessment should focus on the following:

Determination of functional limitations
Medical conditions that contraindicate general strengthening
Degree of client debilitation

Outcome Identification and Planning

Desired Outcomes (sample)
The client will recover general strength and endurance within 6 months.

Special Considerations
Home Health

Many clients seen in their homes have recently been hospitalized or have experienced a decrease in activity, and have lost general strength and endurance. Although their diagnosis may not justify physical therapy, they can benefit from basic exercise.

Have clients who are being prepared for discharge from the acute or rehab setting practice with items of similar weight before discharge (or have family bring cans they plan to use from home for practice).

Cost-cutting Tip

For basic strengthening, purchased equipment is not necessary. Items found in the home may be used as weights. Such items include cans of soup or vegetables, or bags of flour or sugar.

IMPLEMENTATION

Action	Rationale
1. Evaluate client ambulation ability, upper extremity strength, ability to transfer from sitting to standing.	*Allows the nurse to determine client needs, ability to perform exercises*
2. Discuss benefits of increased upper extremity strength to assist in transfer.	*Indicates to client that exercise has benefits*
3. Discuss importance of ambulation in terms of increased strength, general well-being, increased independence.	*Generates interest on the part of the client in participating in an exercise program*
4. Instruct and demonstrate upper extremity strengthening using small unopened cans of food. Instruct to lift slowly to shoulder level, bending elbows. Have client demonstrate (Fig. 7.21).	*Allows nurse to see client ability and understanding*
5. If appropriate to client, have client lift cans over head to strengthen upper arms.	

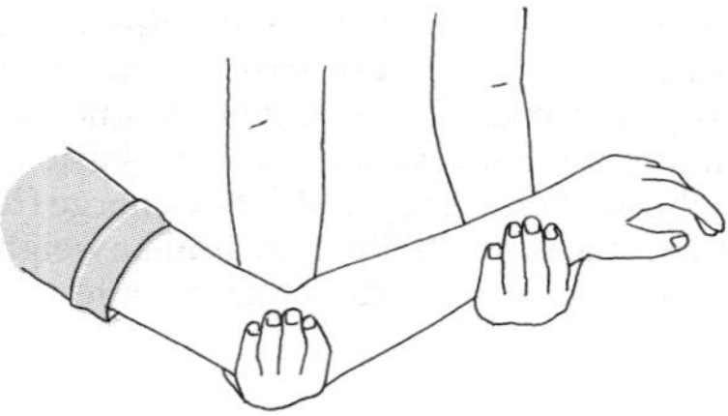

FIGURE 7.21

Action	Rationale
6. Specify number of repetitions and number of times per day to do exercises.	*Promotes client participation by establishing a definite schedule.*
7. Gradually increase size and and weight of cans, and number of repetitions. Note weight of can on label.	*Allows client to see progress*
8. For ambulation, determine client's usual habits (eg, does client spend a lot of time watching TV or reading?). Instruct client to ambulate a specified route (such as to the kitchen and back if at home) during each commercial or after each chapter.	*Connects exercise times with an already established habit and improves client compliance*
9. Gradually lengthen distance ambulated.	*Indicates progress to client*
10. Discuss available out-patient exercise programs, if applicable, after discharge from services, and benefits of regular exercise.	*Promotes ongoing health maintenance activities*

Evaluation

Were desired outcomes achieved?

DOCUMENTATION

The following should be noted on the client's chart or visit note:

- Client limitations
- Exercise program established
- Client progress

SAMPLE DOCUMENTATION

DATE	TIME	
9/6/02	1100	Difficulty rising to a standing position, ambulates only 4 feet. General debilitation noted due to previous hospital bed rest exceeding 3 days. Instructed in basic strengthening, use of soup cans for upper extremities 4 times/day, 5 reps each arm. Instructed to stand and ambulate around room at each TV commercial. Return demonstration of instructions by client. (Will evaluate next visit and increase weight, reps, and ambulation distance, if indicated—home health note addition).

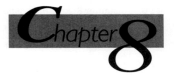

Rest and Comfort

OVERVIEW

► Each person's perception of pain is unique.

► Cultural background may have a great impact on a client's pain threshold and pain tolerance, as well as on the client's expression of pain. The nurse must consider cultural impacts on the pain experience when planning care.

► Heat and cold may have special cultural significance for some clients (Asians or Hispanics, for example) who classify conditions accordingly and expect corresponding treatments. (Table 8.1).

► Nurses must be sensitive to alternative pain relief measures used by clients and the cultural significance of those measures. Efforts should be made to reconcile religious rituals, herbal remedies, or other alternate treatments with the established medical plan to facilitate culturally sensitive care.

► The assessment of pain should include its location, duration, intensity, and precipitating, alleviating, and associated factors.

► Appropriate duration of treatment is essential for the therapeutic use of heat and cold.

TABLE 8.1	Hot and Cold Conditions*
Hot Conditions	**Cold Conditions**
Fever	Arthritis
Infections	Colds
Diarrhea	Indigestion
Constipation	Joint pain
Rashes	Menstrual period
Tenesmus	Ear ache
Ulcers	Cancer
Kidney problems	Tuberculosis
Skin ailments	Headache
Sore throat	Paralysis
Liver problems	Teething
	Rheumatism
	Pneumonia
	Malaria

*The usual treatment for a hot or cold condition is thought to be the use of a food or substance of the opposite temperature.

▶ Cold therapy causes vasoconstriction; reduces local metabolism, edema, and inflammation; and induces local anesthetic effects.
▶ Heat therapy causes vasodilatation, relieves muscle tension, stimulates circulation, and promotes healing.
▶ DANGER—ADDITIONAL TISSUE DAMAGE CAN RESULT IF:
  - Excessive temperature is used (hot or cold)
  - Overexposure of site to treatment occurs
  - Electrical equipment is not checked for safety
▶ Some major nursing diagnostic labels related to rest and comfort are altered comfort, risk of altered comfort, and anxiety.

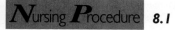

Aquathermia Pad

EQUIPMENT

- Aquathermia module (K-module) with pad (K-pad)
- Overbed or bedside table
- Disposable gloves
- Pillowcase
- Distilled water
- Tape

Purpose

Stimulates circulation, thus providing nutrients to tissues
Reduces muscle tension

Assessment

Assessment should focus on the following:

Treatment order
Client's tolerance of last treatment
Status of treatment area (redness, tenderness, cleanliness, and
 dryness)
Temperature, pulse rate, and rhythm
Degree of pain and position of comfort, if any
Mental status of client
Adequate functioning of heating device for proper functioning

Nursing Diagnoses

The nursing diagnoses may include the following:

Altered comfort related to joint pain

Outcome Identification and Planning

Desired Outcomes (sample)

Client verbalizes increased comfort after treatment.
Client demonstrates increased mobility of affected extremity after treatment.

Special Considerations

Make sure lamp functions accurately and safely. DO NOT USE IF CORD IS FRAYED OR CRACKS ARE NOTED.

Schedule procedure when client can be assessed frequently. IF A CLIENT IS CONFUSED OR UNABLE TO REMAIN ALONE WITH A HEATING DEVICE ON, REMAIN WITH THE CLIENT OR FIND SOMEONE TO DO SO.

Clients with decreased peripheral sensory perception, such as diabetics, must be monitored closely for heat overexposure.

Pediatric and Geriatric

Pediatric and elderly clients may be extremely sensitive to heat therapy. Assess more frequently because their skin is fragile.

Home Health

If a homebound client will be using a K-module when a nurse is not present, teach the client or family how to use the module safely.

 Transcultural

Determine cultural perspective regarding use of heat to treat the condition.

Discuss objections and incorporate hot/cold perception of illness and treatment.

Omit treatment if client objects, and consult physician.

Delegation

Generally, this procedure may be delegated to unlicensed assistive personnel. Check agency policy. Emphasize importance of monitoring local skin area and maintaining time limits for therapy.

IMPLEMENTATION

Action	Rationale
1. Wash hands and organize equipment.	*Reduces microorganism transfer* *Promotes efficiency*
2. Explain procedure to client.	*Decreases anxiety and promotes cooperation*
3. Place heating module on bedside or overbed table at a level above the client's body level (Fig. 8.1).	*Facilitates flow of fluid*
4. Fill module two thirds full with distilled water.	*Enables unit to function properly*

Action	Rationale

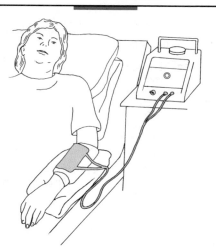

FIGURE 8.1

5. Turn module on low setting and allow water to begin circulating throughout the pad and tubing.

Detects leakage of fluid or improper functioning before initiating therapy

6. After water is fully circulating through the pad and tubing, check the pad with your hands to ascertain that it is warming.

Checks for proper functioning and heating of unit

7. Don disposable gloves, if indicated.

Decreases exposure to secretions

8. Place pillowcase over the heating pad and position pad on or (if an extremity) around treatment area.

Prevents direct skin contact with pad, minimizing danger of burn injury

9. If placement of pad needs to be secured, use tape. DO NOT USE PINS.

Prevents water leakage from possible puncture to pad

Action	Rationale
10. After 60 sec, assess for heat intolerance by: - Observing client's facial expression - Asking if heat is too high - Noting any dizziness, faintness, or palpitations - Removing pad and assessing for redness or tenderness; readjust temperature if necessary	*Prevents burn injury and complications of heat therapy*
11. Replace pad and secure with tape, if needed.	*Resumes treatment*
12. Instruct client NOT to alter placement of pad or heating module and to call if heat becomes too intense.	*Promotes client cooperation and continued optimum functioning of unit* *Prevents burn injury*
13. Leave call light within reach.	*Permits client communication*
14. Recheck client every 5 min.	*Prevents burn injury*
15. After 20 min, turn module off and place pad on table with module.	*Terminates treatment*
16. Reposition client.	*Facilitates comfort*
17. Return equipment.	*Maintains organized environment*
18. Remove gloves and wash hands.	*Reduces microorganism transfer*

Evaluation

Were desired outcomes achieved?

Documentation

The following should be noted on the client's chart:

- Appearance of treatment area
- General response of client (weakness, faintness, palpitations, diaphoresis, extreme tenderness, if any)
- Duration of treatment
- Status of pain

SAMPLE DOCUMENTATION

DATE	TIME	
12/3/02	1400	K-module applied to right calf for 20 minutes. No redness, warmth, or tenderness to touch at treatment area. Vital signs stable during and after treatment.

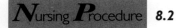

 Heat Therapy: Commercial Hot Pack/ Moist, Warm Compresses

EQUIPMENT

- Prepackaged heat pack
- Tape
- Small towel or washcloth
or
- Warm compress
- Warmed solution, 43°C (110°F)
- Petroleum jelly
- Heating pad or aquathermia pad (optional)
- Distilled water (for aquathermia pad)
- Towel
- Plastic-lined underpad
- Clean basin
- Bath thermometer
- Pack of 4 × 4-inch gauze pads
- Bath blanket
- Two forceps (optional)
- Two pairs of nonsterile gloves

Purpose

Promotes comfort
Warm compress stimulates circulation and promotes localization
   of purulent matter in tissues

Assessment

Assessment should focus on the following:

Treatment order, type of solution to be used, and response of
   client to previous treatments
Appearance of treatment area (edema, local bleeding)
Status of pain
Sensitivity of skin to heat treatment.

Nursing Diagnoses

The nursing diagnoses may include the following:

Altered comfort related to inflammation at IV infiltration site
Decreased wound healing related to wound infection

Outcome Identification and Planning

Desired Outcome (sample)

Client verbalizes that pain is decreased within 1 hr after treatment.

Special Considerations

Schedule application of heat therapy when the client can be assessed at frequent intervals.

Determine with client the best body position for comfort and alignment.

If applying warm compresses, check heating device for safety and proper functioning.

If using aquathermia pad for warm compress, set up heating device according to the guidelines in Nursing Procedure 8.1.

Home Health

Warn client that a clothing iron should never be used as a heat source for a warm compress.

Schedule the treatment when the client can be checked every 5 to 10 min.

Do not use on clients with peripheral sensory deficits.

Pediatric and Geriatric

Pediatric and elderly clients may require more frequent checks because skin may be more fragile.

Transcultural

Determine cultural perspective regarding hot/cold perception of illness and appropriateness of treatment (Procedure 8.1, Table 8.1).

Incorporate client preference when possible.

Omit treatment if client objects, and consult physician.

Delegation

Generally, this procedure may be delegated to unlicensed assistive personnel. Check agency policy. Emphasize importance of monitoring local skin area.

IMPLEMENTATION

Action	Rationale

1. Explain procedure to client.

Decreases anxiety and promotes cooperation

2. Wash hands and organize equipment.

Decreases microorganism transfer

Promotes efficiency

For Commercial Hot Pack

3. Remove heat pack from outer package, if present.

Provides access to pack

4. Break the inner seal: hold pack tightly in the center in upright position and squeeze. DO NOT USE PACK IF LEAKING IS NOTED (CHEMICAL BURN MAY OCCUR).

Activates chemical ingredients to form "heat" pack

5. Lightly shake pack until the inner contents are lying in the lower portion of the pack.

Localizes activated chemicals

6. Proceed to application.

For Warm, Moist Compress

7. Place gauze into basin half-filled with ordered solution.

Promotes efficiency

Saturates gauze with solution

8. Assist client into position.

Facilitates compress placement

9. Place plastic pad under treatment area.

Prevents soiling of linens

10. Drape client.

Provides privacy

11. Wring one layer of wet gauze until it is dripless.

Removes excess solution

12. Proceed to application steps.

Application Steps

13. Don gloves.

Reduces microorganism transfer

14. Remove and discard old dressings, if present.

Provides access to treatment site

15. Remove and discard old gloves and don new gloves.

Reduces microorganism transfer

16. If necessary, clean and dry treatment area.

Facilitates effectiveness of treatment

17. Place the hot pack lightly against treatment area.

Allows for gradual initiation of dilatory effect

Action	Rationale
18. Remove pack and assess client for redness of skin or complaint of burning after 30 sec.	*Prevents burn injury*
19. Replace pack snugly against the area if no problems are noted and secure placement with tape (go to step 8).	*Resumes treatment* *Stabilizes heat pack*

For Moist Compress

Action	Rationale
20. Place compress on the wound for several seconds.	*Initiates vasodilatation therapy*
21. Pick up edge of compress to observe initial skin response to therapy.	*Allows assessment of skin for adverse responses to therapy* *Promotes safety*
22. Replace compress gauze every 5 min, or as needed, to maintain warmth, assessing treatment area each time.	*Provides for reassessment of treatment area*
Place towel over compress (a heating device, if available, may be placed over towel); instruct client not to alter settings of heating device (proceed to step 8).	*Maintains heat of warm compress* *Promotes safety*
23. Place call light within reach and raise side rails.	*Facilitates client–nurse communication*
24. Reassess treatment area every 5 min by lifting the corners of the pack.	*Monitors effects of treatment over time*
25. After 20 min, terminate treatment and dry skin.	*Prevents local injury due to overexposure to treatment*
26. Apply new dressing over wound, if necessary.	*Promotes wound healing*
27. Reposition client and raise side rails.	*Facilitates comfort and safety*
28. Remove all equipment from bedside, remove gloves, and wash hands.	*Maintains clean environment and facilitates asepsis*

Evaluation

Were desired outcomes achieved?

Documentation

The following should be noted on the client's chart:

- Size, location, and appearance of treatment area
- Status of pain
- Duration of treatment
- Client tolerance to treatment

SAMPLE DOCUMENTATION

DATE	TIME	
12/3/02	1300	Warm compress applied to right wrist for 20 minutes. Redness decreased from 2 to 1 cm. Site slightly warm to touch after treatment, capillary refill 3 seconds. Client reports relief of pain.

Heat Cradle and Heat Lamp

EQUIPMENT

- Heat lamp (with adjustable neck and 60-watt bulb)
  or
- Heat cradle (25-watt bulb)
- Disposable gloves
- Washcloth
- Towels
- Soap
- Warm water

Purpose

Increases circulation
Promotes wound healing
Promotes general comfort
Assists with drying of wet cast

Assessment

Assessment should focus on the following:

Treatment order and response of client to previous treatment
Skin and appearance of wound (presence of edema, redness, heat, drainage)
Pulse and temperature
Mental status of client
Ability of client to maintain appropriate position without assistance
Degree of pain
Proper functioning and safety of heating device

Nursing Diagnoses

The nursing diagnoses may include the following:

Altered skin integrity related to episiotomy
Altered comfort related to disruption of skin integrity
Decreased tissue perfusion related to edema

Outcome Identification and Planning

Desired Outcomes (sample)
Site is clean, with no redness, edema, or drainage, within 48 hr.
Within 24 hr after beginning treatment, client verbalizes that pain
  is relieved or decreased.

Special Considerations
Make sure lamp functions accurately and safely. DO NOT USE IF
  CORD IS FRAYED OR CRACKS ARE NOTED.
Schedule timing of procedure so client can be checked every 5
  min. Do not leave confused clients unattended with heating ap-
  paratus.
Be sure hands are THOROUGHLY DRY when handling electrical
  equipment.

Pediatric and Geriatric
Assess pediatric and elderly clients frequently because of the
  fragile nature of their skin.
If client must be attended (as with many elderly clients) during
  treatment, FIND SOMEONE TO STAY WITH CLIENT DUR-
  ING TREATMENT.

Home Health
At home, a mechanic's trouble light with appropriate wattage
  bulb may be used as a heat lamp. Teach client/family safety
  precautions for using light.

 Transcultural
See note in Nursing Procedure 8.1, Table 8.1.

Delegation
Generally, this procedure may be delegated to trained unlicensed
  assistive personnel. Check individual agency policy. Emphasize importance of monitoring local treatment area closely.

IMPLEMENTATION

Action	Rationale
1. Explain procedure to client.	*Reduces anxiety and promotes cooperation*
2. Wash hands and organize equipment.	*Reduces microorganism transfer* *Promotes efficiency*
3. Don disposable gloves.	*Prevents contamination from secretions*

Action	Rationale
4. Position client for comfort and for optimum exposure of treatment area.	*Facilitates optimum treatment results*
5. With lamp turned off, place lamp 18 to 24 inches from wound to be treated.	*Prevents accidental burns from placing lamp too close*
6. Turn lamp on and observe client's response to the heat for 1 min: - Observe facial and body gestures. - Observe wound area for redness. - Ask client if heat is too high.	*Determines initial response to treatment*
7. Replace covers while keeping treatment area well exposed to the lamp; for heat cradle, place top sheet over cradle and client (Fig. 8.2).	*Provides privacy*
BE SURE THAT NEITHER CLOTHING NOR COVERS ARE TOUCHING THE BULB OF THE LAMP.	*Reduces electrical hazard*

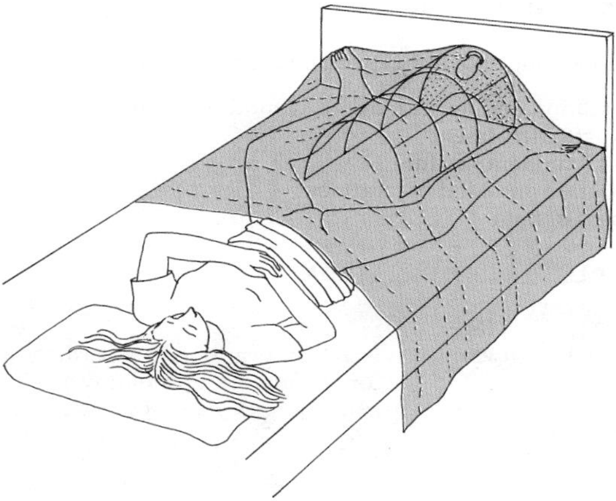

FIGURE 8.2

Action	Rationale
8. Remove disposable gloves and wash hands; don gloves again, as needed (ie, when direct contact with body secretions is possible).	*Prevents microorganism transfer*
9. Place call light within reach.	*Permits communication* *Promotes prompt response to client needs*
10. Assess client response to heat every 5 min.	*Prevents complications to treatment*
11. Remove lamp after 20 min.	*Terminates treatment* *Prevents local burn injury from overexposure to heat*
12. Reposition client and replace covers.	*Promotes comfort and safety*
13. Remove equipment from bedside and wash hands.	*Prevents hazards and microorganism transfer*

Evaluation

Were desired outcomes achieved?

Documentation

The following should be noted on the client's chart:

- Condition and appearance of wound or treatment area before and after treatment
- Pulse and temperature
- Duration and kind of treatment
- Status of pain

SAMPLE DOCUMENTATION

DATE	TIME	
12/3/02	1600	Heat lamp applied to perineal area for 20 minutes. Episiotomy site intact and dry, with slight redness and 1-cm edema. Client reports no perineal pain.

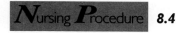
 Cold Therapy: Ice Bag/ Collar/Glove/Commercial Cold Pack/Moist Cold Compresses

EQUIPMENT

- Ice bag/collar/glove or prepackaged cold pack *or* for cold compress
- Plastic-lined linen saver
- Clean basin
- Bath thermometer
- Pack of 4 × 4 gauze pads
- Solution cooled with ice, 15°C (59°F)
- Cotton swab stick
- Tape
- Disposable gloves (2 pairs)
- Small towel or washcloth
- Ice chips

Purpose

Reduces local edema, bleeding, and hematoma formation
Decreases local pain sensation

Assessment

Assessment should focus on the following:

Treatment order and client's response to previous treatment, if used
Condition and appearance of treatment area (edema, local bleeding)
Status of pain

Nursing Diagnoses

The nursing diagnoses may include the following:

Altered comfort related to sprained right wrist

Outcome Identification and Planning

Desired Outcomes (sample)

Client states that pain is reduced or relieved after treatment.
No bleeding or hematoma is noted at treatment site.

Special Considerations

Schedule the procedure when the client can be checked frequently.

Pediatric and Geriatric

Young pediatric and elderly clients may require more frequent
checks because skin may be fragile.

Home Health

In the home, a self-sealing plastic bag may be used as an ice bag,
if necessary.

 Transcultural

Consider cultural perspective and preference for cold therapy.
See Nursing Procedure 8.1, Table 8.1.
Consult physician if client objects to planned therapy.

Delegation

Generally, this procedure may be delegated to unlicensed assistive personnel. Check agency policy.
Monitor local treatment area closely.

IMPLEMENTATION

Action	Rationale
1. Explain procedure to client.	*Decreases anxiety*
2. Wash hands and organize equipment.	*Reduces microorganism transfer* *Promotes efficiency*
For Ice Pack With Bag/Collar/Glove	
3. Fill bag/collar/glove about three fourths full with ice chips.	*Provides cold surface area*
4. Remove excess air from bag/collar/glove: - Place bag/collar/glove on flat surface. - Gently press until ice reaches the opening.	*Improves functioning of pack*
5. Contain ice securely by fastening end of the bag or collar; for plastic glove, tie end of glove itself.	*Prevents water seepage*

Action	Rationale
6. Cover with small towel or washcloth (if bag is made of a soft cloth exterior, this is not necessary).	*Promotes comfort*
7. Proceed to application steps.	

For Commercial Cold Pack

8. Remove ice pack from outer package, if present.	*Promotes efficiency* *Provides access to pack*
9. Break the inner seal; hold pack tightly in the center in upright position and squeeze. DO NOT USE PACK IF LEAKING IS NOTED (CHEMICAL BURN MAY OCCUR).	*Activates chemical ingredients to form "cold" pack*
10. Lightly shake pack until the inner contents are lying in the lower portion of the pack.	*Localizes activated chemicals*
11. Proceed to application steps.	

For Moist, Cold Compresses

12. Place gauze into basin half-filled with ordered solution.	*Promotes efficiency* *Saturates gauze with solution*
13. Assist client into position.	*Facilitates compress placement*
14. Place plastic pad under treatment area.	*Prevents soiling of linens*
15. Drape client.	*Provides privacy*
16. Wring one layer of wet gauze until it is dripless.	*Removes excess solution*
17. Proceed to application steps.	

Application Steps

18. Don gloves.	*Reduces microorganism transfer*
19. Remove and discard old dressings, if present.	*Provides access to treatment site*
20. Remove and discard old gloves and don new gloves.	*Reduces microorganism transfer*
21. If necessary, clean and dry treatment area.	*Facilitates effectiveness of treatment*
22. Place the pack lightly against treatment area.	*Allows for gradual initiation of vasoconstrictive effect*

Action	Rationale
23. Remove pack and assess client for redness of skin or complaint of burning after 30 sec.	*Prevents burn injury*
24. Replace pack snugly against the area if no problems are noted, and secure placement with tape (proceed to step 28).	*Resumes treatment* *Stabilizes cold pack*

For Moist Compress

Action	Rationale
25. Place compress on the wound for several seconds.	*Initiates vasoconstrictive therapy*
26. Pick up edge of compress to observe initial skin response to therapy.	*Allows assessment of skin for adverse responses to therapy*
27. Replace compress gauze every 5 min, or as needed, to maintain coolness, assessing treatment area each time.	*Promotes safety* *Provides for reassessment of treatment area*
28. Place call light within reach and raise side rails.	*Facilitates client–nurse communication*
29. Reassess treatment area every 5 min by lifting the corners of the pack.	*Monitors effects of treatment over time*
30. After 20 min, terminate treatment and dry skin.	*Prevents local injury due to overexposure to treatment*
31. Apply new dressing over wound, if necessary.	*Promotes wound healing*
32. Reposition client and raise side rails.	*Facilitates comfort and safety*
33. Remove all equipment from bedside, remove gloves, and wash hands.	*Maintains clean environment and facilitates asepsis*

Evaluation

Were desired outcomes achieved?

Documentation

The following should be noted on the client's chart:

- Size, location, and appearance of treatment area
- Status of pain
- Duration of treatment
- Client tolerance to treatment

SAMPLE DOCUMENTATION

DATE	TIME	
12/3/02	1300	Ice bag applied to right wrist for 20 minutes. Edema decreased from 2 to 1 cm. Site slightly cool to touch after treatment, capillary refill 3 seconds. Client reports relief of pain.

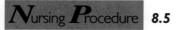

 Sitz Bath

EQUIPMENT

- Clean bathtub filled with enough warm water to cover buttocks (or portable sitz tub, if available)
- Bath towel
- Bath thermometer, if available
- Rubber tub ring
- Bathroom mat
- Gown
- Small footstool
- Nonsterile gloves

Purpose

Promotes perineal and anorectal healing
Reduces local inflammation and discomfort

Assessment

Assessment should focus on the following:

Baseline vital signs
Appearance and condition of treatment area
Client's knowledge of benefits of sitz bath
Client's inability to remain unattended in bathtub (eg, confusion, weakness)
Status of pain

Nursing Diagnoses

The nursing diagnoses may include the following:

Altered skin integrity related to episiotomy
Altered comfort related to disruption of skin integrity
Decreased tissue perfusion related to edema

Outcome Identification and Planning

Desired Outcomes (sample)
Client verbalizes relieved or decreased pain after treatment.

Within 48 hr, site is clean, without redness, edema, or drainage.

Special Considerations

Schedule the procedure when the client can be checked frequently.

If client is confused or unable to remain alone, plan to remain with client or find someone to do so.

Geriatric

Vasodilatation from exposure to warm water could cause severe changes in blood pressure and cardiac function in elderly clients with compromised cardiovascular status. Duration and temperature of sitz bath might need to be decreased, and clients must be watched closely for adverse reactions.

Home Health

Instruct client and family regarding the procedure. Emphasize the importance of a family member's checking on the client frequently if a potential safety hazard (such as falling in tub or on floor) exists.

 Transcultural

See overview regarding hot/cold conditions and Nursing Procedure 8.1, Table 8.1.

Discuss therapy with client and relate objections to physician.

Delegation

Generally, this procedure may be delegated to unlicensed assistive personnel. Stress the importance of monitoring water temperature before contact with patient's skin.

IMPLEMENTATION

Action	Rationale
1. Explain procedure to client.	*Promotes relaxation and compliance*
2. Wash hands, organize equipment, and don gloves.	*Reduces microorganism transfer to client or nurse* *Promotes efficiency*
3. Check temperature of water with thermometer (105°F to 110°F [40.5°C to 43°C]); if thermometer is unavailable, test water with your wrist (water should be warm).	*Prevents skin damage from high water temperature*
4. Place rubber ring at bottom of tub and bathmat on floor.	*Prevents accidental falls*

Action	Rationale
5. Assist client to bathroom.	
6. Close door and assist client with undressing.	*Provides privacy*
7. Assist client into tub, using footstool if necessary.	*Prevents accidental injury*
8. Seat client on the rubber ring.	
9. Ascertain client's stability in the tub alone and assess reaction to the heat: - Observe facial expressions and body motions for signs of discomfort. - Ask if heat is too high. - Watch for dizziness, faintness, profuse diaphoresis. - Note any rapid increase or irregularity of pulse.	*Prevents complications from falling or unusual reaction to therapy*
10. Instruct client on use of call light and place light within reach.	*Facilitates client–nurse communication and immediate response to emergency*
11. Recheck client every 5 to 10 min.	*Allows assessment of unusual reactions*
12. After 15 to 20 min, help client out of the tub.	*Terminates treatment*
13. Assist client with drying and dressing; then place linens in hamper.	*Prevents chilling*
14. Return client to room or bed.	*Promotes comfort*
15. Remove equipment and clean tub.	*Reduces microorganism transfer to others using tub*
16. Remove gloves and wash hands.	*Reduces microorganism transfer*

Evaluation

Were desired outcomes achieved?

Documentation

The following should be noted on the client's chart:
- Appearance of treatment area before and after treatment
- Any unusual reactions to treatment, such as profuse diaphoresis, faintness, dizziness, palpitations, or pulse changes
- Duration of sitz bath
- Status of pain

SAMPLE DOCUMENTATION

DATE	TIME	
12/3/02	1500	Sitz bath to perineal area for 20 minutes. Client states pain decreased after treatment. No drainage from open perineal wound. No complaints of dizziness.

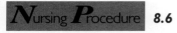

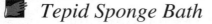 *Tepid Sponge Bath*

EQUIPMENT

- Thermometer (oral or rectal)
- Basin of cold water
- Gown
- Plastic-lined pads
- Bath blanket
- Six or seven washcloths
- Two towels
- Nonsterile gloves

Purpose

Provides controlled reduction of body temperature

Assessment

Assessment should focus on the following:

Doctor's order and client's response to previous treatment
Condition and appearance of skin
Pulse and temperature
Level of consciousness

Nursing Diagnoses

The nursing diagnoses may include the following:

Elevated body temperature related to sepsis
Risk for injury related to elevated temperature

Outcome Identification and Planning

Desired Outcomes (sample)
Client maintains temperature within normal or acceptable limits (specified by physician).
Client tolerates treatment with no adverse changes in status or vital signs.

Special Consideration

If an alcohol bath is ordered, use equal parts of alcohol and water and assess client more frequently. Body temperature is decreased more rapidly by alcohol than by water.

Pediatric and Geriatric

The body temperature of pediatric and elderly clients is less stable than that of adult clients and may require more frequent assessment.

To lower a child's temperature, try placing the child in a cool bath and splashing water over the body, or place the child on a wet towel and cover groin and axillary areas with wet washcloths for 20 min. This technique may effectively reduce the temperature by 1°F.

Home Health

Instruct client and family on the procedure and precautions of the tepid sponge bath, and recommend that a thermometer be secured for the home.

 Transcultural

Note overview regarding hot/cold conditions and Nursing Procedure 8.1, Table 8.1.

Adhere to cultural idiosyncracies regarding same-sex or opposite-sex care providers; family member should be instructed on procedure for sponge bath if preferred by client.

Delegation

Generally, this procedure may be delegated to unlicensed assistive personnel.

IMPLEMENTATION

Action	Rationale
1. Explain procedure to client.	*Reduces anxiety and promotes compliance*
2. Close windows and doors.	*Eliminates drafts, thus preventing chilling*
3. Wash hands and organize equipment.	*Reduces microorganism transfer Promotes efficiency*
4. Undress client, covering body with bath blanket and rolling topsheet to the bottom of bed.	*Prevents chilling and protects privacy*
5. Place washcloths and one towel in basin of water.	*Cools cloths and towel*

ction	Rationale
6. Place plastic pads under client.	*Prevents linen soilage*
7. Wring washcloths and place one in each of the following areas: - Over forehead - Under armpits - Over groin	*Promotes rapid cooling due to increased vascularity of these regions*
8. Rewet and replace washcloths as they become warm.	*Maintains coolness of cloths*
9. Wring the wet towel and place around client's arm (Fig. 8.3).	*Promotes decreased temperature in extremity*
10. Wring a washcloth and sponge the other arm for 3 or 4 min. Repeat steps 9 and 10 with the opposite arm.	*Facilitates gradual cooling of extremity*
11. Remove towel from arm and place in basin, dry both arms thoroughly, and replace blanket.	*Prepares towel for future use* *Prevents chilling*
12. Check client's temperature and pulse: - If temperature is above 100°F (37.7°C), proceed with bath.	*Prevents complications related to overcooling*

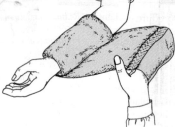

FIGURE 8.3

Action	**Rationale**
- *If temperature is at or below 100°F (37.7°C),* terminate the procedure by skipping to step 17.	
- *If pulse is significantly increased,* terminate procedure for 5 min and recheck; if it remains significantly elevated, terminate procedure and notify physician.	
13. Repeat temperature and pulse check.	*Assesses effectiveness of treatment*
14. Continue by sponging and drying the following areas for 3 to 5 min: • Chest • Left leg • Back • Abdomen • Right leg • Buttocks	*Facilitates cooling by expanding the body surface area being treated*
15. You may use steps 9 to 11 when sponging legs.	
16. STOP EVERY 10 MIN TO REASSESS TEMPERATURE AND PULSE.	*Assesses effectiveness* *Prevents overcooling*
17. Remove all cloths and towels and dry client thoroughly.	*Terminates treatment* *Promotes comfort*
18. Replace gown.	*Restores privacy*
19. Reposition client and raise side rails.	*Promotes comfort and safety*
20. Remove and properly discard all washcloths, towels, plastic pads, and wet linens. (If necessary, obtain dry linens and remake bed.)	*Maintains cleanliness of environment*
21. Remove and discard gloves.	*Reduces microorganism transfer*

Evaluation

Were desired outcomes achieved?

Documentation

The following should be noted on the client's chart:

- Pulse and temperature before and after bath
- Client mentation and general tolerance of the bath
- Untoward reactions to the treatment
- Length of the treatment and percentage of body sponged

SAMPLE DOCUMENTATION

DATE	TIME	
12/25/02	0100	Tepid sponge bath administered for 20 minutes because client's temperature is 104.7°F. Temperature after bath, 102.6°F; pulse, 118 and regular; respirations, 28 and regular; blood pressure, 110/62. Client dozing quietly in bed. Doctor notified of status. Tylenol suppository grains XX given.

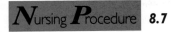

Transcutaneous Electrical
Nerve Stimulation Unit

 EQUIPMENT

- Transcutaneous electrical nerve stimulation (TENS) unit
- Lead wires
- Electrodes
- Water (optional)
- Fresh 9-volt battery

Purpose

Controls pain by delivering electrical impulse to nerve endings, which blocks pain message along pathway and prevents brain reception

Reduces amount of pain medication required to maintain comfort

Allows client to remain mentally alert, active, and pain free

Assessment

Assessment should focus on the following:

Status of pain (location and degree; alleviating and aggravating factors)

Type and location of incision, if applicable

Previous use of and knowledge level regarding TENS unit

Presence of skin irritation, abrasions, or breakage

Nursing Diagnoses

The nursing diagnoses may include the following:

Altered comfort related to incisional pain

Outcome Identification and Planning

Desired Outcomes (sample)

Client ambulates in hallway with minimal complaint of pain.
Client requests pain medication less frequently.

Decreased dosages of medication are needed.

Special Considerations

Apply electrodes to clean, unbroken skin only.

If sensitivity to electrode adhesive is noted, notify doctor before application. If skin irritation is noted during TENS usage, remove electrodes and notify doctor.

Client should be informed that TENS unit may not totally relieve pain but should reduce discomfort.

Geriatric

Check skin frequently for tenderness and sensitivity.

If client is confused and electrical stimulation increases irritation, decrease or stop stimulation and notify doctor.

Delegation

Specially-trained personnel may apply TENS units in some agencies. Note individual agency policy.

IMPLEMENTATION

Action	Rationale
1. Wash hands and organize equipment.	*Reduces microorganism transfer* *Promotes efficiency*
2. Explain procedure to client.	*Promotes relaxation and compliance*
3. Wash, rinse, and dry skin thoroughly.	*Facilitates electrode adhesion*
4. Prepare electrodes as described in package insert.	
5. Place electrodes on body areas directed by doctor or physical therapist (often along incision site or spinal column or both, depending on location of pain).	*Places electrodes in position for optimal results*
6. Plug lead wires into TENS unit (Fig. 8.4).	
7. Turn unit on and regulate for comfort:	
- Work with one lead (set) at a time.	*Ensures proper stimulation of each area addressed*
- Before beginning, ask client to indicate when stimulation is felt.	

Action	Rationale

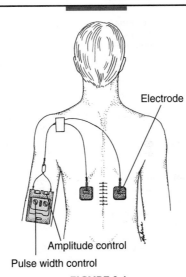

FIGURE 8.4

- Beginning at 0, increase level of stimulation until client indicates feeling of discomfort (muscle contraction under electrode area).

  Achieves maximum stimulation to block pain sensation

- When client indicates discomfort, reduce stimulation level slightly.

  Prevents continued contraction of muscles at pain site or around incision

- Try to maintain highest tolerable level of stimulation.
  Repeat above steps with other lead (set).

  Promotes maximum blockage of pain sensations

- Note color of blinking light on unit and change battery as needed.

  Indicates that unit is functional (red light may indicate low battery)

8. Stabilize unit for client mobility, using one of the following methods:

Action	Rationale
- Clamp unit to pajama bottom or gown (may place tape around unit and pin to gown with safety pin).	
- Place in pants pocket or clip to belt if client is ambulatory.	
9. Monitor client for comfort level with vital signs assessment; check for increased respiratory rate, pulse, or blood pressure.	*Indicates effectiveness of unit* *Indicates need to adjust stimulation due to increased discomfort*
10. Be alert for malfunctions and correct them; the following guidelines should be used for general management of the TENS unit:	*Prevents injury to client and damage to TENS unit*
- Client should remove unit before a shower or bath.	*Prevents shock to client*
- If client complains of increased or sudden pain sensation, check TENS connections and perform general assessment of incision, dressing, and client.	*Verifies function of unit and detects possible causes of increased discomfort*
- TENS unit should be off whenever removing or applying leads. If lead becomes disconnected, TURN UNIT OFF, RECONNECT LEAD, THEN INCREASE STIMULATION LEVEL FROM 0.	*Prevents shocking sensation*
- NEVER turn unit on when set at maximum stimulation: always start at 0 and gradually increase level.	*Prevents client discomfort at shocking sensation*

Action	Rationale
- If client complains of "shocking sensation" or muscle contraction, decrease stimulation level.	*Prevents excessive stimulation*
- Check battery status frequently.	

Evaluation

Were desired outcomes achieved?

Documentation

The following should be noted on the client's chart:

- Type and location of incision, if applicable
- Time and date of TENS application
- Level of stimulation of each lead (set)
- Area stimulated by each lead (set)
- Pain location, level, aggravating and alleviating factors
- Client teaching done and accuracy with which client repeats instructions

SAMPLE DOCUMENTATION

DATE	TIME	
1/2/02	1200	TENs unit applied for lumbar back pain. Electrodes applied to lumbar area with setting of 5.5 on lead 1 and 6.0 on lead 2. Client verbalized understanding of unit function and states that minimum pain is felt at present.

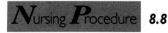

 Patient-Controlled Analgesia and Epidural Pump Therapy

EQUIPMENT

- Patient-controlled analgesia (PCA) infuser
- PCA administration set (pump tubing)
- IV tubing and fluid as applicable
- PCA infuser key
- PCA flow sheet or appropriate form
- Epidural pump setup
- Ordered narcotic analgesic vial bag or syringe (mixed by pharmacy)
- Vial injector (accompanies vial)
- Client information booklet
- IV start kit (unless venous access is already available)

Purpose

Allows client to control delivery of pain medication in a safe, consistent, effective, and reliable manner

Assessment

Assessment should focus on the following:

Any contraindication for epidural analgesia, such as allergy to any proposed medication; any coagulopathy due to disease process or administration of systemic anticoagulants (anticoagulants in combination with nonsteroidal anti-inflammatory drugs (NSAIDs) increases risk of epidural hematoma); localized infection or inflammation of the area of the epidural catheter, diagnosis of meningitis, or central nervous system infection; history of increased intracranial pressure

Doctor's orders for type of analgesic, loading dosage, concentration of analgesic mixture, lock-out interval (minimum time allowed between doses), and supplemental medication or bolus for uncontrolled pain

Type of illness or surgery

Pain (type, location, character, intensity, aggravating and alleviating factors)

Level of consciousness and orientation

Venous access (patency of IV line, if present; skin status if IV is to be started)

Ability to learn and comprehend

Reading ability

Urinary retention (obtain an order for bladder scan or straight catheterization or to reinsert Foley catheter if indicated)

Respiratory rate (if <10/min, stop infusion and notify physician)

Nursing Diagnoses

The nursing diagnoses may include the following:

Altered comfort: pain related to thoracic incision site

Anxiety related to lack of pain control

Outcome Identification and Planning

Desired Outcomes (sample)

Client states that pain is relieved within 2 hr of PCA initiation.

Adequate relief from chronic pain is achieved.

There is an increase in the patient's activity that is currently limited due to constant pain.

Special Consideration

Pain is very subjective; for pain management to be effective, it must meet individual patient's needs.

Geriatric

The analgesic may have an adverse effect on some elderly clients (eg, changes in level of orientation).

Pediatric

PCA therapy is usually used in adolescents or adults. When it is used with a pediatric client, instruct the parents as well as the child.

Considerations

Do not remove epidural catheter immediately after a dose of antithrombotic. Wait 12 hr after subcutaneous low molecular weight (LMW) heparin (enoxaparin [Lovenox], dalteparin [Fragmin]), remove within first 24 hr of initiating warfarin (Coumadin). You may resume anticoagulant/antithrombotics 2 hr after removal.

Home Health

Teach family members how to recognize signs of overdosage in the homebound client.

Only preservative-free (nonbacteriostatic) opioid solutions or anesthetics are administered through an epidural catheter.

There are many varied types of pumps for use with pain control in the home. Discuss the specific pump applications with the client or care provider.

Naloxone must be readily available, and a plan for emergencies must be discussed with the client and caregiver.

Economic: Portable infusion pumps are not necessarily trouble free or less expensive for the client. The cost/benefit ratio must be considered when discussing this method of controlling pain in the home setting.

Hint: Educate and assist the client in implementing nonpharmacologic methods of pain relief, as well as administration of medications. Often, these techniques have synergistic effects with the medication that increase the home client's tolerance of activities of daily living.

Refer client and family to home health agency for additional education and follow-up assessment of pain management effectiveness.

Delegation

PCA pumps and epidural catheters are managed by the RN and not delegated to others.

Other personnel should be instructed on management of the client related to positioning and moving.

IMPLEMENTATION

Action	Rationale
1. Wash hands and organize equipment.	*Reduces microorganism transfer* *Promotes efficiency*
2. Explain use of system to client and provide written literature; assess accuracy of client's understanding.	*Decreases anxiety* *Promotes compliance*
3. Prepare analgesic for administration:	*Ensures delivery of appropriate medication and dosage*
- Check five rights of drug administration: client, drug, dosage (concentration), route, room.	

For PCA Setup

- Connect injector to pre-filled vial or syringe (Fig. 8.5).
- Hold vial vertically and push injector to remove air.

Action	Rationale

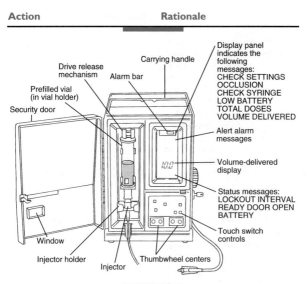

Drive release mechanism

Alarm bar

Carrying handle

Prefilled vial
(in vial holder)

Security door

Display panel
indicates the
following
messages:
CHECK SETTINGS
OCCLUSION
CHECK SYRINGE
LOW BATTERY
TOTAL DOSES
VOLUME DELIVERED

Alert alarm
messages

10.0

Volume-delivered
display

Status messages:
LOCKOUT INTERVAL
READY DOOR OPEN
BATTERY

Touch switch
controls

Window

Injector holder   Injector   Thumbwheel centers

FIGURE 8.5

- Connect PCA administration set to vial, prime tubing, and close tubing clamp.
- Plug machine into electrical outlet and use PCA infuser key to open pump door.
- Load vial into machine according to equipment operation booklet.
4. Prepare primary IV fluid and tubing (see Procedure 5.3).
5. Attach primary IV tubing to Y-connector line of PCA tubing.

Provides fluid to keep vein open between medication doses

6. Open primary tubing clamp and prime lower portion of PCA tubing.

Removes air from tubing

7. Close clamp on primary IV.

Action	Rationale
8. Prepare venous access: - Insert IV catheter (see Procedures 5.2 and 5.4); or, if venous access (IV lock or central line) is already present, verify patency, and connect PCA tubing directly to IV catheter. - Release clamps on PCA and primary tubing. - Regulate primary IV to infuse at keep-vein-open (or ordered) rate (see Procedures 5.5 and 5.6).	*Maintains patency of vein between medication doses*
9. Administer loading dose if ordered: - Verify ordered dosage. - Set lock-out interval on pump at 00 minutes. - Set volume to be delivered, using dose-volume thumbwheel control. - Press and release loading-dose control switch.	*Delivers dose of analgesic to initiate pain relief*
10. Set parameters for dosage control: - Calculate volume of medication needed to deliver ordered dose (available dose per volume divided by ordered dose equals volume); often vials contain 200 mg per 20-ml vial of Demerol or 30 mg morphine per 30-ml vial. - Set *dose volume*, using thumbwheel control for desired volume for each dose.	*Determines volume that will deliver ordered dose* *Delivers 10 mg per 1-ml dose* *Delivers 1 mg per 1-ml dose* *Sets amount of fluid and medication to be delivered for each dose*

Action	Rationale
- If patient is receiving a continuous infusion (basal rate), set the basal rate as ordered using the touchpad control.	*Delivers continuous rate of medication and allows patient-controlled supplement*
- Set *lock-out interval*, using thumbwheel control to set the desired time interval.	*Sets minimum time between allotted doses* *Prevents medication overdose*
- To set 4-hr limit, push control switch to display current limit; if different limit is desired, depress again and hold switch until desired limit is reached; then release switch.	*Limits total volume to be infused over any consecutive 4-hr period*
- Close and lock security door using infuser key; READY message should appear indicating that PCA infuser is in client-control mode and first dose can be administered.	
- Place key with narcotic keys (or per agency policy).	*Secures narcotic and parameters set into machine*
11. Instruct client on administration of dose; inform client of the following information:	
- When pain is experienced, press and release control button.	*Delivers set dose of analgesic*
- Medication will be delivered, and infuser will enter a lock-out period during which no additional medication can be delivered.	
- A "ready" message will appear when next dose can be delivered.	
12. For maintenance of PCA therapy, *every 1 to 2 hr:*	*Allows for monitoring of dosages received by client*

Action	Rationale

- Press TOTAL DOSE switch and note number of client doses administered during past period.

For Epidural Pain Management

- Check pump function and notify physician of any need for changes in therapy.	*Assesses adequate control and physical response to medication level (high pain scores require reassessment)*
- Record temperature, pulse, respirations, pain relief level, mobility, sensation, and any observations.	*Excessive sedation and any indication of respiratory depression require pump reprogramming*
- At each assessment, monitor insertion site for erythema, inflammation, or drainage.	*Continuously assesses infection potential*
- For epidural pump (each assessment): Press "enter" button and record volume remaining.	

For PCA and Epidural Therapy

- Monitor client's respiratory rate, level of sedation (alert to sleeping), and pain level (pain free to severe pain).	*Monitors for oversedation*
- Document above volumes and observations on flow sheet, and calculate total volume in appropriate column.	*Identifies total volume infused and remaining in vial*
Every 8 hr (or per policy):	*Complies with federal narcotic administration laws*
- Check volume of medication delivered; if agency policy, open pump door with infuser key and verify volume remaining in analgesic vial/bag (volume should equal initial volume minus total volume infused).	

Action	Rationale
13. If you are oncoming shift nurse, check drug infusing, dose volume, and lock-out interval with doctor's order.	*Verifies accuracy of infusion*

14. Change vial/bag and injector (when nearly empty or at end of 24-hr period, if agency policy):
  - Assemble new vial/bag and injector.
  - Clear air from vial/bag and close tubing clamp.
	Provides fresh medication

For PCA
- Use infuser key to unlock and open PCA pump door.
- Press on/off switch.
- Close clamp to old vial and primary fluid tubing.
- Remove empty vial (or old vial) and administration set from pump (see equipment operation booklet).
- Attach new vial and injector to PCA administration set and prime to remove air.
- Attach primary IV to Y-connector of new PCA administration set.
- Insert administration set into pump (see equipment operation booklet).
- Close and lock pump door.
- Release tubing clamps.
- Press on/off switch.   *Initiates client-control mode*
- Record vial change on PCA flow sheet.   *Identifies current volume of analgesic in PCA pump*
- Send previous vial and tubing to pharmacy (per agency protocol).

Action	Rationale
15. To discontinue PCA therapy, follow step 14, omitting preparation of new vial; remove PCA tubing from IV catheter and replace with primary fluid tubing or infusion plug.	
16. Send vial and tubing to pharmacy (check agency policy).	*Adheres to federal regulations for narcotic control*
17. Discontinue epidural therapy per hospital policy. See Special Considerations.	*Reduces risk of hematoma*

Evaluation

Were desired outcomes achieved?

Documentation

The following should be noted on the client's chart:
- Name and dosage of medication being infused
- PCA parameters (hourly dose, lock-out interval, and 4-hr limit)
- Level of consciousness (on scale of 1 to 5)
- Pain level (on scale of 1 to 5)
- Status of respirations
- Amount of medication (analgesic) used each hour
- Number of client attempts to obtain dose (if agency policy)

For epidural catheters, the following should ALSO be noted on the visit record:

- Condition of insertion site
- Dressing changes
- Client or caregiver education activities

SAMPLE DOCUMENTATION

DATE	TIME	
1/2/02	1200	Client received from recovery room after total hip replacement. PCA therapy initiated, with 5 mg morphine given IV as loading dose. Dose volume set at 2 ml (2 mg), lock-out interval set at 60 minutes, and 4-hr limit set at 8 mg. Client alert and oriented. States pain measures 2 on a scale of 1 to 5, with 5 indicating severe pain. Return-demonstrated procedure for obtaining dose with 100% accuracy.

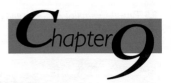

Hygienic Care

OVERVIEW

▶ Hygiene is usually a private matter; consider the client's preference in timing, family assistance, and toiletries.

▶ Clients should be encouraged to perform as much hygienic care as possible within prescribed limitations.

▶ Maintaining good hygiene can promote the following:
  - Healthy skin, by preventing infections and skin breakdown
  - Improved circulation
  - Comfort and rest
  - Nutrition, by improving the appetite
  - Self-esteem, by improving the appearance
  - Sense of well-being

▶ Some major nursing diagnostic labels related to hygienic care are bathing/hygienic self-care deficit, dressing/grooming self-care deficit, risk of impaired skin integrity, and anxiety.

Cost-cutting Tip

When appropriate, teaching family members hygienic care techniques and encouraging them to assist with or perform this care provides an effective teaching experience and conserves staff time during the course of the client's debilitation.

Delegation

All of these hygienic care procedures may be delegated to unlicensed assistive personnel. The care of clients with special needs related to special positioning or transfer during care, prevention of aspiration, or other care concerns may require additional instruction or supervision.

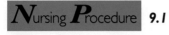

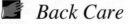 *Back Care*

EQUIPMENT

- Lotion
- Soap
- Towel
- Washcloth
- Warm water

Purpose

Promotes comfort
Stimulates circulation
Relieves muscle tension
Facilitates therapeutic interaction

Assessment

Assessment should focus on the following:

Client's desire for back rub
Client's knowledge of purpose of back rub
Blood pressure and pulse rate/rhythm if there is a history of cardiac or vascular problems
Skin and bony prominences
Client's ability to tolerate prone or lateral position
Client's allergy to ingredients of lotion

Nursing Diagnoses

The nursing diagnoses may include the following:

Pain related to muscle tension, decreased mobility, or impaired circulation
Risk of impaired skin integrity related to immobility or decreased circulation
Anxiety related to fear of the unknown (tests, back rub)

Outcome Identification and Planning

Desired Outcomes (sample)

Client expresses feelings of comfort and falls asleep or has calm, relaxed facial expression.

Client verbalizes concerns during back rub.

Special Considerations

Many clients may prefer baby oil or powder rather than lotion.

Care should be taken to use only light pressure for clients with back disorders; a doctor's order is required for a back rub for these clients.

Geriatric

Baby oil or oil-based lotion may be best for the skin of elderly clients.

Pediatric

Total body massage with gentle conversation may be soothing and calming for a child and may serve to reduce the stress of hospitalization.

Home Health

Teach the procedure to a family member as a possible method of potentiating the effects of, or decreasing the need for, pain or sleeping medication.

🛑 *Cost-cutting Tip*

Teach family members back care techniques and encourage them to perform care.

IMPLEMENTATION

Action	Rationale
1. Explain procedure to client.	*Promotes relaxation and compliance*
2. Maintain a quiet, relaxing atmosphere (temperature at a comfortable setting, lighting dim, room neat, noise eliminated, door closed).	*Promotes relaxation*
3. Wash hands and organize equipment.	*Reduces microorganism transfer* *Promotes efficiency*

Action	Rationale
4. Warm lotion bottle and hands with warm water.	*Cold lotion and hands increase discomfort and cause muscle spasms*
5. Place client in prone or side-lying position.	*Comfortable, relaxing position provides easy access to back*
6. Drape with sheet or bath blanket.	*Provides warmth and privacy*
7. Wash back with soap and water; rinse and dry thoroughly.	*Removes dirt and/or perspiration*
8. Pour lotion into hands and rub hands together.	*Facilitates even lotion distribution*
9. Encourage client to take slow, deep breaths as you begin.	*Facilitates relaxation*
10. Place palms of hands on sacrococcygeal area. ONCE HANDS HAVE BEEN PLACED, DO NOT REMOVE HANDS FROM CLIENT'S BACK UNTIL BACK RUB IS COMPLETED.	*Upward massage facilitates circulation* *Continuous contact with skin is essential for maximum soothing effect*
11. Make long, firm strokes up center of back, moving toward shoulders, and back down toward buttocks, covering the lateral areas of the back; repeat this step several times.	*Stimulates circulation and release of muscle tension (it may be helpful to imagine a large heart on the client's back in accomplishing this step)*
12. Move hands up center of the back toward the neck and rub nape of neck with fingers; continue rubbing outward across the shoulders.	*Releases tension in neck muscles and promotes relaxation*
13. Move hands downward to scapula areas and massage in a circular motion over both scapulae for several seconds.	*Stimulates circulation around pressure points*
14. Move hands downward to the buttocks and massage in a figure-eight motion	*Stimulates circulation around pressure points*

Action	Rationale

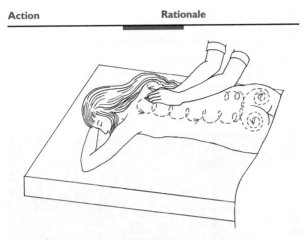

FIGURE 9.1

over the buttocks; continue this step for several seconds (Fig. 9.1).

15. Lightly rub toward the neck and shoulders, then back down toward the buttocks for several strokes (using lighter pressure and moving laterally with each stroke).

Ends back rub with a calming, therapeutic effect

16. Remove excessive lotion with towel.

Excessive moisture leads to skin breakdown and bacterial growth

17. Reposition client and replace covers.

Promotes comfort and provides warmth

18. Raise side rails and place call light within reach.

Facilitates client–nurse communication
Promotes safety

Evaluation

Were desired outcomes achieved?

Documentation

The following should be noted on the client's chart:

- Client's response to back rub
- Condition of skin and bony prominences
- Blood pressure and pulse before and after procedure, if applicable

SAMPLE DOCUMENTATION

DATE	TIME	
12/3/02	2200	Back rub given; activity tolerated without excessive fatigue, shortness of breath, or changes in vital signs. Client now in lateral-recumbent position, with call light within reach. Bilateral side rails up. Stated back rub was relaxing.

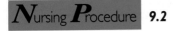

Bed Preparation Techniques

 EQUIPMENT

- Bottom sheet (fitted, if available)
- Top sheet (regular sheet)
- Draw sheet (may use second regular sheet)
- Pillowcase for each pillow in the room
- Gloves to remove old linens
- Gown and gloves, if client has draining wound or is in isolation

Purpose

Prepares bed covers to promote client's comfort

Assessment

Assessment should focus on the following:

Doctor's order for activity, impending surgery, or procedure
Need, if any, for assistance in turning client
Bladder and bowel continence
Presence of surgical wound or drains
Plans for client absence from room for a day or anticipation of
   new admission

Outcome Identification and Planning

Desired Outcomes (sample)
Client verbalizes comfort when assisted into bed.
Client experiences minimum discomfort during turning.

Special Considerations
A bed should be made after the client's bath is completed. You
   may need assistance to turn the client if you are making an oc-
   cupied bed.
If client has low activity tolerance and is fatigued, plan a rest period after the bath, then get assistance with the bed change to
   decrease client energy expenditure during the process.

Cost-cutting Tip

If client discharge is anticipated, do not apply fresh linen to bed.

IMPLEMENTATION

Action	Rationale
1. Assist client to chair for meal or to use bedside commode.	*Provides easy access to bed for changing*
2. Don gloves, remove old linen, and place in pillow-case or a linen bag; if bed is soiled or new client is due, spray or wash mattress with germicidal agent. If an egg crate mattress is used, place it on bed. Remove gloves and wash hands.	*Reduces microorganism transfer*
3. Apply bottom sheet:	
- Place bottom sheet over mattress as evenly as possible, leaving 1 inch or less hanging over bottom edge.	
- Tuck sheet at top and miter corners.	
- Move along the side of the bed, tucking the sheets securely and pulling tightly to remove wrinkles.	*Ensures snug fit on mattress*
- If fitted sheets are supplied, pull each corner of the mattress up slightly and slip it into a corner of the fitted sheet (pin the last two corners of sheet to undersides of mattress to keep sheets smooth).	
4. Place a draw sheet or pull sheet on bed:	*Assists in repositioning client*
- Fold full-sized sheet into thirds (Fig. 9.2).	

Action	Rationale

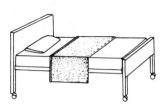

FIGURE 9.2

- Place sheet across bed 2 feet from the top, tucking it in or not, depending on activity level of client, agency policy, or preference.

Places sheet under shoulders and hips of the client

5. The top sheet should be placed over bed with top edge 2 inches over top of the mattress; if blanket is used, place on top of sheet, tuck and miter bottom corners of both but make small fold or pleat at bottom edge of top linen.

Provides room for feet

6. Place a clean pillowcase on each pillow in room.
7. Assist client to bed and position for comfort or finish bed in appropriate manner for circumstances:

Closed bed
- Place pillow on bed with open end facing the wall or place pillow on the bedside table.

Preserves bed when client is out of room for extended period or when new client is expected

Open bed
- Pull top of sheet (and blanket) to head of bed.
- Fanfold both back neatly to bottom third of bed.

Prepares bed for client when return is expected momentarily

Action	Rationale

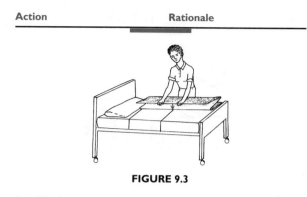

FIGURE 9.3

Surgical bed

Action	Rationale
- Make an open bed but do not tuck top sheet and blanket.	*Facilitates moving client from stretcher to bed without prolonged exposure or draft*
- Leave top sheet and blanket fanfolded to the side of bed opposite door (Fig. 9.3).	*Prevents interference of client transfer to bed by bed linens*
- After client is transferred to bed, pull covers across bed and tuck and miter at bottom.	*Covers client easily* *Secures linen on bed*
8. Discard or restore linen appropriately.	*Promotes clean environment*

Evaluation

Were desired outcomes achieved?

Documentation

The following should be noted on the client's chart:

- Bed linens changed
- Status of client (expected from surgery, discharged, or in bed)

SAMPLE DOCUMENTATION

A bed change is not usually documented in note form. You may indicate with brief note on activity checklist if patient tolerance of procedure is being monitored.

DATE	TIME	
12/3/02	1000	Discharged home on 1-day pass. Room cleaned and linens changed. Bed in closed position.

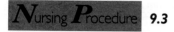

Nursing Procedure 9.3

Shampoo for the Bedridden Client

 EQUIPMENT

- Shampoo
- Washcloth
- Shampoo board (or other assistive device)
- Two towels
- Nonsterile gloves
- Wash basin or plastic-lined trash can
- Water pitcher
- Linen saver or plastic trash bag
- Hair dryer (safety-approved and approved by agency)

Purpose

Improves appearance and self-esteem
Facilitates comfort and relaxation
Stimulates circulation to scalp
Relaxes client

Assessment

Assessment should focus on the following:

Client need or desire for shampoo
Client's knowledge of procedure of bed shampoo
Blood pressure and pulse rate/rhythm if there is a history of cardiac or vascular problems
Neurostatus (eg, increased intracranial pressure or other contraindications to manipulation of head)
Client's ability to tolerate prone or side-lying position
Client's allergy to ingredients of shampoo or need for medicated shampoo

Nursing Diagnoses

The nursing diagnoses may include the following:

Pain related to unclean scalp
Risk of impaired skin integrity related to inadequate circulation at scalp area

Outcome Identification and Planning

Desired Outcomes (sample)

Client verbalizes increased comfort and expresses interest in further grooming.

Scalp is warm, with brisk capillary refill and no irritation.

Special Considerations

Some clients require more frequent shampooing than others; treat each case individually. See basic hair-care techniques in Procedure 9.4 for considerations based on ethnic-cultural diversity.

Avoid aerosol sprays if patient has respiratory condition or tracheostomy.

Geriatric

In the elderly client, skin is often thin and hair is brittle.

Check scalp for irritation before shampooing.

Pediatric

Shampoo that is less harsh and less irritating to the eyes than regular shampoo may be obtained for children.

Assistance may be needed when shampooing the hair of infants and children to avoid excessive movement and wetting of covers.

Home Health

Teach proper hair-care techniques to family members for continued care. If client has lice, instruct family on need to treat all family members for lice, as well as need to clean home, linens, and personal items to prevent further spread.

 Cost-cutting Tip

Encourage family members to perform hair-care techniques when acceptable to client.

IMPLEMENTATION

Action	Rationale
1. Prepare room environment (warm temperature and draft free).	*Avoids discomfort from chills*
2. Obtain doctor's orders for medicated shampoo, if needed.	*Provides scalp treatment*
3. Explain procedure to client and family members.	*Facilitates cooperation*

Action	Rationale
4. Wash hands and organize equipment.	*Reduces microorganism transfer* *Promotes efficiency*
5. Remove pillow from under client's head.	*Prevents soiling of pillow*
6. Place linen saver or plastic bag under shoulders and head of client.	*Avoids wetting of linens*
7. Place towel on top of linen saver.	*Absorbs water overflow*
8. Place shampoo board under client's neck and head.	*Facilitates drainage of water*
9. Position wash basin or trash can in direct line with spout of shampoo board (Fig. 9.4).	*Provides reservoir for water*
10. Fill the pitcher with warm water (105°F to 110°F [40.5°C to 43.3°C]); check with thermometer or test for comfortable temperature with your inner wrist.	*Promotes scalp circulation* *Prevents chilling or skin injury from excess heat*

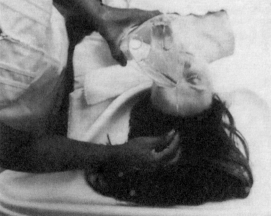

FIGURE 9.4

Action	Rationale
11. Ask client to hold wash-cloth over eyes during procedure.	*Prevents pain from shampoo in eyes*
12. Lower head of bed (infants may be held in lap, with shampoo board under head); place supplies and sufficient water within easy reach.	*Facilitates downward flow of water* *Prevents delays in procedure*
13. Pour warm water over hair and moisten thoroughly.	*Facilitates action of shampoo*
14. Don gloves and place small amount of shampoo in palms; massage shampoo into hair at front and back of head, working shampoo into a lather.	*Provides lather for removal of dirt and oils*
15. Massage lather over entire head in a slow, kneading motion.	*Cleans hair and scalp* *Promotes scalp circulation*
16. Rinse hair by pouring warm water over head several times.	*Removes shampoo and debris*
17. Repeat application of shampoo and massage hair and scalp vigorously with fingers for a longer period of time.	*Promotes thorough cleaning of hair and scalp*
18. Rinse thoroughly using several pitchers of water.	*Removes remaining residue of shampoo*
19. If desired, apply a de-tangling conditioner to hair and leave on for 3 to 5 minutes per package instructions, then rinse thoroughly.	
20. Support client's head in hand and remove shampoo board from bed.	*Clears area for completion of procedure* *Prevents inadvertent injury*
21. Position client's head on the towel and cover head with it.	*Absorbs water from hair*
22. Briskly massage hair with towel.	*Removes water*

Action	Rationale
23. Replace wet towel with dry one and continue to rub hair.	*Promotes drying of hair*
24. Leave hair covered with towel until ready to use dryer.	*Provides for continued absorption of moisture and prevents chilling*
25. Thoroughly dry hands.	*Promotes safety in next steps*
26. Elevate head of bed to desired or prescribed angle.	*Promotes access to hair*
27. Turn on dryer to warm setting; feel heat to be sure it is not excessive.	*Prevents injury from dryer heat*
28. Blow hair until thoroughly dry; concentrate on one section of hair at a time, moving fingers or comb through hair while drying.	*Facilitates thorough drying of hair* *Removes tangles and ensures drying of all parts of hair*
29. Brush or comb hair to remove all tangles.	
30. Oil or spray hair, as desired, and style.	*Facilitates styling*
31. Remove linen saver, linens, and other equipment from bedside.	*Provides clean environment*
32. Assist client to position of comfort, with side rails raised and call light within reach.	*Promotes safety* *Facilitates communication*

Evaluation

Were desired outcomes achieved?

Documentation

The following should be noted on the client's chart:

- When shampoo was done and if completed
- Client's response to activity
- Condition of hair and scalp
- Blood pressure, pulse, and neurostatus before and after procedure, if applicable

SAMPLE DOCUMENTATION

DATE	TIME	
12/3/02	0900	Shampoo performed in bed. Client tolerated supine position and procedure without distress. No scalp irritation noted. Client resting quietly, lying on left side

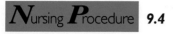

Hair Care Techniques

EQUIPMENT (varies with hair style desired)

- Comb (teeth size varies with coarseness of hair)
- Setting gel and rollers with rolling papers (optional)
- Hair dryer with dome or heat cap (optional)
- Brush
- Hair net (optional)
- Moisturizers, oils (optional)
- Rubber bands, hair pins, clamps
- Nonsterile gloves

Purpose

Improves client's appearance and self-esteem
Increases client's sense of well-being
Stimulates circulation to hair and scalp
Relaxes client
Provides opportunity for therapeutic communication

Assessment

Assessment should focus on the following:

Contraindications to excessive movement and lowering or elevating head (eg, skull fractures, neck injury)
Knowledge of procedure for care
Type of hair care needed or style desired
Activity level and positions of comfort
Allergy to ingredients of hair-care products
Status of hair and scalp (presence of tangles, dandruff, lice, or need for shampoo)

Nursing Diagnoses

The nursing diagnoses may include the following:

Impaired skin (scalp) integrity due to inadequate or excessive hair oils
Risk of self-esteem disturbance due to inability to perform grooming procedures

Risk of infection related to scratching of scalp and head-lice infestation

Outcome Identification and Planning

Desired Outcomes (sample)

Client requests mirror to observe appearance of hair and suggests other self-care activities.
Scalp is warm, with good capillary refill and no irritation.
Hair is clean and comfortable, without tangles.

Special Considerations

DO NOT place braids or knots from rubber bands or hair nets under the head. Check for pressure spots or irritation to the scalp and loosen or release braids in irritated areas.

Geriatric

The elderly client's skin is often thin, dry, and fragile, and the hair is brittle. Use a gentle technique when performing care, avoid tightly binding hair, and assess scalp for irritation frequently.

Pediatric

Pediatric clients can't always express the discomfort caused by hair that is too tightly bound or braided. Bind hair loosely and assess frequently for irritation or discomfort.

 Cost-cutting Tip

Encourage family member to perform hair-care techniques when acceptable to client.

 Transcultural

Clients of different ethnic and cultural origins require shampoos with different frequencies and use different forms of basic hair care. Black clients usually shampoo every 1 to 2 weeks and often add oils or moisturizers; white clients may shampoo daily or every other day to avoid buildup of hair oils. WHEN IN DOUBT REGARDING HAIR PRACTICES, CONSULT CLIENT OR FAMILY MEMBERS.

IMPLEMENTATION

Action	Rationale
1. Explain procedure to client.	*Increases cooperation and assistance*

Action	Rationale
2. Allow 15 to 30 min of uninterrupted time for hair care.	*Avoids rush and possible injury to client*
3. Check and clean comb and brush before beginning (particularly if not client's personal property).	*Prevents passing of head lice or infection to client*
4. Wash hands and organize equipment.	*Reduces microorganism transfer* *Promotes efficiency*
5. Lower side rail.	*Allows easier access*
6. Assist client into position: - Supine position, with head of bed elevated and pillows under back - Bedside chair, if able, with towel on shoulders - Side-lying position, with towel under head, *or* - Prone position	*Allows head to move freely and provides access to hair and towel under head*
7. Don gloves (if broken skin present) and comb hair through with fingers.	*Prevents body-fluid contact* *Assesses degree of tangling*
8. Massage scalp and observe status.	*Increases circulation*
9. Shampoo and dry hair, if needed and allowed (see Procedure 9.3).	*Improves appearance of hair* *Promotes scalp circulation*
10. Brush hair to remove as many tangles as possible: - Hold hair with one hand and brush with the other (Fig. 9.5). - If hair is coarse and kinky, processed for curls, or naturally curly, a comb may be more effective for removing tangles.	*Decreases discomfort of hair care*
11. Divide hair into sections with comb and fingers.	*Provides for easier handling*
12. Comb one section through at a time: - Gently and slowly comb tangles loose from scalp.	*Removes tangles*

Action	Rationale

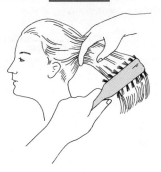

FIGURE 9.5

- Hold hair section stable (near the scalp) with one hand.
- Comb through hair with other hand (as when brushing).

Prevents pulling during combing
Decreases pain to client

13. Keep hair loose at the scalp.

Counteracts pulling from comb

Evaluation

Were desired outcomes achieved?

Documentation

The following should be noted on the client's chart:

- Response to hair care
- Condition of hair and scalp
- Blood pressure, pulse, and neurostatus before and after procedure, if applicable

SAMPLE DOCUMENTATION

DATE	TIME	
12/3/02	1300	Hair combed with assistance of client. Client took active interest in grooming. Makeup applied by client. Scalp warm, with brisk capillary refill.

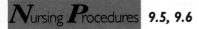

 Oral Care Techniques (9.5)

 Denture Care Techniques (9.6)

EQUIPMENT

- Soft toothbrush (or denture brush for dentures)
- Toothpaste
- Toothettes or swabs
- Emesis basin
- Nonsterile gloves
- Towel or linen saver and washcloth
- Cup of warm water
- Mouthwash (alcohol free)
- Denture cream
- Denture cup
- Denture cleanser
- Dental floss (optional)
- Suction and catheter (if client is unconscious)

Purpose

Decreases microorganisms in mouth and on teeth or dentures
Decreases cavities and mouth disease
Decreases buildup of food residue on teeth or dentures
Improves appetite and taste of food
Facilitates comfort
Stimulates circulation to oral tissues, tongue, and gums
Improves appearance and self-esteem

Assessment

Assessment should focus on the following:

Client's desire and need for oral care
Client's usual routine for oral hygiene (method, frequency)
Client's knowledge of purpose and procedure
Client's ability to understand and follow instructions (eg, to expectorate instead of swallowing mouthwash and toothpaste)
Presence of dentures
Status of palate, floor of mouth, throat, cheeks, tongue, gums and teeth (eg, presence of lesions, cavities)

Nursing Diagnoses

The nursing diagnoses may include the following:

Altered oral mucous membranes related to inadequate denture cleaning

Outcome Identification and Planning

Desired Outcomes (sample)

Oral intake increased from 10% to 50%.
Mucous membranes and lips are intact.
Oral passage and teeth or dentures are clean.

Special Considerations

Clients on anticoagulation therapy will require use of a soft toothbrush or Toothette only.
Clients with oral lesions or sensitive oral tissues may require dilution of mouthwash.

Cost-cutting Tip

Encourage client to perform as much oral care as possible and encourage family members to assist, when necessary.

IMPLEMENTATION

Action	Rationale

Procedure 9.5 Oral Care Techniques

Action	Rationale
1. Wash hands and organize equipment.	*Reduces microorganism transfer* *Promotes efficiency*
2. Provide explanation of procedure to client.	*Reduces anxiety* *Promotes compliance*
3. Lower side rail and position client in one of the following positions:	*Promotes drainage of mouthwash from mouth*
- Supine at an angle greater than 45 degrees, if not contraindicated, *or*	*Decreases risk of aspiration*
- Side-lying, *or*	
- Prone with head turned to side	
4. Don gloves.	*Prevents exposure to body fluids*

Action	Rationale
5. Drape towel under client's neck and assist client to rinse mouth with water.	*Catches secretions* *Facilitates removal of secretions* *Facilitates self-care*
6. Assist client in brushing teeth: - Provide a glass of water, toothbrush and toothpaste. - Moisten toothbrush with water. - Apply toothpaste to brush. - Allow client to brush teeth, if able.	
7. **If client is unable to perform own care:** - Prepare toothbrush as in step 6. - Apply brush to back teeth and brush inside, top, and outside of teeth (brush from back to front, using an up-and-down motion) (Fig. 9.6). - Repeat these steps, brushing teeth on opposite side of mouth. - Allow client to expectorate or suction excess secretions. - Instruct client to clench teeth together, or grasp the mandible and press lower teeth to upper teeth; brush outside of front teeth and side/back teeth. - Open mouth and brush top and insides of teeth.	*Permits cleaning back and sides of teeth* *Removes toothpaste and oral secretions* *Exposes front teeth for brushing*

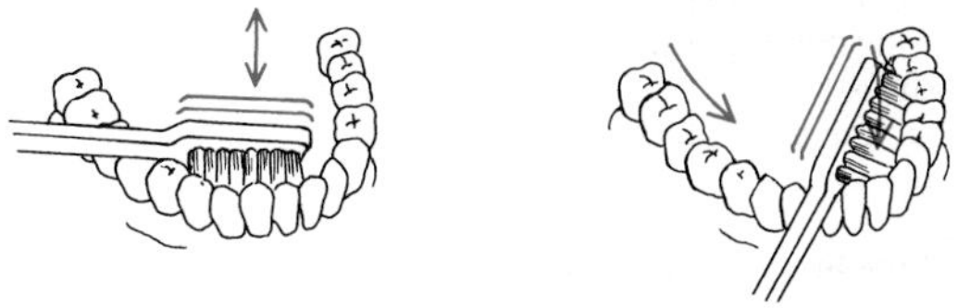

FIGURE 9.6

Action	Rationale
- Rinse toothbrush and brush tongue.	
- Rinse toothbrush and brush teeth again.	*Removes residual toothpaste*
- If use of dental floss is desired, provide care at this time.	*Cleans between teeth*
8. Assist client in cleansing oral cavity:	
- Provide mouthwash-soaked Toothette.	*Freshens mouth*
- Encourage client to swab inner cheeks, lips, tongue, and gums, or perform these actions for client, if needed.	*Decreases microorganism growth in mouth*
- Instruct client to rinse with mouthwash and expectorate, or irrigate mouth with mouthwash and suction excess fluid.	
- Rinse with water.	
- Have client expectorate or suction excess.	
9. **If working with an unconscious client:**	
- Don gloves.	*Reduces microorganism transfer*
- Brush teeth with tooth-brush and toothpaste, as in step 7.	
- Irrigate mouth with small amounts of water, suctioning constantly.	*Removes water and avoids pooling*
- Swab mouth with Toothette moistened with mouthwash.	
- Beginning with inside of cheeks and lips, proceed to swab tongue and gums. Rinse.	
- Suction excess toothpaste, mouthwash, and secretions.	
- Wipe lips with wet wash-cloth.	

Action	Rationale

- Apply petroleum jelly or mineral oil to lips.

10. Discard gloves and soiled materials; restore supplies in proper place. — *Promotes clean environment*

11. Position client for comfort with call button within reach. — *Promotes safety, comfort, and communication*

Procedure 9.6 Denture Care Techniques

1. Wash hands and organize supplies. — *Reduces microorganism transfer* / *Promotes efficiency*

2. Explain procedure to client and encourage participation, if able. — *Promotes compliance*

3. Don gloves. — *Prevents contact with saliva*

4. Assist client with denture removal:
   - Half fill denture cup with cool water.
   - Put denture cleanser into water per instructions.
   - Instruct client to hold water in mouth and "float" dentures loose. — *Prevents breaking of dentures when removing*
   - Allow client to remove dentures, or gently rock dentures back and forth until free from gums. — *Breaks seal created with dentures*
   - Lift bottom dentures up to remove, pull top dentures down. — *Prevents undue pressure and injury to oral membranes*
   - Place dentures in denture cup to soak. — *Facilitates removal of microorganisms*

5. Assist client with cleansing of oral cavity: — *Facilitates removal of microorganisms*
   - Provide mouthwash-soaked Toothette.
   - Encourage client to swab inner cheeks, lips, tongue, and gums.
   - Instruct client to swirl mouthwash in mouth and expectorate.
   - Follow with water, as desired.

Action	Rationale

6. Cleanse dentures:
  - Use same procedure as when brushing teeth but may use denture cleaner (see Procedure 9.5).
  - Thoroughly rinse paste from dentures with cool water.	

7. Reinsert dentures:
  - Apply denture cream to gum side of denture plate.
  - Insert upper plate and press firmly to gums.
  - Repeat with lower plate.
  - Instruct client to swirl mouthwash in mouth, expectorate, and rinse with water.
	Facilitates intake of solid foods

8. Apply petroleum jelly or mineral oil to client's lips.	*Maintains skin integrity of lips*
9. Remove towel from client's chest.	
10. Discard gloves and soiled materials.	*Maintains clean environment*
11. Position client for comfort, with side rails raised and call button within reach.	*Promotes comfort, safety, and communication*
12. Place personal hygiene items in client's drawer or on bedside table.	*Provides an orderly environment*

Evaluation

Were desired outcomes achieved?

Documentation

The following should be noted on the client's chart:

- Amount of care done by client
- Client's response to activity
- Condition of oral cavity and lips

SAMPLE DOCUMENTATION

DATE	TIME	
12/3/02	1000	Care of dentures performed with assistance of client. Client fatigued after brushing back teeth but expressed interest in grooming activity. Makeup applied by client after rest period. Mucous membranes moist. Lips moist, skin intact.

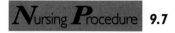

Contacts and Artificial Eye Care Techniques

 EQUIPMENT

- Container for lenses or prosthesis
- Saline solution
- Nonsterile gloves

Purpose

Prevents corneal damage
If prosthesis, prevents damage to tissue

Assessment

Assessment should focus on the following:

Client/family ability to understand and perform procedure

Outcome Identification and Planning

Desired Outcomes (sample)

Tissues of eye and socket will be maintained.
Client/caregiver will demonstrate ability to perform procedure.

Special Considerations

If at all possible, have the client perform the procedure as per the client's routine. If needed, make suggestions as to how to improve techniques.

Home Health

This can be a difficult procedure for the nurse to perform in the home setting. If the client and/or family are unable to remove a prosthesis or contact lens, and the nurse has any doubt about his or her ability to perform the procedure, every attempt should be made to arrange a rapid referral to an ophthalmologist.

IMPLEMENTATION

Action	Rationale
1. Assemble and organize supplies.	*Promotes efficiency*
2. Teach, perform, or observe good handwashing.	*Reduces microorganism transfer*
3. Discuss procedure with client and encourage participation, if able, and assist as client requires or desires.	*Promotes compliance*
4. If anyone other than client is performing procedure, don gloves.	*Prevents contact with bodily fluids*
5. If wearing gloves, rinse with saline.	*Removes powder from gloves*
6. Position client in recumbent position, stand on right side to remove right contact or prosthesis.	*Improves access to eye*
7. Position left thumb on upper eyelid, right thumb on lower eyelid, and gently pull apart.	*Improves visualization*
8. If lens is visible, proceed. If lens cannot be seen, arrange for ophthalmologist to see client.	*Prevents probing and possible damage to the eye*
9. For hard lens or prosthesis, gently open the eye beyond the edges of the lens or prosthesis, and apply gentle pressure on the eyeball with the right thumb.	*Releases the suction holding the lens or prosthesis in*
10. Gently slide the lens or prosthesis out.	
11. If soft lens, perform steps 1 through 7. Once lens is seen, gently pinch between thumb and forefinger and remove.	
12. Inspect the eye tissues for any damage.	
13. Place lenses or prosthesis in appropriate container and perform cleaning.	*Reduces transmission of microorganisms* *Maintains clean lens or prosthesis*

Action	Rationale

14. If necessary, repeat steps for left eye.
15. Replace prosthesis or lens, if needed or desired.
16. Dispose of soiled gloves appropriately; wash hands.

Evaluation

Were desired outcomes achieved?

DOCUMENTATION

The following should be noted on the client's chart:

- Condition of eye and surrounding tissue
- Ability of client or caregiver to properly perform procedure

SAMPLE DOCUMENTATION

DATE	TIME	
9/6/02	1100	Left eye prosthesis removed. Eye socket cleaned as per physician's order and prosthesis replaced. Client instructed on procedure, including handwashing before and after procedure, cleaning of eye socket, storage and cleaning of prosthesis. Verbalized understanding of procedure.

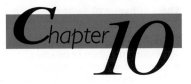

*C*hapter *10*

Biologic Safety Needs

OVERVIEW

▶ The chain of infection requires that six links be present:
  - Infectious agent in sufficient amount to cause an infection
  - Place for the agent to multiply and grow
  - Point at which the agent can exit the growth area
  - Method of transportation from the growth area to other sites
  - Available access or entrance to another site
  - Susceptible host or medium for agent growth
▶ The aim of all isolation procedures (standard precautions as well as disease-specific, category-specific, or body-substance isolation) is to decrease exposure to and the spread of

microorganisms and disease; all actions are aimed at breaking the chain of infection by eliminating the links.

▶ Gloves should be worn whenever exposure to body secretions is likely. ALWAYS WEAR GLOVES WHEN EMPTYING DRAINAGE CONTAINERS.

▶ If the sterility of materials, gloves, or gowns is in doubt, treat them as nonsterile.

▶ Some major nursing diagnostic labels related to biologic safety are risk for infection, impaired tissue integrity, risk of altered biologic safety, acute pain knowledge deficit, and anxiety.

▶ Unlicensed assistive personnel should be trained in safety protocols that prevent exposure to microorganisms such as application of gowns and gloves, use of isolation protocols, and disposal of wastes. In general, procedures such as dressing changes are performed by the registered or licensed practical nurse. For less complex dressings, some agencies train special personnel to assist with the dressing change. ALL ASSESSMENT AND THE MANAGEMENT OF COMPLEX DRESSING CHANGES AND WOUND MANAGEMENT ARE THE RESPONSIBILITY OF THE LICENSED NURSE. See agency policy concerning delegation of specific procedures listed in this chapter to unlicensed assistive personnel.

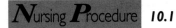

 Venipuncture for Blood Specimen

EQUIPMENT

- Nonsterile gloves
- Alcohol pads
- Tourniquet (or blood pressure cuff)
- Povidone-iodine (Betadine) pad (optional)

Vacutainer Method
- Blood-collecting device or vacutainer holder with double-point needle
- Appropriately colored test tube or vacutainer (consult agency laboratory manual):
  - Striped (red/black, green/black, or other), used for chemical or drug studies and containing a preservative
  - Solid red, used for blood bank
  - Purple, used for complete blood count
  - Blue or lavender, used for coagulation
- Blood culture bottle(s) (optional)

Syringe Method
- Sterile needles
  - 20 or 21 gauge
  or
  - Scalp vein (butterfly) catheter
- Sterile syringe of appropriate size

Purpose

Provides blood specimen for analysis

Assessment

Assessment should focus on the following:

Type of lab test ordered
Time for which test is ordered
Adequacy of client preparation (eg, fasting state, medication withheld or given)
Client's ability to cooperate

Nursing Diagnoses

The nursing diagnoses may include the following:

Altered level of consciousness: lethargy related to drug overdose
Risk of infection related to incision site

Outcome Identification and Planning

Desired Outcomes (sample)

Blood is drawn with minimal discomfort to client.
Blood is placed in appropriate tubes and sent to lab.

Special Considerations

Do not perform venipuncture on arm.

Geriatric

The elderly often have veins that appear large and dilated. Use a
blood pressure cuff instead of a tourniquet to prevent excessive
stress on the vessel and subsequent collapse or rupture.

Pediatric

Enlist an assistant to restrain a child during venipuncture to prevent injury from resistance.
Use a butterfly catheter with syringe to avoid excessive suction on
the vein.

Home Health

A blood pressure cuff may be used instead of a tourniquet (maintain a pressure greater than the client's diastolic pressure).

Delegation

Blood drawing should not be delegated to unlicensed assistive
personnel, unless specific training is completed through the
agency. However, as a general rule, this procedure is not delegated to unlicensed assistive personnel in nursing. Consult
agency policy.

IMPLEMENTATION

Action	Rationale
1. Wash hands and organize equipment; explain procedure and cooperation required to client.	*Reduces microorganism transfer* *Promotes efficiency* *Promotes relaxation and compliance*

Action	Rationale
2. Lower side rail and assist client into a semi-Fowler's position; raise bed to high position.	*Provides easier access to veins* *Promotes comfort during procedure* *Facilitates good body mechanics*
3. Open several alcohol and Povidone pads.	*Provides fast access to cleaning supplies*
4. Screw needle into blood collection device, if used (Fig. 10.1).	
5. Place towel under extremity.	*Prevents soiling of linens*
6. Locate largest, most distal vein (see Procedure 5.2); place tourniquet on extremity 2 to 6 inches (5–15 cm) above venipuncture site or inflate blood pressure cuff.	*If insertion attempt fails, vein can be entered at a higher point* *Restricts blood flow, distending vein*
7. Don gloves.	*Reduces microorganism transfer*
8. Clean vein area, beginning at the vein and circling outward to a 2-inch diameter.	*Maintains asepsis*
9. Encourage client to take slow, deep breaths as you begin.	*Facilitates relaxation*
10. Remove cap from needle and hold skin taut with one hand while holding syringe or vacutainer	*Stabilizes vein and prevents skin from moving during insertion*

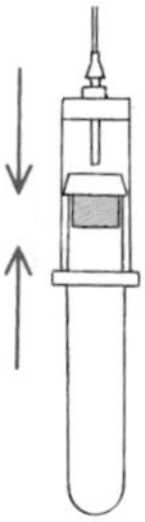

FIGURE 10.1

Action	Rationale
holder with other hand (with butterfly catheter, pinch "wings" together).	*Decreases pain during needle insertion*
11. Maintaining needle sterility, insert needle, bevel up, into the straightest section of vein; puncture skin at a 15- to 30-degree angle.	*Provides clear area for puncture* *Provides for downward movement toward vein*
12. When needle has entered skin, lower needle until almost parallel with skin.	*Decreases risk of penetration of both walls of the vein*
13. Following path of vein, insert needle into wall of vein.	
14. Watch for backflow of blood (not noted with vacutainer); push needle slightly further into vein.	*Indicates that needle has pierced vein wall*
15. Gently pull back syringe plunger until adequate amount of blood is obtained.	
16. If using blood collection device, put tube or blood culture bottle into device and push in until needle punctures rubber stopper and blood is pulled into tube by vacuum; keep tube in device until it is three fourths full or until culture medium is blood-colored; remove tube and replace with new tube if additional specimens are needed.	*Connects needle with tube* *Allows suction in tube to pull blood into tube*
17. Place alcohol pad or cotton ball over needle insertion site and remove needle from vein while applying pressure with pad or cotton ball.	*Facilitates sealing of vein* *Decreases bleeding from site*

Action	Rationale
18. Hold pressure for 2 to 3 min (5–10 min if client is on anticoagulant therapy); check for bleeding and apply pressure until bleeding has stopped.	*Facilitates clotting*
19. Position client for comfort with call light within reach.	*Promotes comfort and communication*
20. Attach properly completed identification label to each tube, affix requisition, and send to lab.	*Tests should be performed properly* *Incorrect labeling can cause diagnostic error*
21. Dispose of and store equipment properly (unscrew needle from device and save tube holder portion).	*Maintains clean and organized environment*
22. Remove gloves and wash hands.	*Reduces microorganism transfer*

Evaluation

Were desired outcomes achieved?

Documentation

The following should be noted on the client's chart:

- Time blood is drawn
- Test to be run on specimen
- Client's tolerance to procedure
- Status of skin (eg, bruising, excessive bleeding)

SAMPLE DOCUMENTATION

DATE	TIME	
1/2/02	1500	Blood drawn for complete blood count and electrolytes. Specimen sent to laboratory. Needle insertion site intact. Procedure tolerated well.

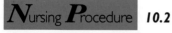
 Sterile and Nonsterile Dressing Change

EQUIPMENT

- Sterile dressing tray (forceps, scissors, gauze pads [optional])
- Sterile gauze dressing pads (2 × 2-inch, 4 × 4-inch, or surgical [ABD] pads, depending on drainage and size of area to be covered), or transparent dressing
- Sterile bowl
- 2-inch tape or Montgomery straps (paper tape, if allergic to others)
- Sterile gloves (for sterile dressing change)
- Nonsterile gloves
- Towel or linen-saver pad
- Cotton balls and cotton-tipped swabs (optional)
- Sterile irrigation saline or sterile water
- Cleaning solution as ordered
- Bacteriostatic ointment
- Overbed table or bedside stand
- Trash bag

Purpose

Removes accumulated secretions and dead tissue from wound or incision site

Decreases microorganism growth on wound or incision site

Promotes wound healing

Assessment

Assessment should focus on the following:

Doctor's orders regarding type of dressing change, procedure, and frequency of change

Type and location of wound or incision

Time of last pain medication

Allergies to tape or solution used for cleaning

Nursing Diagnoses

The nursing diagnoses may include the following:

Impaired tissue integrity related to pressure ulcer
Risk of infection related to impaired skin integrity

Outcome Identification and Planning

Desired Outcome (sample)
Wound healing noted with no signs of infection.

Special Considerations
Dressing changes are often painful. Assess pain needs and medicate client 30 min before beginning the procedure.

Pediatric and Geriatric

Clients are often immunosuppressed and have decreased resistance; strict asepsis is needed to minimize exposure to microorganisms.

Home Health

Newspaper should be used to cover the table surface before arranging the work field. Animals in the home should be barred from the area during the procedure.

Delegation

In general, procedures such as dressing changes are performed by the registered or licensed practical nurse. For less complex dressings, some agencies train special personnel to assist with the dressing change. ALL ASSESSMENT AND THE MANAGEMENT OF COMPLEX DRESSING CHANGES AND WOUND MANAGEMENT ARE THE RESPONSIBILITY OF THE LICENSED NURSE. See agency policy concerning delegation of specific procedures listed in this chapter to unlicensed assistive personnel.

IMPLEMENTATION

Action	Rationale
1. Wash hands and organize equipment.	*Reduces microorganism transfer* *Promotes efficiency*
2. Explain procedure and assistance needed to client.	*Decreases anxiety* *Promotes cooperation*

Action	Rationale
3. Assess client's pain level and wait for medication to take effect before beginning.	*Decreases discomfort of dressing change*
4. Place bedside table close to area being dressed.	*Facilitates management of sterile field and supplies*
5. Prepare supplies:	
- Place supplies on bedside table.	*Promotes swift dressing change*
- Tape trash bag to side of table.	*Facilitates easy disposal of contaminated waste*
- Open sterile gloves and use inside of glove package as sterile field.	*Facilitates use of supplies without contamination*
- Open gauze-pad packages and drop several onto sterile field; leave some pads in open packages if in plastic container (if not, place some pads into sterile bowl).	*Permits wetting of some pads*
- Open dressing tray and bowl.	
- Open liquids and pour saline on two gauze pads and pour ordered cleaning solution on four gauze pads (more if wet-to-dry dressing).	*Prevents transmission of organisms from table to supplies*
- Place several sterile cotton-tipped swabs and cotton balls on sterile field (use gauze instead if staples are present because cotton may catch on edges of staples).	
6. Don nonsterile gloves.	
7. Place towel or pad under wound area.	
8. Loosen tape by pulling toward the wound and remove soiled dressing (note appearance of dressing and wound).	*Permits observation of site and exposes site for cleaning*

Action	Rationale

SOAK DRESSING WITH
SALINE IF IT ADHERES
TO WOUND, THEN
GENTLY PULL FREE.
9. Place dressing in trash bag.
10. Discard gloves and wash
hands.

Sterile Dressing Change
11. Don sterile gloves and
face mask (optional).
12. Pick up saline-soaked
dressing pad with forceps
and form a large swab.
13. Cleanse away debris and   *Prevents contamination of*
drainage from wound,   *wound from organisms on*
moving from center   *skin surface*
outward and using a new   *Maintains sterility of supplies*
pad for each area cleaned
(Fig. 10.2); discard old
pads away from sterile
supplies.
14. Wipe wound with pads   *Reduces microorganism transfer*
soaked with ordered
cleansing solution, moving *Avoids cross-contamination*
from center of wound
outward; discard forceps.
15. Assess need for frequent *Prevents infection due to soiled*
(every 4–6 h) dressing   *dressings*
changes and effect of tape *Prevents skin injury*
on skin, and apply

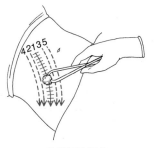

FIGURE 10.2

Action	Rationale

Montgomery straps to hold dressing:
- Place 8-inch strip of tape on table, sticky side up, and cover with 4-inch strip of tape, sticky side down.
- Place sticky side of tape on client, with nonsticky end reaching across half of wound area.
- Repeat process on other side of wound; if wound is long, apply straps to upper and lower portions.
- Place dressings over wound and secure by pinning, banding, or tying Montgomery straps together (the tying method may be used when frequent dressing changes are anticipated) (Fig. 10.3).

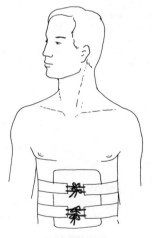

FIGURE 10.3

Action	Rationale
16. Dress the wound or incision in the following manner: - Pick up dressing pads by edge saline-soaked, if wet-to-dry dressing). - Place pads over wound or incision site until site is totally covered. - Cover with surgical pad (if wet-to-dry). - Secure dressing with tape along edges or use Montgomery straps.	*Prevents contamination of dressing or wound*
17. Write the date and time of dressing change on a strip of tape and place tape across dressing.	*Indicates last dressing change and need for next change within 24 to 48 h*
18. Dispose of gloves and materials and store supplies appropriately.	*Decreases spread of micro-organisms* *Maintains organized environment*
19. Position client for comfort with call light within reach.	*Facilitates comfort and communication*
20. Wash hands.	*Decreases spread of micro-organisms*

Clean Dressing Change

21. Follow steps 11 to 18 but forceps and gloves need not be sterile.	*Allows handling of dressing without sterile instruments*

Evaluation

Were desired outcomes achieved?

Documentation

The following should be noted on the client's chart:

- Location and type of wound or incision
- Status of previous dressing
- Status of the wound/incision site
- Solution and medications applied to wound
- Client teaching done
- Client's tolerance of procedure

SAMPLE DOCUMENTATION

DATE	TIME	
1/12/02	0600	Abdominal wound saturated with serous drainage. Wound bed is red with erythema around wound edges. Wound cleansed with normal saline, dressed with saline-moistened 4 × 4 gauze and covered with ABD pad secured with 2-inch paper tape.

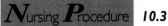

 Blood Glucose Testing

EQUIPMENT

- Blood glucose machine (optional)
- Chemical strips for blood glucose with color chart (on container or insert)
- Nonsterile gloves
- Lancets (or 19- or 21-gauge needle)
- Autoclix or lancet injector (optional)
- Cotton balls
- Alcohol pads (or bottle of alcohol)
- Watch with second hand or stop watch
- Needle disposal unit

Purpose

Determines level of glucose in blood
Promotes stricter blood glucose regulation

Assessment

Assessment should focus on the following:

Doctor's orders for frequency and type of glucose testing and sliding scale for insulin coverage
Client's knowledge of procedure and of diabetic self-care
Response to previous testing

Nursing Diagnoses

The nursing diagnoses may include the following:

Self-care knowledge deficit related to newly diagnosed diabetes

Outcome Identification and Planning

Desired Outcomes (sample)
Blood glucose elevation is noted and treated promptly per sliding scale.
Blood glucose is maintained within acceptable range.

Special Considerations

An ideal time for client teaching is during the blood glucose testing procedure.

Geriatric

If vision disturbances are present, use of a glucose-monitoring
machine may be preferable to a visual-comparison chart.

Pediatric

Consider developmental stage and assess the child's ability to understand and perform the procedure. For reinforcement of
teaching, include family members in teaching.

Home Health

An egg timer may be used to time the reaction of the blood-glu-
cose testing procedure.

Delegation

In most areas, this procedure may be delegated to unlicensed assistive personnel; however, the individual must have had specific training for the procedure on the specific machine being
used for glucose testing. Assistive personnel should be instructed to report all results and indicators of machine mal-
function immediately to avoid unnecessary oversights. The
nurse must check test results and treat patient using sliding
scale, if ordered. Any unusually high or low readings should be
verified by the nurse.

IMPLEMENTATION

Action	Rationale
1. Wash hands and organize equipment.	*Reduces microorganism transfer* *Promotes efficiency*
2. Explain procedure to client and inquire about preference of finger and use of lancet injector.	*Facilitates cooperation and promotes sense of involvement in and control of own care*
3. Calibrate glucose machine, if used: - Turn machine on. - Compare number/code on machine or strip in machine with number on bottle of chemical strips (Fig. 10.4).	

Action	Rationale

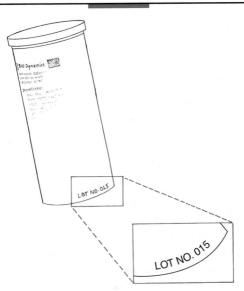

FIGURE 10.4

- Perform procedures to ready machine for operation; consult user's manual for steps and readiness indicator.
- Machine accuracy should be validated daily, or per laboratory policy, with sample low- and high-glucose solutions to ensure accuracy.

4. Remove chemical strip from container and place it in the glucose testing machine (according to manufacturer's instructions).

Prevents delay
Prevents damage to indicator
Prepares machine for reading

5. Load lancet in injector, if used, and set trigger.

Prepares injector to push lancet into finger

6. Don gloves.

Prevents exposure to blood

Action	Rationale
7. Hold chosen finger down and squeeze gently from lower digits to fingertip, or wrap finger in warm, wet cloth for 30 sec or longer. (If using arm lancet device, dangle arm for about 1 min.)	*Facilitates flow of blood to finger for easy sampling* *Facilitates blood flow to injection area*
8. Wipe intended puncture site with alcohol pad.	*Removes dirt and skin oils* *Decreases microorganisms*
9. Place injector against side of finger (where there are fewer nerve endings) and release trigger, or stick side of finger with lancet or needle using a darting motion. (If using arm lancet device, puncture arm site area with lancet device.)	*Obtains a large drop of blood with minimal pain stimulation*
10. Hold chemical strip under puncture site and squeeze gently until drop of blood is large enough to drop onto strip and cover indicator squares. If using arm lancet devices, hold strip close to blood drop after appropriate amount of blood (according to manufacturer's instructions) has formed.	*Ensures that indicator squares are covered with blood* *Prevents uneven exposure of indicators*
11. Push timer button on machine as soon as blood has covered indicator squares, or note position of second hand on watch. *Note:* Some machines automatically begin timing and require no action to start timing once blood makes contact with strip.	*Determines when to remove excess blood from strip and when to read color change*
12. Apply pressure to puncture site until bleeding stops (or have client do so) and place lancet in needle disposal unit.	

Action	Rationale
13. When timer or watch indicates that appropriate number of seconds have passed, perform reading of glucose value. If manual or machine indicates, remove excess blood from strip.	*Removes blood cells and facilitates accurate reading*
14. Put strip inside (or insert into) machine with indicator patch facing reading window (see manufacturer's instructions).	*Facilitates accurate reading*
15. Alternatively, compare colors on strip with color chart, (Fig. 10.5), if comparison chart is available.	

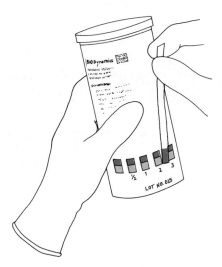

FIGURE 10.5

Action	Rationale
16. Discard soiled materials and gloves in proper container.	*Prevents exposure to blood-soiled materials*
17. Record results on glucose flow sheet and administer insulin, if indicated.	*Maintains record of glucose levels and insulin coverage*
18. Position client for comfort, with call light within reach.	*Promotes comfort and communication*

Evaluation

Were desired outcomes achieved?

Documentation

The following should be noted on the client's chart:
- Method of glucose testing
- Level of glucose
- Insulin coverage provided and route
- Teaching done and demonstration of client understanding, if necessary

SAMPLE DOCUMENTATION

DATE	TIME	
1/2/02	1200	Fingerstick blood glucose testing performed by client after teaching and demonstration by nurse. Client's technique good, with good asepsis noted. Results showed 256 mg glucose/dl. Five (5) units regular human insulin given in abdominal area by client with good technique.

Sterile Gown Application (10.4)

Sterile Glove Application (10.5)

📇 EQUIPMENT

- Sterile gown
- Sterile gloves
- Bedside table

Purpose

Preserves sterile field during sterile procedure

Assessment

Assessment should focus on the following:

Client's ability to cooperate and not contaminate sterile gown or gloves

Nursing Diagnoses

The nursing diagnoses may include the following:

Risk of infection related to incision site

Outcome Identification and Planning

Desired Outcome (sample)
Procedure is performed with no apparent exposure to microorganisms.

Special Consideration
Pediatric
If a child is restless or too young to understand the importance of maintaining a sterile field, restrain the child's arms and legs

527

with linen or soft restraints during the medical procedure. Encourage a parent to sit at child's bedside during the procedure, if possible.

IMPLEMENTATION

Action	Rationale

Procedure 10.4 Sterile Gown Application

1. Wash hands and organize equipment; apply mask, if needed; enlist assistant to tie gown.

   Reduces microorganism transfer
   Promotes efficiency

2. Remove sterile gown package from outer cover and open inner covering to expose sterile gown; place on bedside table, touching only outsides of covering. Spread covering over table; open outer glove package and slide inside glove cover onto sterile field.

   Maintains sterility of gown

   Provides sterile field
   Places gloves in convenient location and on sterile field

3. Remove gown from field, grasping inside of gown and gently shaking to loosen folds; hold gown with inside facing you (Fig. 10.6).

   Prepares gown for application

4. Place both arms inside gown at the same time and stretch outward until hands reach edge of sleeves; don sterile gloves (see Procedure 10.5).

   Preserves sterility of gown

5. Have assistant pull tie from back of gown and fasten to inside tie; have assistant pull outside tie around with sterile tongs or sterile gloves. Grasp tie, pull around to front of gown, and secure to front tie.

   Secures gown without contamination of outer portion

   Secures gown

6. IF GLOVE OR GOWN BECOMES CONTAMINATED, DISCARD AND REPLACE WITH STERILE GARB.

Action	Rationale

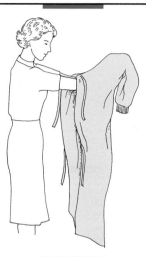

FIGURE 10.6

Procedure 10.5 Sterile Glove Application

1. Don gown, if needed; otherwise, open glove package, place on bedside table, and remove inner glove covering; open inner package, using sterile technique, and expose gloves.
2. Pick up one glove by cuff and slip fingers of other hand into glove (keep gown sleeve inside glove if applicable); pull glove over hand and sleeve.
3. Place gloved hand inside cuff of remaining glove and lift slightly; slide other hand into glove and pull cuff over hand, wrist, and sleeve of gown, if applicable (Fig. 10.7).

Facilitates placing glove on hand without contaminating glove or gloved hand

Stabilizes gown sleeve and creates continuous sterile hand-to-arm connection

Action	Rationale

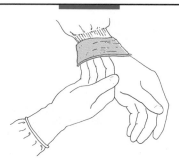

FIGURE 10.7

DO NOT TOUCH SKIN
WITH GLOVED HAND.

4. Pull gloves securely over
   fingers and adjust for fit,
   using one hand to fix the
   other.

*Places fingers deeply into gloves
while maintaining sterility*

5. Proceed to sterile field,
   maintaining hands above
   waist; do not touch non-
   sterile items. IF GLOVE OR
   GOWN BECOMES
   CONTAMINATED,
   DISCARD AND REPLACE
   WITH STERILE GARB.

Prevents contamination of gloves

Evaluation

Were desired outcomes achieved?

Documentation

The following should be noted on the client's chart:

- Sterile procedure performed
- Sterile garments used

SAMPLE DOCUMENTATION

DATE	TIME	
1/2/02	1200	Temporary pacemaker inserted by Dr. Jones, with sterile technique used. Client tolerated procedure with no reports of unusual discomfort.

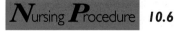

*N*ursing *P*rocedure 10.6

Principles of Medical Asepsis

EQUIPMENT

- Soap and warm running water
- Nonsterile gloves
- Clean gown
- Mask
- Waste disposal materials: trash can, bags (isolation bags optional)
- Isolation stickers
- Linen bags
- Specimen bags, as needed

Purpose

Prevents the growth and spread of pathogenic microorganisms to one individual from another individual or from the environment

Assessment

Assessment should focus on the following:

Data from medical history and physical or diagnostic studies indicating susceptibility to or presence of infection (fever, cloudy urine, positive culture, decreased white blood count, history of immunosuppression or steroid intake)
Doctor's orders or agency policy regarding isolation procedures
Client's or nurse's allergy to soap or bacteriostatic solutions
Client's assignment (ward, double or single room)
Client's knowledge of principles of asepsis
Ability of client to cooperate and not contaminate sterile field

Nursing Diagnoses

The nursing diagnoses may include the following:

Risk of altered biologic safety: infection related to abdominal abscess
Risk of infection related to immunosuppressive therapy for renal transplant

Outcome Identification and Planning

Desired Outcomes (sample)

Client shows no signs of infection or of additional infection.
Medical procedures are performed with no evidence of exposure
to microorganisms.

Special Consideration

Keep your fingernails short and filed. Dirt and secretions that
lodge under fingernails contain microorganisms. Long fingernails can scratch client's skin.

Geriatric

If a client is disoriented and restless, restrain the client during procedures that require maintenance of sterile or clean materials.

Pediatric

If a child is restless or too young to understand the importance of
maintaining a sterile field, restrain the child with linen or soft
restraints during the medical procedure.

Home Health

Bar pets from the room in which a medical procedure is being performed.

Most procedures are performed with clean rather than sterile
technique.

IMPLEMENTATION

Action	Rationale

Hand Washing—Medical

1. Perform 2- to 4-minute
hand washing:

Action	Rationale
	Reduces microorganisms on hands
- Remove rings (often may retain wedding band) and chipped nail polish; move watch to position high on wrist.	*Removes sources that harbor and promote growth of micro-organisms*
- Wet hands from wrist to fingertips under flowing water.	*Cleans from least to most dirty* *Aids in removal of micro-organisms*
- Keep hands and forearms lower than elbows during washing.	*Hands are the most contami-nated parts to be washed* *Water flows from least to most contaminated area*

Action	Rationale
- Place soap, preferably bacteriostatic, on hands and rub vigorously for 15 to 30 sec, massaging all skin areas, joints, fingernails, between fingers, and so forth; slide ring up and down while rubbing fingers (if unable to remove).	*Creates friction to remove organisms* *Permits cleaning around and under ring*
- Rinse hands from fingers to wrist under flow of water.	*Washes dirt and organisms from cleanest to least clean area*
- Repeat soaping, rubbing, and rinsing until hands are clean.	
- Dry hands with paper towel, moving from fingers to wrist to forearm.	*Dries hands from cleanest to least clean area*
- Turn off faucet with paper towel.	*Prevents recontamination of hand*
2. Management of contaminated materials:	
- Don gloves when contact with body fluids or infected area is possible. Use specimen bags for any specimens collected.	*Prevents contamination of hands* *Prevents contact with secretions* *Prevents exposure to specimens*
- Don mask if organism can be transmitted by airborne route through contact with mucous membranes.	*Prevents exposure to airborne microorganisms or projectile body fluids*
- Don gown if contact with body secretions or contaminated area is likely, if client has highly contagious condition, or if client is immunosuppressed.	*Avoids contact with potentially infectious material* *Avoids spread of infection* *Protects client from exposure to microorganisms*
- Place disposable contaminated materials in bag before leaving bedside; place in dirty utility room or send for waste disposal personnel; or place in isolation bag or mark "Isolation" on bag; use	*Provides added protection against exposure to body fluids or infectious materials* *Alerts housekeeping department to dispose of materials properly*

Action	Rationale
double bagging, if agency policy.	
- Reusable items should be bagged, labeled "Isolation," and sent to central supply unit for sterilization or to appropriate department for cleaning; items too large to bag should be sprayed with disinfectant and sent for thorough cleaning.	*Decreases spread of micro-organisms on used medical equipment*
- Linens should be placed in linen bags before leaving bedside and placed in central hamper or linen chute (agency may require double bagging).	
- Clean stethoscope between use for different clients with soap and water and wipe with alcohol swab (if used in an infected area or with an infected client, thorough disassembly and cleaning may be needed); use a separate stethoscope for an infected client, if possible.	*Decreases spread of micro-organisms on stethoscope* *Limits exposure to infection*
- Sphygmomanometers, thermometers, ECG leads, or similar daily-use items should be sprayed or wiped with a bacteriostatic substance between use with different clients.	*Decreases exposure to potentially infectious medium* *These items provide a good medium for organism growth*
- Used syringes and needles, scalpels, and other sharp disposables should be placed in appropriately marked container.	*Prevents accidental stick and contact with client's blood*
DO NOT REPLACE CAPS ON NEEDLES.	*Prevents accidental sticks during attempts to recap needle*

Action	Rationale
- Discard gown, gloves, and mask before leaving client's room.	*Prevents spread of infection*
3. Handling of personal effects of patients with infection:	
- Items should be placed in bags and sent home with family; if client is discharged and does not want certain items, dispose of these as in step 2. NEVER SHARE PERSONAL-CARE ITEMS BETWEEN CLIENTS.	*Prevents general spread of infection*
- If papers, books, or other items become soiled with infectious material, items should be discarded unless sterilization is possible and desired.	
4. Room assignment:	
- A private room is preferable but is required only when a highly virulent or infectious microorganism is present, the microorganism is airborne, or the client is highly suceptible to infection.	*Protects other clients or client from cross-contamination*
- A semiprivate room may be used when the microorganism is limited to one body area; however, good medical asepsis must be maintained by staff, client, family, and visitors to prevent spread of infection.	
5. Room cleaning:	
- Room should be cleaned with disinfectant daily.	*Reduces microorganisms in the environment*
- If soiled materials spill on floor, clean area with disinfectant or bacteriocidal agent specific to organism, if known.	

Action	Rationale
- When client with known infection is discharged, is transferred, or dies, room should be cleaned and disinfected thoroughly and allowed to remain vacant for 12 to 24 h. (See Procedure 12.3 for post-mortem care and Procedure 10.8 for additional information on isolation techniques.)	*Promotes thorough removal of microorganisms*

Evaluation

Were desired outcomes achieved?

Documentation

The following should be noted on the client's chart:
• Status of source of infection/potential infection (wound, dressing, breath sounds, secretions)
• Procedure performed
• Protective garments used
• Client teaching completed

SAMPLE DOCUMENTATION

DATE	TIME	
1/2/02	1200	Abdominal abscess site dressed. Site clean and without redness. Drains intact. Client tolerated procedure without complaint of unusual discomfort. States understands dressing change process and would like to change dressing in morning. Wound and drainage precautions maintained.

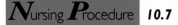

 *Principles of Surgical
Asepsis
(Aseptic Technique)*

EQUIPMENT

- Bacteriocidal or antimicrobial soap
- Sink with side or foot pedal
- Surgical scrub brush
- Sterile gloves
- Sterile gown
- Mask
- Hair covering and booties (optional)
- Sterile materials (dressing, instruments)
- Sterile sheets or towels (occasionally found in dressing tray)
- Waste disposal materials: trash can, bags (isolation bags optional)

Purpose

Avoids the introduction of microorganisms onto a designated field

Assessment

Assessment should focus on the following:

Data from medical history and physical or diagnostic studies indicating susceptibility to infection (decreased leukocyte count, history of immunosuppression, or steroid intake)

Doctor's orders or agency policy regarding dressing changes and isolation procedures

Client's or nurse's allergy to soap or bacteriostatic solutions

Client's room assignment (ward, double or single room)

Date of expiration and sterility indicator on sterile supplies and solutions

Client's knowledge of principles of asepsis

Client's ability to cooperate and not contaminate sterile field

Agency policy regarding surgical scrub procedure

Nursing Diagnoses

The nursing diagnoses may include the following:

Risk of altered biologic safety: infection related to central line insertion and total parenteral nutrition (TPN) therapy

Risk of infection related to immunosuppression from renal transplant therapy

Outcome Identification and Planning

Desired Outcomes (sample)

Client shows no signs of infection or of additional infection.

Procedures are performed with no evidence of exposure to microorganisms.

Special Considerations

Variations in sterile technique (eg, the omission of some protective coverings [hair cover, booties, mask]) may be used in performing some procedures. CONTINUE TO USE ASEPTIC PRINCIPLES TO GOVERN ACTIONS DURING A PROCEDURE.

IF UNSURE OF STERILITY OF MATERIAL, GLOVE, OR FIELD, CONSIDER IT CONTAMINATED.

Geriatric

If a client is disoriented and restless, restrain the client during procedures requiring maintenance of sterile materials. Enlist assistance for manual restraint of the client or use mechanical restraints (see Procedure 10.12).

Pediatric

If a child is restless or too young to understand the importance of maintaining a sterile field, restrain the child with linen or soft restraints during the procedure. Use a family member to assist in restraining the child and allaying fears, if possible. Provide sedation or pain medication before the procedure to comfort and calm the child.

Home Health

Bar pets from the room in which a sterile or clean procedure is being performed.

Most procedures are performed with clean rather than sterile technique.

Enlist and instruct a family member to serve as an assistant.

IMPLEMENTATION

Action	Rationale
1. A private room is preferable for performance of a sterile procedure; transfer client to treatment room, if necessary.	*Minimizes microorganisms in environment*

Hand Washing—Surgical

Action	Rationale
2. Don mask, hair cover, and booties, if required.	*Prevents introduction of contaminants from mouth, hair, or shoes into environment*
3. Perform 5- to 10-min surgical scrub using counted brush stroke method:	*Reduces organisms on hands* *Counted brush stroke method places emphasis on attention to specific areas and ensures that all skin surfaces are exposed to sufficient friction*
- Remove rings (often must remove wedding band), chipped nail polish, and watch.	*Removes sources that harbor and promote growth of micro-organisms*
- Wet hands and arms from elbows to fingertips under flowing water (use sink with side or foot pedal).	*Cleans from least to most dirty area* *Aids in removal of micro-organisms*
- Place soap, preferably antimicrobial/bacterio-static, on hands and rub vigorously for 15 to 30 sec; use scrub brush gently— do not abrade skin.	*Creates friction to remove organisms*
- Using circular motion, scrub all skin areas, joints, fingernails, between fingers, and so forth (on all sides and 2 inches above elbows); slide ring, if present, up and down while rubbing fingers.	*Permits cleaning around and under ring*
- Continue scrub for 5 to 10 min or per agency policy.	
- Rinse hands from fingers to elbows under flow of water.	*Washes dirt and organisms from cleanest to least clean area*
- Repeat soaping, rubbing, and rinsing until hands and arms are clean.	

Action	Rationale
- Pat hands dry with sterile towel, moving from fingers to wrist.	*Dries hands from clean to least clean area*
- Turn off faucet with side or foot pedal.	*Prevents recontamination of hand*

Sterile Field

4. To create a sterile field:
   - Arrange sterile supplies on overbed table or surgical stand.
   - Never use opened items or items of questionable sterility.
   - Open packages to reveal supplies, using insides of packages to form sterile field; open package's outer flap away from you, open side flaps next, and then pull inner flap toward you (Fig. 10.8); spread edges of package cover over table with fingertips.

   Prevents reaching over exposed materials

   Edges are considered unsterile

5. To add items to sterile field:
   - Drop sterile items onto field, keeping packaging between items and hands (Fig. 10.9); *use sterile forceps or tongs to remove items from package if unable to do so with sterile technique;* if unable to remove item from package without

   Prevents contamination of supplies

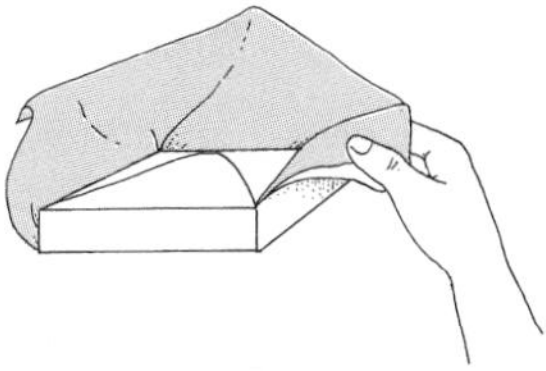

FIGURE 10.8

Action	Rationale

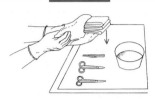

FIGURE 10.9

contamination, wait until
sterile garb is applied,
then place items on
sterile field.

- Use sterile gloves or *sterile
tongs* to remove sterile
towels from field, and
cover field and
supplies if not beginning
procedure immediately.
DO NOT REACH OVER
OPEN STERILE FIELD.

*Sterility will be lost if field is
exposed to air for extended
period of time*

Exposes field to contamination

- Don sterile gown and
sterile gloves (see
Procedures 10.4 and 10.5).

*Prevents exposure of sterile field
to hands or clothing*

- Begin procedure with
hands held above waist.

*Area below waist considered
nonsterile*

6. To maintain a sterile
environment:

- Drape sterile sheets or
towels over area
surrounding site being
treated.

*Decreases chance of exposure to
nonsterile sites*

- *Use tongs or forceps* to
clean site thoroughly with
bacteriocidal agent.

*Maintains sterility of gloves
Reduces microorganisms*

- Discard *tongs* from sterile
field.

Prevents field contamination

- Pour liquids into a sterile
basin held by an assistant
in sterile garb or by
holding bottle over 1-inch
outer parameter of field;
avoid splashing on field.

*Prevents reaching over sterile
field*

Action	Rationale
IF FIELD BECOMES WET, CONSIDER IT CONTAMINATED.	*Water conducts microorganisms from nonsterile area to sterile field*

Maintain Asepsis During Procedure

7. As procedure is performed:
   - Remove soiled equipment from area or sterile field; drop trash in bag or receptacle.
   - Avoid touching nonsterile surfaces.
   - When procedure is complete and dressing is intact, label dressing with date, time, and your initials. — *Indicates when next dressing change is due*
8. Decrease exposure of immunosuppressed clients or burn clients to microorganisms by maintaining sterile environment: — *Limits exposure to microorganisms from other clients*
   - Place client in single room.
   - Use a separate stethoscope, sphygmomanometer, and thermometer for client, if possible.
   - Only hospital gowns, linens, and materials should be used; allow no items from home unless approved and sterilized by hospital. — *Prevents introduction of possible source of contamination*
   - When client is severely immunosuppressed, papers, books, and other personal items should be removed from immediate area unless sterilization is possible.
   - Special food trays, disposable or presterilized, should be used.

Evaluation

Were desired outcomes achieved?

Documentation

The following should be noted on the client's chart:

- Status of wound, dressing, and incision site, with indication of signs of infection, if any
- Procedure performed
- Protective garments used
- Client teaching done regarding maintenance of dressing and sterile protective environment and verbalized understanding by client

SAMPLE DOCUMENTATION

DATE	TIME	
1/2/02	1200	Temporary pacemaker inserted at bedside by Dr. Hope using sterile technique. Site clean and without redness. Client tolerated procedure without complaint of unusual discomfort. Client states understanding of dressing change process and need for sterility.

Isolation Techniques (10.8)

 Biohazardous Waste Disposal (10.9)

EQUIPMENT

- Isolation cart or the following supplies:
  - Masks
  - Gloves (nonsterile or sterile)
  - Gowns
  - Plastic bags (or cloth linen bags)
  - Tape, bag ties, or fasteners
- Isolation card, indicating requirements for type of isolation (see Appendix F)
- Soap and source of water
- Paper towels
- Approved sharps container
- Approved rigid biohazardous waste container
- Approved biohazardous waste bags
- Spill kit or spill cloth

Purpose

Prevents spread of infection from client to others

Decreases exposure of susceptible client to infection

Provides for safe disposal of contaminated items in accordance with safety, laws, and regulations

Assessment

Assessment should focus on the following:

Type of isolation indicated

Site of infection

Kind of restrictions needed in addition to standard precautions

Perceptions of client and family regarding information provided by doctor

Usual duration of infection

Adequate ventilation in room (often door is kept closed)

Associated physical symptoms of client, such as elevated temperature, chills, stiff neck

Items considered to be biohazardous waste
Requirements and methods for safe disposal of biohazardous waste (agency and community)

Nursing Diagnoses

The nursing diagnoses may include the following:

Risk of altered safety related to presence of infection
Risk of sepsis related to decreased resistance to infection
Risk of spread of infection related to knowledge deficit
Impaired skin integrity related to burn

Outcome Identification and Planning

Desired Outcomes (sample)

Infection is cleared, with no spread to other body areas, or to other clients, family, visitors, or staff.
Client demonstrates use of mask, proper disposal of infected tissues, and good hand-washing technique.
Client speaks freely about isolation, with no complaints of a sense of neglect by staff or abandonment.
Client verbalizes three procedures needed to maintain specified isolation by end of day.
Biohazardous waste is collected, transported, and disposed of safely and legally.

Special Considerations

Hand washing is the single most important measure used to prevent the spread of infection. Hands should be washed before entering and upon leaving isolation rooms, as well as between care procedures for different clients.
Most hospital policies require a nurse to obtain a culture from a draining body area and to initiate isolation procedures when positive cultures are reported. Consult the agency policy manual.
A client may become withdrawn, depressed, and feel abandoned due to isolation. Plan frequent visitation times with the client and follow through as promised.

Home Health

An isolation card or information sheet, with clear instructions to family members, should be provided.
See Display 10.1 for various considerations in teaching the client/family regarding infection control and disposal of biohazardous waste in the home. Disposal requirements for biohazardous waste vary by state and by agency. Be sure to consult appropriate policies and procedures manuals.

DISPLAY 10.1 Infection Control in the Home
(Teaching Points)

Desired Outcomes: No transfer of microorganisms will
occur from client to others. No contamination of sterile and
clean supplies by microorganisms will occur.
Special Considerations: Basic infection control practices
should be a basic part of instruction in healthy lifestyle,
particularly in multigenerational families living in one
house.
Note: Handwashing, environmental cleaning and laundry
may have cultural implications. Contact a resource person
before proceeding with teaching.
Hints: Be alert for possibility that poor compliance with
infection control practices may be related to insufficient
funds; contact social service agencies and other community
resources, if necessary. Insect and/or rodent infestation may
be a major obstacle to infection control in the home. If
needed, contact the public health department for advice and
assistance.

Pre-teaching Preparation

---

1. Assessment:	Client/family ability to understand and perform procedures (handwashing, cleaning of environment, avoidance of organism transmission, maintenance of supplies)
	General environmental cleanliness
	Possibility of insect or rodent infestation
	Status of others living in the home
	Specific client conditions that could require special infection control technique
2. Planning:	Gather supplies: nonsterile gloves, gown/apron, masks, goggles, 10% bleach solution, biohazardous waste containers, rigid plastic container (eg, detergent jug), household disinfectant, paper towels.
	Note: Nurse must arrange for pickup of biohazardous waste containers from home.
	Note: All family members and caregivers must be instructed in standard precautions if they are going to be exposed to blood or body fluids.

DISPLAY 10.1	Infection Control in the Home (Teaching Points)

3. Implementation:

Handwashing Steps

a. Turn on water or pour water over hands if no running water is available.

b. Using soap, apply vigorous friction to all skin surfaces for at least 10 sec.

c. Rinse hands under running water and turn off faucet with paper towel; or have water poured over hands.

d. Dry hands with paper towel, not cloth towel used by others.

e. Instruct all family members to perform handwashing before and after doing client care, after using toilet, and whenever handling trash or biohazardous materials, including raw meats.

General Environmental Cleaning

a. Instruct in general household cleaning of
   - Bathroom and kitchen with disinfectant and/or bleach solution
   - Surfaces in client area with disinfectant (avoid strong odors if patient has respiratory condition or arrange for patient to be out of room until odor dissipates).
   - Vacuum and dust as needed (also remove patient from area until completed).

b. Instruct removal of heavy carpet and difficult-to-clean furniture from client area, if possible.

c. Instruct all family members to use own towel, washcloth, and toothbrush.

Infection Control in the Home
(Teaching Points)

Avoidance of Bloodborne Transmission

a. Instruct to wash garments, linens, towels soiled with blood and body fluids:
   - Wear gloves.
   - Rinse all items in cold water.
   - Wash separately from family laundry in washer with hot water and bleach.

b. To dispose of used dressing soiled with blood or body fluids:
   - Wear gloves.
   - Wear other personal protective equipment if splashing is anticipated.
   - Place soiled dressings in an approved biohazardous waste container.

c. If needles are being used, instruct in use of sharps container (heavy plastic jug with lid).
   - Place small amount of bleach solution in jug.
   - Place all used sharps in jug and replace lid each time.
   - Discard when two thirds full.
   - If sharps container exchange program is available in the community, instruct in how to access resource.

d. Instruct in standard precautions as indicated.

Maintenance of Supplies

a. If sterile or clean supplies are to be left in the home for client use:
   - Assist client to locate clean, protected storage area that may be used for supplies only.
   - Cover supplies with clean plastic or towel.

4. Documentation: In the visit note include the infection control instructions given and to whom, special circumstances in the home and activities taken to address.

IMPLEMENTATION

Action	Rationale

Procedure 10.8 Isolation Techniques

1. Clearly explain to client and family the isolation type, reason initiated, how microorganisms are spread, staff and visitor restrictions related to dress and duration of contact (if applicable), and compliance needed; demonstrate procedure for applying sterile mask and gown. THE DOCTOR SHOULD INITIALLY INFORM THE CLIENT OF THE DIAGNOSED INFECTION.

   Increases compliance of client, family, and visitors and decreases anxiety

2. Ensure that isolation cart is complete and that sufficient trash cans and linen bags are in room.

   Promotes proper disposal of contaminated materials

3. Keep sufficient linens and towels in room.

   Avoids unnecessary trips into and out of room
   Decreases spread of micro-organisms
   Promotes hand washing

4. Have housekeeping staff check room daily for sufficient soap and paper towels.

5. Wash hands and organize equipment.

   Reduces microorganism transfer
   Promotes efficiency

6. Note doctor's orders or refer to isolation guidelines adopted by agency for precautions necessary to establish appropriate type of isolation (see Appendix F).

   Provides sufficient protection from microorganisms with minimum stress and restriction on client, visitors, and staff

7. Obtain appropriate isolation card and place on client's door.

   Alerts visitors and staff to follow dress and hand-washing restrictions

8. If card must be filled out, include instructions on hand washing; use of masks, gloves, and gowns; handling of linen and disposable

Action	Rationale

    items; need for private
    room, if appropriate.

9. Review disinfectants needed to eliminate specific microorganisms.

Prepares nurse for environ-mental and client management

10. Inform family members and visitors of necessary isolation precautions.

Allays fears to prevent with-drawal of friends and family from client
Increases compliance

11. Install isolation supplies and cart outside client door.

Facilitates maintenance of isolation

12. Obtain supplies needed for wound care, if required, and keep sufficient supplies in client's room.

Avoids unnecessary trips into and out of room
Decreases spread of micro-organisms

Procedure 10.9 Biohazardous Waste Disposal

1. Don gloves, maintain asep-sis while handling waste.

Prevents contact with bodily fluids

2. Keep disposal equipment readily available for use at all times (eg, if using sharps, take sharps container into the house). Replace sharps container when it is two-thirds full.

Allows for safe disposal of waste even if not anticipated before care.

Prevents needlestick when putting additional sharps in nearly full container.

3. Dispose of used supplies taken into room or place them inside appropriate isolation bag for removal. (Remove biohazardous waste from home each visit.)

Prevents spread of infection from objects used on or by client

4. When removing full sharps container, close securely, (date and label, if agency policy). If transporting in car, place in second rigid-walled container. Log in sharps container for dis-posal per agency policy.

Prevents contamination of supplies in car, adds extra barrier.

5. Use plastic bags for garbage and reusable equipment; Use biohazard bags to bag disposable drainage sys-tems and soiled non-sharps

Prevents spread of infection from contaminated materials

Action	Rationale
bioazardous materials before delivering to agency's disposal unit. If removing to car for disposal, place bags in rigid container in car.	*Keeps biohazardous waste separate from other supplies*
6. Label reusable equipment.	*Indicates date of use and possible replacement time*
7. Place soiled linens in proper linen bags; double bag linens if required by agency. Take linen bags to soiled utility room. (Instruct family to wash soiled linen and clothing separate from family wash.)	*Allows for washing without removing bag*
8. Clean room thoroughly with appropriate anti-microbial agent. If blood or body fluids occur in home, use spill kit or spill cloth.	*Kills virulent organisms* *Prevents exposure of other clients to infection*
9. Leave room unoccupied after client discharge for appropriate time period.	*Minimizes exchange of organisms between clients*
10. Wash hands.	*Reduces microorganism transfer*

Evaluation

Were desired outcomes achieved?

Documentation

The following should be noted on the client's chart:
- Status of client's infection (identity and extent of areas involved)
- Client's, family's, and visitors' understanding of and compliance with isolation and required precautions
- Staff compliance with isolation precautions and biohazardous waste disposal
- Periodic culture reports to establish need for continued isolation

SAMPLE DOCUMENTATION

DATE	TIME	
2/3/02	1400	Lab report obtained on culture of sputum specimen, with results showing pneumococcal pneumonia. Doctor notified. Client and family instructed on isolation procedures; understanding voiced. Respiratory precautions sign placed on door. Masks and gloves placed outside of room. Visitors instructed on use of mask. Understanding verbalized by visitors and compliance noted. Biohazardous waste disposed of properly.

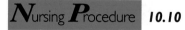

Preoperative Care

EQUIPMENT

- Assessment equipment (eg, blood pressure cuff, stethoscope, pen light)
- Scale
- Teaching materials (films, booklet, sample equipment)
- Preoperative checklist
- Shave and preparation kit (razor, soap, sponge, tray for water) (optional); check agency policy
- Procedure (hospital) gown
- Fingernail polish remover
- Denture cup (optional)
- Envelope for valuables (optional)
- Preoperative medications and administration equipment
- Nonsterile gloves

Purpose

Prepares client physically and emotionally for impending surgery

Assessment

Assessment should focus on the following:

Type of surgery
Preparatory regimen for type of surgery (per doctor's order or agency policy)
Signed consent form on chart before administering preoperative sedation
Client perceptions of previous surgical experiences
Admission history and physical for factors increasing risks of surgery (eg, age, chronic or acute illness, depression, fluid and electrolyte imbalance)
Learning or comprehension ability
Reading ability
Language barriers

Nursing Diagnoses

The nursing diagnoses may include the following:

Knowledge deficit related to postoperative regimen
Anxiety related to impending surgery

Outcome Identification and Planning

Desired Outcomes (sample)

Client verbalizes purpose of postoperative regimen.
Client correctly demonstrates pulmonary and cardiovascular exercise regimens.

Special Considerations

Assess the client's readiness to learn and, if preoperative teaching time is limited, gear teaching toward essential items of concern.
Prior exposure to the postoperative environment, staff, and regimen often decreases the client's anxiety and promotes cooperation postoperatively.

Geriatric

Fear of death may be particularly profound in some elderly clients, especially if this is a first hospitalization or first surgery. Supply clear and thorough explanations of all procedures. Encourage the client to participate in preoperative preparations.

Pediatric

Puppets may be used to explain the surgical procedure, preoperative care, and postoperative regimen. Answer questions simply, providing only necessary information and explanations. Ensure that legal guardian has signed consent form.

Delegation

Preoperative teaching and physical/health assessment are to be performed by a licensed nurse and not delegated to unlicensed assistive personnel.

IMPLEMENTATION

Action	Rationale
1. Wash hands and organize supplies.	*Reduces microorganism transfer* *Promotes efficiency*
2. Assess client's knowledge of impending surgery; reinforce information and correct errors in understanding. *Note:* It is the physician's responsibility	*Determines client's teaching needs* *Corrects misinformation*

Action	Rationale
initially to inform the client about surgery, options, and risks.	
3. Show films and provide booklets regarding surgery and postoperative care; encourage questions; answer questions clearly.	*Reduces anxiety* *Imparts knowledge*
4. Verify that operative permit is signed and on chart. *Note:* It is the physician's responsibility to obtain proper informed consent.	*Avoids error in sending client to surgery without written consent*
5. Verify that ordered lab work and diagnostic studies (x-ray films, ECGs) have been done; check results of diagnostic studies, place copies on chart, and include results on preoperative checklist; alert doctor to abnormal values.	*Assesses client's preparation and readiness for surgery* *Determines if treatment of abnormalities is needed or if surgery must be postponed*
6. Check to be certain pre-operative medications are available.	*Avoids delays for client and surgical team on day of surgery*
7. Obtain client's height and weight; perform head-to-toe assessment, with in-depth assessment of areas related to surgery (see Procedure 3.5).	*Provides baseline data*
8. Instruct client about procedures or equipment that will be used to provide adequate oxygenation:	
- Demonstrate use of oxygen mask/cannula or of endotracheal tube and ventilator.	*Prepares client for postoperative regimen*
- Explain related noises and sensations.	*Decreases anxiety produced by postoperative regimen*
- Arrange introduction to respiratory therapy personnel.	*Facilitates cooperation*

Action	Rationale
- Demonstrate turning, coughing, and deep-breathing exercises, demonstrating use of pillow to splint incision site.	
- Explain techniques of chest physiotherapy, if applicable.	
- Stress the importance of pulmonary toilet in prevention of secretion buildup.	
9. Discuss and demonstrate, if applicable, techniques for maintaining adequate circulation and pain control:	
- Demonstrate range-of-motion and leg exercises and check client's technique.	*Maintains circulation while client is bedridden*
- If transcutaneous electrical nerve stimulation (TENS) unit is to be used, explain procedure to client.	*Prepares client for use of TENS unit postoperatively*
- Arrange for physical therapist to visit client.	*Facilitates postoperative relationship and cooperation*
10. Discuss with client and family the postoperative unit or environment; tour unit and introduce client to staff; inform family of special visitation hours, if applicable; review tentative timetable of surgery and recovery room period; instruct family on agency's methods of communicating status updates during and after surgery.	*Reduces anxiety about unfamiliar setting and caregivers*
11. **On the night before surgery:**	
- Don gloves.	

Action	Rationale
- Shave designated body areas.	*Prevents postoperative infection*
- Instruct client to shower with povidone solution, if ordered or if agency policy.	
- Administer laxative or other medications, if ordered.	*Helps flush bowel to prevent contamination of sterile field*
- Perform enema and check results.	*Evacuates bowel to prevent sterile field contamination*
- Withhold foods and fluids after midnight the night before surgery (clear fluids may often be administered up to 3–4 h before surgery, particularly if no IV fluids are infusing); consult agency policy.	*Prevents sterile field contamination secondary to incontinence* *Prevents bowel and bladder puncture because of distended organs*
- Check chart to determine which, if any, medications are to be given (permit sips of water) and at what time.	*Delivers drugs client needs to maintain therapeutic levels during surgery while eliminating those that may cause compatibility problems with drugs given in surgery*
12. **On day before or morning of surgery, prepare client:**	
- Verify presence of identification band (obtain duplicate band if needed).	*Facilitates identification of client*
- Remove jewelry (may retain wedding ring— wrap with tape); ask client to send valuables and jewelry home with family or place in valuables envelope and store with security department or according to agency policy.	*Prevents loss during surgery* *Secures valuables and belongings*
- Remove nail polish.	*Allows for good visualization of nail beds to monitor oxygenation status*

Action	Rationale
- Remove and label glasses, contact lenses, or other prostheses.	*Prevents loss*
- Remove full or partial dentures and label container (place with family or security department).	*Prevents loss*
- Assist client into hospital gown.	
13. **Thirty to 60 minutes before surgery** (when operating room signals that client's preoperative medication is to be given):	
- Check client identification band.	*Verifies client's identity*
- Encourage client to void.	*Prevents field contamination and accidental bladder puncture*
- Obtain vital signs.	*Provides baseline data*
- Administer ordered medication.	*Induces mild sedation and achieves or maintains therapeutic levels*
- Raise side rails and instruct client to stay in bed.	*Prevents falls after client has been sedated*
- Place call bell within reach and instruct client to call for assistance.	*Facilitates communication and safety*
- Encourage family to sit with client until stretcher arrives.	*Decreases anxiety*
14. **When operating room personnel arrive to take client to surgery:**	*Prepares client for transport*
- Compare client identification band with surgery call slip; note spelling of name and identification number.	*Confirms correspondence of client identity with impending surgical procedure*
- Assist client onto stretcher.	
- Write final note in chart.	

Action	Rationale

- Place chart, stamp plate,
  and ordered medications
  on stretcher with client.
15. Assist family to
    appropriate postoperative
    waiting room, or remain
    in client's room, if ordered
    by doctor.

Evaluation

Were desired outcomes achieved?

Documentation

The following should be noted on the client's chart:

- Presence of signed consent form
- Preoperative teaching done and client response
- Preparation procedures performed (eg, enema, shave)
- Vital signs and other clinical data
- Preoperative medications given
- Disposition of valuables
- Completed preoperative checklist or areas pending completion
- Abnormal test results and time doctor was notified of these
- Further teaching or preparation needed

SAMPLE DOCUMENTATION

DATE	TIME	
1/2/02	1200	Preoperative teaching done with instructions on importance of pulmonary toilet, range-of-motion and calf exercises. Client verbalizes understanding. Preoperative checklist completed except for final vital signs and medication.

Postoperative Care

EQUIPMENT (CONSULT PROCEDURE
MANUAL FOR DETAILED LISTS)

- Assessment equipment (eg, blood pressure cuff, stethoscope, pen light, scale)
- Respiratory therapy equipment (eg, oxygen unit, incentive spirometer, nebulizer)
- Physical therapy equipment (eg, transcutaneous electrical nerve stimulation [TENS] unit, mechanical percussor, vibrator)
- Emesis basin
- IV therapy equipment
- Nasogastric (NG) suction equipment
- Medications and medication administration record
- Teaching materials (films, booklets, sample equipment)
- Sterile gloves

Purpose

Promotes return to state of physical and emotional well-being
Detects complications related to postsurgical status at early stage
Prevents postoperative complications
Facilitates wound healing

Assessment

Assessment should focus on the following:

Type of surgery
Nature of supportive therapy (ventilator, feeding tube, IV therapy)
Medication infusions
Preoperative physiologic status
History of chronic or concurrent illnesses that could delay recovery
Monitoring equipment (eg, telemetry unit, central venous pressure)
Drainage systems (eg, chest tube, wound, NG, or urine drainage systems)
Communication barriers (eg, language barrier, neurologic damage, presence of endotracheal tube)
Level of consciousness and orientation
Family support
Emotional state

Nursing Diagnoses

The nursing diagnoses may include the following:

Knowledge deficit related to postoperative regimen
Anxiety related to postoperative situation
Pain related to surgical incision
Risk of infection related to disruption in skin integrity

Outcome Identification and Planning

Desired Outcomes (sample)

Client verbalizes purpose of postoperative regimen.
Client correctly demonstrates pulmonary and cardiovascular exercise regimen.

Special Considerations

Geriatric

Anesthesia may cause temporary disorientation and personality change. Reorient the client frequently; allow family members to remain with client as much as possible.

Pediatric

Puppets may be used to encourage cooperation with the postoperative regimen. Family members may be effective in persuading client to participate.

Home Health

If client has had outpatient surgery, arrange for follow-up by home health or public health nurse. Teach client and family information needed for safe and complete healing after surgery.

Delegation

Postoperative assessment, teaching, and dressing or wound management are the responsibility of a licensed nurse.
Consult agency policy for assessments that can be performed by registered nurse only.

IMPLEMENTATION

Action	Rationale
1. Wash hands and organize supplies.	*Reduces microorganism transfer* *Provides efficiency*
2. When client is admitted to unit:	

Action	Rationale
- Assist client from stretcher to bed; remove excess linens and cover client with sheet.	*Promotes warmth and privacy*
- Orient to staff and environment, especially location of call button.	*Decreases anxiety* *Promotes client–staff communication*
- Hook up oxygen, connect telemetry, begin drainage systems; position client as ordered or with head of bed elevated 30 to 45 degrees.	*Initiates support therapy* *Facilitates lung expansion*
- Assess respiratory, neurologic and neurovascular status, vital signs, apical pulse, bowel sounds, and ECG tracing from telemetry, as well as other parameters pertaining to specific body systems affected by surgery.	*Provides baseline data on postoperative status*
- Assess incisional dressings and surgical wound drainage systems.	
- Note urine output and output from drainage systems, as well as diaphoresis, emesis, and diarrhea.	*Enables early detection of fluid imbalances or systemic changes*
3. Allow family members at bedside as soon as possible.	*Reassures family* *Facilitates client comfort and orientation*
4. Review postoperative orders:	*Updates nurse on postoperative therapy program*
- Contact departments to schedule ordered lab work, x-ray films, ECGs, and other diagnostic tests.	*Facilitates early detection of complications*
- Note medications given after surgery and in recovery room and arrange medication schedule at appropriate intervals.	*Returns client to routine medication regimen*

Action	Rationale
- Administer initial medication doses and treatments as soon as appropriate (if oral medication is needed, wait until client is able to tolerate fluids).	*Prevents gastrointestinal upset from decreased peristalsis related to anesthesia*
- Monitor for nausea or vomiting and return of bowel sounds.	*Indicates activity of bowel and possible ileus development*
5. Monitor vital signs as indicated by client status or as ordered by routine post-operative protocol (eg, every 1½ h times 2, every hour times 2, then every 2–4 h if vital signs are stable).	*Facilitates early detection of post operative complications*
6. Assess pain level and medicate as ordered; en-courage client to request pain medication before onset of severe pain; medicate client 30 min before exercises and pulmonary toilet.	*Promotes deep breathing and effective coughing* *Decreases the pain of turning*
7. Begin pulmonary toilet immediately (if not contraindicated).	*Prevents buildup of secretions*
- Turn, deep breathe, and cough/suction client every 2 h.	
- Instruct client in use of incentive spirometry equipment and encourage use every hour.	*Facilitates lung expansion* *Mobilizes secretions*
8. Initiate range-of-motion and leg exercises, as well as chest physiotherapy, if applicable; if TENS unit is to be used, apply and turn on (see Procedure 8.7).	*Maintains circulation while client is bedridden* *Facilitates removal of accumulated secretions* *Promotes comfort by blocking pain reception of nerves*
9. Monitor surgical dressing and change or reinforce as needed and permitted.	*Promotes sense of well-being* *Increases self-esteem and sense of self-control*

Action	Rationale
MANY DOCTORS PREFER TO REMOVE INITIAL DRESSING.	
10. Help client to resume a normal state of personal grooming and hygiene:	
- Obtain glasses, contact lenses, dentures, or other prostheses and apply, if appropriate and client desires.	
- Obtain valuables from security when client is fully awake and requests them.	
- Assist client in personal hygiene and grooming, when desired and not prohibited.	*Increases self-esteem*

Evaluation

Were desired outcomes achieved?

Documentation

The following should be noted on the client's chart:

- Time of admission of client to room and area admitted from
- Complete assessment with emphasis on abnormal findings
- Status of operative dressings, tubes, drains, and incisions
- Support equipment initiated
- Procedures performed
- Client's tolerance of therapy
- Abnormal test results noted and time doctor is notified
- Medications administered
- Client's and family's concerns
- Teaching needs noted

SAMPLE DOCUMENTATION

DATE	TIME	
1/2/02	1200	Client admitted from recovery room after right thoracotomy. Alert and oriented. Vital signs obtained every 1–2 hour, with stable results. Skin warm and dry. Respirations deep and regular, at rate of 16. Denies pain, epidural PCA functioning. Mediastinal tube to 20 cm H_2O suction. Serosanguineous drainage (50 ml) noted in Pleurevac. Chest dressing clean, dry, and intact.

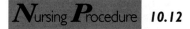

Use of Protective Devices: Limb and Body Restraints

EQUIPMENT

- Restraint appropriate for limb or body area (ie, wrist, ankle, vest or waist restraint)
- Wash cloths for each limb restraint
- Lotion and powder (optional)
- Kerlix gauze (3- or 4-inch roll)
- 2-inch tape

Purpose

Prevents injury to client from falls, wound contamination, and tube dislodgment

Prevents injury to others from disoriented or hostile client when other methods of control have been ineffective

Assessment

Assessment should focus on the following:

Specific client behaviors and circumstances indicating need for protective devices

Client's orientation and level of consciousness

Alternative activities attempted to avoid use of restraints (unless part of care standard or protocol)

Effectiveness of other safety controls and precautions

Availability of staff or family members to sit with client

Doctor's order (obtain if not on chart)

Agency policy regarding use of restraints

Skin and circulatory status in areas requiring restraint

Nursing Diagnoses

The nursing diagnoses may include the following:

Risk of injury related to confusion and disorientation

Outcome Identification and Planning

Desired Outcomes (sample)

Client experiences no falls or injury while under nurse's care.

Skin and circulation remains intact at and below the site of restraint.

Special Considerations

Because restraints may actually cause injury instead of preventing it, use alternative protective measures specific to the problem resulting in the use of restraints, whenever possible (eg, minimize use of invasive treatments, disguise tubings or keep out of client's view, wrap infusion sites in stockinette or bandage and use abdominal binder for dressings to prevent disruption of lines or wounds).

A doctor's order must be obtained before applying restraints, unless an approved protocol or standard is in place.

The doctor must be notified of the time when restraints were initiated so a face-to-face evaluation can be performed within 1 h of restraint use as required by Joint Commission on Accreditation of Healthcare Organizations (JCAHO) and the Health Care Financing Administration (HCFA).

Learn standards and protocols and agency policy regarding use of restraints (some agencies require that restraints be used in certain situations, such as presence of an endotracheal tube). Note that JCAHO standards limit restraint use to emergent dangerous client actions; addictive disorders; adjunct to planned care; component of an approved protocol, or in some cases as part of standard practice.

During the period a client is in restraints, assessments must be performed every 15 min or, in some agencies, 1:1 supervision of the client is required for the entire period.

Geriatric

The skin of elderly clients is often very sensitive, and the blood vessels are easily collapsed. Restrain such clients loosely with linen or soft restraints and check the circulation frequently. Remove restraints frequently to check the skin beneath them.

Pediatric

Mittens may be preferable to wrist restraints because they are less restrictive and permit growth and developmental activities.

Home Health

Sheets may be used to tie client securely to a bed or chair to prevent falls. Socks or other soft pieces of cloth may be fashioned into wrist restraints, and mittens may be used to prevent pulling of tubes.

Delegation

All unlicensed assistive personnel who apply restraints must be
trained before applying restraints.

Training focuses on appropriate application and client monitoring. Monitoring physical status remains the primary responsibility of the nurse.

IMPLEMENTATION

Action	Rationale
1. Wash hands and organize equipment.	*Prevents microorganism transfer* *Promotes efficiency*
2. Explain procedure to client and state why restraints are needed.	*Promotes cooperation* *Reduces anxiety*
3. Place client in a comfortable position with good body alignment.	
4. Wash and dry area to which restraint will be applied; massage area and apply lotion if skin is dry; apply powder, if desired.	*Facilitates circulation to skin* *Decrease friction on skin from dirt and dead skin cells*
5. To apply wrist or ankle restraints: - Use 10-inch strip of Kerlix gauze folded to 2-inch width; wrap strip in a figure eight (Fig. 10.10)	

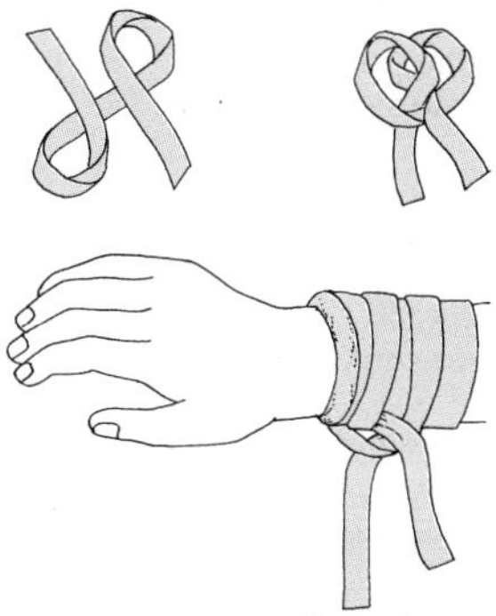

FIGURE 10.10

Action	Rationale
and fold the circles of the figure over one another; slip wrist or ankle through loop.	
- To use commercial restraints, wrap padded portion of restraint around wrist or ankle, thread tie through slit in restraint, and fasten to second tie with secure knot, or apply Velcro as indicated on package.	*Holds restraint intact around wrist/ankle*
- Secure ends of ties to bed frame. DO NOT SECURE TO BED RAILS (with some two-part restraints, the wrist section snaps into a separate section that is secured to bed frame).	*Prevents accidental pull on limb with movement of bed rail* *Allows removal of restraint for skin care without removal of portion secured to bed*
6. Vest restraint:	*Prevents client from getting out of bed without restricting arm and hand mobility*
- Place vest on client with opening in front.	
- Pull tie on end of vest flap across chest and slip through slit in opposite side of vest.	
- Wrap other end of flap across client and around chair or upper portion of bed.	*Secures vest to client*
- Fasten ends of ties together behind chair or to sides of bed frame.	
- Check respiratory status for distress related to restriction from vest.	
- Reposition client for minimal pressure on chest.	
7. Waist restraint:	*Prevents client from getting out of bed without binding chest*
- Wrap restraint around waist.	
- Slip end of one tie through slit in restraint.	
- Secure ends of ties to bed frame.	

Action	Rationale
- Monitor for complaints of nausea or abdominal distress.	*Indicates possible restriction on abdomen*
8. Hand mittens:	*Prevents pulling of tubes*
- Wrap Kerlix gauze around hand until totally covered.	*Allows mobility of limb*
- Fold hand into fist and continue to wrap fist.	
- Put tape around fist to secure gauze; cover with sock or stocking.	*Minimizes pulling of gauze and disruption of mitt*
9. When a client is in restraints:	
- Remove restraint every 2 to 4 h, as well as when staff or family are at bedside to prevent injury.	*Decreases continuous pressure on skin*
- Massage skin beneath restraint and apply lotion or powder; wrap folded washcloth around limb and place restraint on top of cloth.	*Increases circulation to skin* *Decreases friction and skin irritation*
- Monitor the extremity distal to the restraint every 15 min for color, temperature, and capillary refill.	*Determines adequacy of circulation below restraint* *Identifies need for removal*
- Monitor for skin irritation.	
- Check every 15 min for added pull on restraints and limb, tangled ties, or pressure points from knots; remove and adjust restraint to eliminate problem.	*Prevents loss of skin integrity due to excessive pressure*
- Offer client fluids and mouth care hourly.	
- Assist client with activities of daily living.	
- Offer opportunities for elimination on regular schedule.	

Action	Rationale
10. Continually assess client's orientation and continued need for restraints and remove as soon as safe to do so.	*Decreases risk of disruption of skin integrity* *Restores sense of self-control*

Evaluation

Were desired outcomes achieved?

Documentation

The following should be noted on the client's chart:

- Reason for restraint application (per JCAHO standard in overview)
- Activities taken to attempt to avoid use of restraint
- Time physician's order obtained or protocol/standard activated
- Time of restraint and type of restraint applied
- Time doctor notified of restraint application
- Time of doctor's visit
- Client's response to restraints
- Frequency of checks of client and restraint site
- Status of restraint site and distal circulation
- Frequency of removal of restraints
- Skin care performed

SAMPLE DOCUMENTATION

DATE	TIME	
1/2/02	1200	Admission history reveals pulling of tubes and disruption of wound during recent stay at nursing home. Client diagnosed with senile dementia, anorexia, and severe dehydration. IV and feeding tube inserted. Bilateral wrist restraints applied after use of bandage wrap around IV and use of mitts failed to keep client from pulling. Client monitored q15 minutes, circulation and skin integrity intact. Dr. Knowles notified and will see client in 30 minutes. No family available at this time.

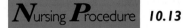

Pressure Ulcer Management

EQUIPMENT

- Dressing change materials as needed; multipack gauze in plastic container (forceps, scissors, transparent dressing, skin prep, tape—paper tape if allergic to other types of tape)
- Nonsterile gloves and sterile gloves
- Towel or linen saver pad
- Sterile irrigation saline
- Topical-care agents (may vary from agency to agency, case to case).
- Moist wound barrier/transparent wound dressing or topical antibiotics, if ordered
- Overbed table or bedside stand
- Waterproof trash bag (adhering to specific guidelines for wound/drainage disposal materials)
- Pressure relief pad (static or dynamic support surface such as air or fluid mattress pad)

Purpose

Removes accumulated secretions and dead tissue from wound or incision

Decreases microorganism growth on wounds or incision site

Promotes wound healing

Assessment

Assessment should focus on the following:

Doctor's order regarding type of dressing change, procedure, and frequency of change

Stage, size, appearance, and location of the pressure ulcer (Fig. 10.11)

Client factors contributing to development of the pressure ulcer (eg, prolonged immobility, poor circulation, nutritional status, incontinence, seepage of wound drainage onto skin)

Risk assessment for development of the pressure ulcer (using standardized tool such as the Braden or Norton scale—or agency-approved risk-assessment tool)

Time of last pain medication

Allergies to tape or medication ordered

Sample pressure ulcer assessment guide

Patient Name: _____   Date: _____   Time: _____

Ulcer 1:			Ulcer 2:		
Site _____			Site _____		
Stage[a] _____			Stage[a] _____		
Size (cm)			Size (cm)		
Length _____			Length _____		
Width _____			Width _____		
Depth			Depth		
	No	Yes		No	Yes
Sinus tract			Sinus tract		
Tunneling			Tunneling		
Undermining			Undermining		
Necrotic Tissue			Necrotic Tissue		
Slough			Slough		
Eschar			Eschar		
Exudate			Exudate		
Serous			Serous		
Serosanguineous			Serosanguineous		
Purulent			Purulent		
Granulation			Granulation		
Epithelialization			Epithelialization		
Pain			Pain		
Surrounding Skin:					
Erythema			Erythema		
Maceration			Maceration		
Induration			Induration		
Description of Ulcers(s):					

Indicate Ulcer Sites:

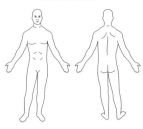

Anterior   Posterior

(Attach a color photo of the pressure ulcer(s) [Optional])

[a] Classification of pressure ulcers:

Stage I: Nonblanchable erythema of intact skin, the heralding lesion of skin ulceration. In individuals with darker skin, discoloration of the skin, warmth, edema, induration, or hardness may also be indicators.

Stage II;   Partial thickness skin loss involving epidermis, dermis, or both.

Stage II: Full thickness skin loss involving damage to or necrosis of subcutaneous tissue that may extend down to, but not through, underlying fascia. The ulcer presents clinically as a deep crater with or without undermining adjacent tissue.

Stage IV: Full thickness skin loss with extensive destruction, tissue necrosis, or damage to muscle, bone, or supporting structures (e.g., tendon or joint capsule).

FIGURE 10.11

Protective bed support (static or dynamic)
Client's activity regimen (frequency of turning, getting out of bed)
Client knowledge regarding factors contributing to development
   of a pressure ulcer
Potential complications (eg, sinus tract or abcess)

Nursing Diagnoses

The nursing diagnoses may include the following:

Impaired tissue integrity related to pressure ulcer
Risk of infection related to decreased skin integrity

Outcome Identification and Planning

Desired Outcomes (sample)

Client regains skin integrity within 3 weeks.
Client demonstrates no signs of infection or of further infection
   during confinement.

Special Considerations

The focus of ulcer care, in some instances, includes débridement,
   as well as wound cleansing, nutritional support, and other ad-
   junctive care. The primary rule is to keep the ulcer tissue moist,
   as well as the surrounding intact skin dry. Care of pressure ulcers is often very painful. Assess the client's pain needs and provide medication 30 min before beginning the procedure. A
   sterile, instead of clean, dressing change may be ordered. Pressure ulcer care tends to vary among agencies; consult the
   agency manual for guidelines.

Geriatric

Debilitation and decreased activity often accompany advanced
   age. Family members should be informed of the importance of
   preventing pressure to certain skin areas for extended periods
   of time.

Home Health

Newspaper should be used to cover the table surface during a
   dressing change, and animals in the home should be barred
   from the area during the procedure.

Delegation

Pressure ulcer management is the responsibility of the nurse. Unlicensed assistive personnel should be instructed in prevention
   techniques such as patient turning and repositioning, use of positioning devices, and the importance of meticulous skin care.

IMPLEMENTATION

Action	Rationale
1. Wash hands and organize equipment.	*Reduces microorganism transfer* *Promotes efficiency*
2. Explain procedure and assistance needed from client.	*Promotes cooperation*
3. Assess pain level; deliver medication, if needed, and wait for medication to take effect before beginning.	*Decreases discomfort of dressing change*
4. Place bedside table close to area being dressed and prepare supplies: - Place supplies on bedside table.	*Facilitates management of sterile field and supplies*
- Tape trash bag to side of table.	*Facilitates easy disposal of contaminated waste*
- Open sterile gloves and use inside of glove package as sterile field. - Open gauze-pad packages and leave gauze pads in plastic container. - Open dressing tray. - Open liquids and pour saline on the gauze pads. - Lower side rails.	*Promotes use of supplies without contamination and prepares work field*
5. Don nonsterile gloves.	*Prevents exposure to drainage*
6. Place towel or pad under wound area.	
7. Loosen tape by pulling toward the pressure ulcer and remove soiled dressing; note appearance of dressing and wound. MOISTEN DRESSING WITH NORMAL SALINE IF IT ADHERES TO WOUND AND THEN GENTLY PULL FREE.	*Exposes site for cleaning* *Permits assessment of site*
8. Place soiled dressing in trash bag.	*Prevents spread of organisms*
9. Discard gloves in trash bag and wash hands. (Be Sure to provide for client safety when away from bed.)	

Action	Rationale
10. Don new pair of gloves.	
11. Pick up saline-soaked dressing pad with forceps and form a large swab.	
12. Cleanse away debris and drainage from the pressure ulcer, moving from center outward; use a new pad for each area cleaned, discarding the old pads.	*Prevents contamination of wound from organisms on skin surface* *Maintains sterility of supplies*
13. Use a dry pad to dry the wound and surrounding skin and a skin prep on the surrounding skin; do not allow skin prep to touch broken skin areas. Discard forceps.	*Facilitates adherence of dressings/pads* *Decreases microorganisms*
14. Place ordered topical agent into pressure ulcer or onto dressing, as appropriate for type of wound. DO NOT OVERPACK WOUND.	*Provides necessary medication* *Minimizes exposure to infectious agents and promotes moisture* *Overpacking may result in additional tissue damage from excessive pressure* *Prevents additional exposure to microbes.*
15. Dress the pressure ulcer by covering with a transparent wound dressing or other dressing as indicated by wound care protocol. Secure dressing with a window or frame of tape.	*Secures dressing*
16. Write date and time of dressing change on a strip of tape and place tape across top of dressing.	*Indicates last dressing change and need for next change*
17. Dispose of gloves and materials and store supplies appropriately.	*Decreases spread of microorganisms*
18. Position client for comfort using additional support devices as needed.	*Promotes comfort* *Support devices reduce pressure, friction, and sheer*
19. Raise side rails and place call bell within reach.	*Promotes safety and communication*
20. Wash hands.	*Decreases spread of microorganisms*

Evaluation

Were desired outcomes achieved?

Documentation

The following should be noted on the client's chart:

- Materials and procedure used for pressure ulcer management
- Location, size, and type of wound or incision
- Solution and medications applied to wound
- Frequency of turning and repositioning client
- Support devices applied and to what areas
- Client teaching done and additional learning needs
- Client's tolerance of procedure

SAMPLE DOCUMENTATION

DATE	TIME	
1/2/02	0600	Pressure ulcer site cleaned with saline. Sacral pressure ulcer approximately 3 cm in diameter, pink, with slightly granulated edges; no drainage or foul odor noted. Wound covered with saline-soaked pads and transparent dressing. Client turned to side with positioning pillow at back and is on Clinitron bed. Tolerated care with minimal discomfort.

Wound Irrigation

EQUIPMENT

- Irrigation solution
- Sterile irrigation set, including sterile syringe with sterile tubing (or catheter) attached
- Sterile basin
- Gauze pads
- Materials for dressing change, if applicable (see Procedure 10.2)
- Linen saver
- Large towel
- Waste receptacle
- Sterile gloves

Purpose

Facilitates removal of secretions and microorganisms from wound

Assessment

Assessment should focus on the following:
Doctor's order regarding irrigation
Type and location of wound
Irrigant (type of medication added, if applicable)
Pain status and time of last pain medication

Nursing Diagnoses

The nursing diagnoses may include the following:

Risk of infection related to open abdominal incision line

Outcome Identification and Planning

Desired Outcomes (sample)
Client regains skin integrity within 1 month.
Client demonstrates no signs of infection during confinement.

Special Consideration

Wound irrigation can be painful; medicate client 30 min before beginning the procedure.

Pediatric

Child may contaminate the sterile field, gown, or gloves accidentally. Restrain child with linen or soft restraints during the procedure, if needed. Encourage a parent to sit with the child during the procedure, if possible, to provide reassurance and to help calm the child.

Home Health

Newspaper should be used to cover the table surface during wound irrigation, and animals in the home should be barred from the area during the procedure.

Delegation

In general, this procedure is performed by the registered or licensed practical nurse. See agency policy concerning delegation to unlicensed specially trained assistive personnel.

IMPLEMENTATION

Action	Rationale
1. Assess pain level; deliver medication, if needed, and wait for medication to take effect.	*Decreases discomfort during procedure*
2. Wash hands and organize supplies.	*Reduces microorganism transfer* *Promotes efficiency*
3. Explain procedure and assistance needed from client; provide privacy.	*Facilitates cooperation* *Decreases anxiety*
4. Place bedside table near wound area and open supplies (arrange for dressing change in addition to wound irrigation).	*Permits replacement of dressing after wound irrigation*
5. Don nonsterile gloves and remove dressing.	
6. Place linen saver and towel under wound.	*Catches overflow of irrigant*
7. Discard nonsterile gloves, wash hands, and don sterile gloves.	*Maintains sterility of process*

Action	Rationale
8. Place basin beside wound and tilt client to side toward basin.	*Facilitates drainage of irrigation into basin*
9. Irrigate wound: - Insert irrigation tubing into upper portion of wound (or above cleanest portion of wound so fluid flows from cleanest to dirtiest portion of wound; Fig. 10.12). - Attach syringe to tubing or catheter and pour in irrigant; continue to pour irrigant until wound debris and drainage are washed into basin. - Move catheter to different part of wound and repeat irrigation until total wound area has been irrigated and all irrigant has been used.	*Flushes debris and contaminants from wound*
10. Use sterile pads, if needed, to remove additional debris; pack wound with gauze pads, if ordered; apply sterile dressing.	

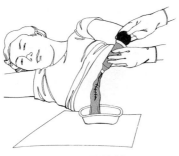

FIGURE 10.12

Action	Rationale
11. Write the date and time of dressing change on a strip of tape and place tape across dressing.	*Indicates last dressing change and need for next change*
12. Dispose of gloves and materials and store supplies appropriately.	*Decreases spread of micro-organisms*
13. Position client for comfort with call bell within reach.	*Promotes comfort and communication*
14. Wash hands.	*Decreases spread of micro-organisms*

Evaluation

Were desired outcomes achieved?

Documentation

The following should be noted on the client's chart:

- Location, appearance, and type of wound or incision
- Status of previous dressing
- Solution and medications applied to wound
- Client teaching done
- Client's tolerance of procedure

SAMPLE DOCUMENTATION

DATE	TIME	
1/12/02	0600	Gaping abdominal incisional wound irrigated with sterile saline. Incision about 8 inches in length and gapes open at 2 cm crosswise along entire length of incision. No purulent drainage from wound. Open area pink, with whitish yellow edges. Wound packed with moist saline gauze. Client turned to side with pillow at back. Tolerated procedure with minimal discomfort.

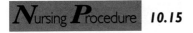

Wound Drain Management (includes Penrose drains, Hemovacs, Jackson-Pratt/ bulb drains, and t-tubes)

EQUIPMENT

- Graduated container
- Sterile dressing tray (forceps, scissors, gauze pads [optional])
- Sterile gauze dressing pads (2 × 2-inch, 4 × 4-inch, or surgical [ABD] pads, depending on drainage and size of area to be covered), or transparent dressing
- Sterile bowl
- 2-inch tape or Montgomery straps (paper tape if allergic to others)
- Sterile gloves
- Nonsterile gloves
- Towel or linen-saver pad
- Cotton balls and cotton-tipped swabs (optional)
- Sterile irrigation saline or sterile water
- Cleansing solution as ordered
- Bacteriostatic ointment
- Overbed table or bedside stand
- Trash bag (appropriate for type of disposal)
- Additional gauze pads

Purpose

Removes accumulated secretions and dead tissue from wound or incision

Decreases microorganism growth on wounds or incision site

Promotes wound healing

Assessment

Assessment should focus on the following:

Type of drain

Doctor's order or agency policy regarding frequency of drainage measurement

Type, appearance, and location of wound or incision

Time of last pain medication
Client allergies to tape or solution used

Nursing Diagnoses

The nursing diagnoses may include the following:

Impaired tissue integrity related to draining abscess
Potential infection related to decreased skin integrity

Outcome Identification and Planning

Desired Outcomes (sample)

Client regains skin integrity within 3 weeks.
Client demonstrates no signs of infection in wound.

Special Consideration

Dressing changes and drain manipulation are often painful. Assess client's pain needs and medicate, if needed, 30 min before beginning procedure.

Pediatric

It may be necessary to have a parent assist while the procedure is being performed.
Using dolls may be helpful in explaining to the child what drain management entails.

Home Health

Newspaper should be used to cover the table surface before arranging a sterile field. Animals in the home should be restricted from the area during the procedure.

Delegation

In general, this procedure is performed by the registered or licensed practical nurse. See agency policy concerning delegation to unlicensed specially trained assistive personnel.

IMPLEMENTATION

Action	Rationale
1. Wash hands and organize equipment.	*Reduces microorganism transfer* *Promotes efficiency*
2. Explain procedure and assistance needed from client; provide privacy.	*Promotes cooperation* *Avoids embarrassment*

Action	Rationale
3. Assess pain level and administer pain medication, if needed; wait for medication to take effect before beginning.	*Decreases discomfort of dressing change*
4. Place bedside table close to area being dressed.	*Facilitates management of sterile field and supplies*
5. Place towel or pad under wound area.	*Eliminates drainage onto surrounding skin*
6. Perform dressing change (see Procedure 10.2); during wound cleaning, note condition of drain-insertion site (intactness of sutures, presence of redness or purulent drainage).	
7. Clean wound with solution-soaked pads or swabs, moving from drain outward in a circular motion; place gauze dressing around drain-insertion site (Fig. 10.13).	*Prevents contamination of wound with microorganisms* *Decreases skin irritation from drainage*
8. Check that tubings are not kinked, twisted, or dislodged.	
9. Continue procedure by performing steps appropriate for type of drain used; then proceed to steps 18 through 20 for completion of procedure.	

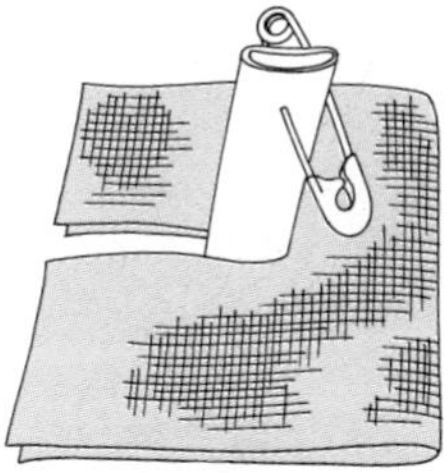

FIGURE 10.13

Action	Rationale

Penrose drains

10. Place extra 4 × 4-inch pads over drain.

Facilitates absorption of drainage

11. Cover with one or two surgical pads and tape securely.

Hemovac

12. Apply and secure dressing; note drainage color and amount; empty if half full or more by opening pouring spout, holding it inverted over graduated container, and squeezing hemovac gently.

Assesses drainage

Empties drain to prevent over filling and applying tension on suture areas

Facilitates flow of clots and drainage

13. Compress evacuator after emptying:
    - Place palm of hand on top of evacuator and press flat with top of spout open.
    - Replace stopper to spout while holding evacuator flat (Fig. 10.14).
    - Remove hand from evacuator and check that it remains flat.

Activates suction needed to maintain drainage evacuation

14. When assessing wound, drainage, and drain, check to be sure evacuator is still compressed; if not, empty drain and recompress.

Maintains suction pressure

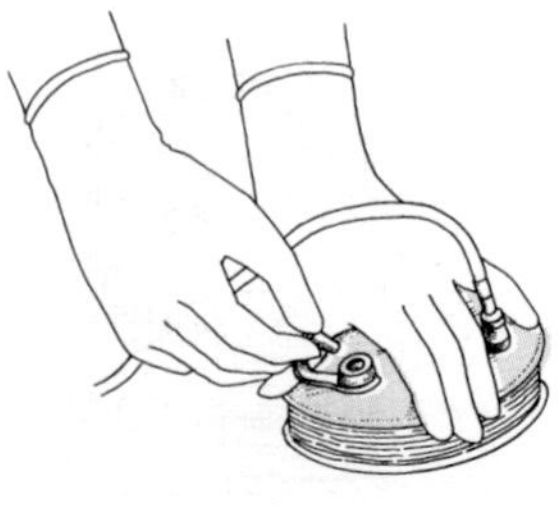

FIGURE 10.14

Action	Rationale

Jackson-Pratt (bulb drain)

15. Apply and secure dressing; note drainage color and amount; empty if half full or more by opening pouring spout, inverting over graduated container, and squeezing bulb.

    Assesses drainage
    Prevents overfilling and tension pull on suture line
    Releases contents from the bulb drain

16. After emptying, recompress bulb by squeezing bulb in palm of hand with top of spout open, then closing spout and releasing bulb.

    Initiates suction needed for drainage evacuation

17. When assessing wound, drainage, and drain, check to be sure evacuator is still compressed; if not, empty drain and recompress.

    Maintains suction pressure

T-tube

18. Apply and secure dressing; hang bag off trunk of body.

    Facilitates use of gravity for drainage

19. To empty, open pouring spout, tilt to side with spout positioned over graduated container, pour, and recap spout.

    Prevents overfill of tube and tension on suture line

20. Dispose of gloves and materials and store supplies appropriately.

    Decreases spread of microorganisms

21. Position client for comfort with call bell within reach.

    Promotes comfort and communication

22. Wash hands.

    Decreases spread of microorganisms

Evaluation

Were desired outcomes achieved?

Documentation

The following should be noted on the client's chart:

- Location and type of wound or incision
- Status of previous dressing
- Status of the wound or incision site and drain
- Type and amount of drainage
- Solution and medications applied to wound
- Client teaching done
- Client's tolerance of procedure

SAMPLE DOCUMENTATION

DATE	TIME	
1/12/02	0600	Abdominal wound dressing saturated with serous drainage. Dressing removed. Penrose drain intact, with moderate drainage. Area surrounding drain intact without redness. Site cleaned with saline solution. Dressing change performed. Client tolerated dressing change with minimal discomfort.

Chapter 11

Medication Administration

OVERVIEW

▶ Medication administration is one of the procedures most frequently performed by the nurse.
▶ Precision is essential in administering medication; otherwise, fatalities may occur.
▶ To administer drugs safely, the nurse must make decisions regarding alterations in technique based on the age, developmental stage, weight, physiologic status, mental status, educational level, and past physical history of the client.

▶ Legal liability remains a major concern in medication administration; however, using a few basic guidelines can significantly decrease the nurse's risk of involvement in a lawsuit:
  - Know the medication being administered.
  - Know the correct technique for administration.
  - Know the client in relation to factors that might affect administration methodology (see above).
  - Know the agency policy on administering drugs by any technique.
  - Know the client's rights in relation to medication administration.
  - REMEMBER THE FIVE RIGHTS OF MEDICATION ADMINISTRATION EACH TIME DRUGS ARE ADMINISTERED: THE RIGHT CLIENT, DRUG, ROUTE, TIME, AND AMOUNT.
  - Document administration immediately after giving medication.
  - If you are unsure about any aspect of drug therapy or administration, ASK!

▶ Generally, medications given by parenteral routes act faster and have more reliable results than drugs given by other routes. Because errors in parenteral medication can quickly become debilitating or lethal, USE EXTREME CAUTION!

▶ Medications given orally are least expensive, but the oral route is the least dependable route of administration.

▶ Although exposure to blood is often minimal during parenteral medication administration, gloves are recommended.

▶ Administration of parenteral medications often requires manipulation of needles, placing the nurse at risk for a needlestick injury. When available, the nurse should use a needleless methodology and equipment for medication administration.

▶ Before administering ordered medication, be sure no folk medications or over-the-counter medications have been ingested that may result in a drug interaction.

▶ The nursing diagnostic labels applicable to medication administration vary greatly with type of drug and route. However, some of the more common diagnoses are acute pain, chronic pain, knowledge deficit, and anxiety.

▶ Delegation: As a basic standard, medication preparation, teaching, and administration are done by a licensed registered or vocational nurse. Some drugs may be given by registered nurses only. Policies vary by agency and state. BE SURE TO NOTE SPECIFIC AGENCY POLICIES FOR A GIVEN ROUTE AND DRUG BEFORE DELEGATING ADMINISTRATION!

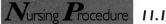

Principles of Medication Administration

EQUIPMENT

- Physician's order
- Medication administration record
- Ink pen
- Disposable gloves
- Medication to be administered
- Drug reference book
- Medicine tray

Optional, depending on route of administration

- Syringes with appropriate-size needles
- Alcohol swabs
- Medication cups
- Cup of water
- Drinking straw
- Medication labels
- Calculator
- Lubricant
- Medicine dropper
- Needleless system equipment (access pins, caps, etc.)

Purpose

Uses basic safety factors of drug administration in preparing and administering medications
Avoids client injury due to drug errors

Assessment

Assessment should focus on the following:
Clarity and legibility of physician's order
Age and weight of client
Lighting in medication preparation area

Outcome Identification and Planning

Desired Outcome (sample)

Client received correct drug and dosage at the correct time without injury.

Special Considerations

Consult a drug reference manual or pharmacist for information on drugs with which you are unfamiliar.

Pediatric

Infants and children often require very small dosages of medications.

Use a syringe instead of a medication cup for the most accurate measurement of liquid medications.

Home Health and Geriatric

See Display 11.1 for home health and geriatric considerations.

Delegation

As a general standard, *only* licensed nurses may administer medications. In most agencies, drugs administered by intravenous (IV) route may only be administered by registered nurses. POLICIES VARY BY AGENCY AND STATE, HOWEVER. BE SURE TO CONSULT SPECIFIC AGENCY POLICIES FOR DELEGATION OF DRUG ADMINISTRATION FOR A GIVEN ROUTE AND/OR DRUG. Registered nurses generally administer IV push medications and medications given through central line catheters and peripherally inserted central catheter (PICC) lines. IV sedation drugs are given by registered nurses. In many facilities, selected IV piggyback medications and peripheral IV saline flush may be given by licensed vocational nurses.
BE SURE TO CHECK AGENCY POLICY BEFORE DELEGATING *ANY* DRUG ADMINISTRATION TO OTHER PERSONNEL!

IMPLEMENTATION

Action	Rationale
1. Wash hands.	*Reduces microorganism transfer*
2. Gather equipment and unlock medication cart or cabinet.	*Promotes efficiency*

Action	Rationale

DISPLAY 11.1 **Principles of Management, Storage, and Disposal of Medications in the Home Setting**

- Administer medications only to the client admitted to the home-health service (ie, not to a spouse or relative).
- Administer only those drugs prescribed by the attending physician.
- Prepare a written schedule of medications that is developed based on client's schedule of activities and sleeping patterns.
- Posting a schedule on the refrigerator may remind the client of medication administration times.
- For elderly and other clients at home who have problems with memory, use devices that remind them when drugs must be taken (eg, calendars, daily pill dispensers).
- Single pills taped to a piece of cardboard (out of reach of children) may increase client recognition and understanding of each medication and its appropriate administration.
- A color code or notation on each pill bottle may be helpful. A 7-day pill administration box may be helpful.
- If working with a client to use a medication box that is set up once a week, there must be a family member or caregiver who can continue to set up the medication box after the client has been discharged from nursing services to meet requirements of some insurance companies for coverage.
- Review the schedule of administration on each visit and with each change in medication.
- Instruct clients to store medications in original labeled containers, with containers for current medications grouped close together.
- Highlighting the number of refills on a prescription bottle with a marker may assist the client in timely reordering of medications.
- If refrigeration is needed, store medications away from food items in an area of limited access.
- Teach how to determine expiration dates.
- Instruct to flush old pills down toilet and discard bottle.

Action	Rationale
3. Compare medication administration record to physician's order, adhering to principles of the five rights of drug administration; use these principles throughout preparation and administration. Check for the right: - *Client*—includes checking name, identification number, room number, prescribing doctor's name on the order, medication administration record, medication cards, and client identification band - *Drug*—includes ascertaining that generic names are compatible with brand names (if both are used) and that client has no allergies to ingredients of ordered medications; includes checking drug labels with medication administration records or cards. - *Dosage*—includes determining that dosage ordered is within usual dosage range for route of administration, weight, and age of client; checking dosages on drug labels for compatibility with dosages written on medication administration record or cards; and performing accurate dose calculations. - *Time*—includes checking that medication administration frequency (eg, "every 12 hours" [q12 h] or "three times a day"	*Promotes safety* *Avoids client injury related to wrong dose, drug, route, time, or client*

Action	Rationale

[tid]) is compatible with times (eg, 6 AM and 6 PM or 10 AM, 2 PM, and 6 PM) listed on medication administration record or medication cards.

- *Route*—includes checking drug label to ascertain if medication can be administered by ordered route and checking that route recorded on medication administration record and cards corresponds to the doctor's order.

4. If client has allergy to any ordered medication, notify physician.

Prevents unnecessary allergic reactions and injury

5. Focusing on one medication at a time, begin label checks by comparing the actual drug labels to the order, as transcribed on the medication administration record; if using a medication administration record, begin at the top and systematically move down the page; if using cards, group the cards according to route of administration (eg, oral medications, intramuscular [IM] medications) and focus on one card at a time.

Prevents error in preparation
Promotes systematic preparation

6. Comparing drug labels with the orders on the medication administration record or cards, determine if dosage calculations are necessary.

7. Perform calculations using one of the following formulas:

Action	Rationale

$$\frac{\text{DESIRED DOSAGE}}{\text{AVAILABLE DOSAGE}} \times \frac{\text{VEHICLE}}{\text{(ML, TABLET)}} = \frac{\text{CORRECT DOSAGE}}{\text{(ML, TABLETS, MINIMS)}}$$

Example: Doctor's order: 15 mEq potassium per liter of D_5W
Available dose: 40 mEq potassium per 20-ml vial
(2 mEq per ml) (inject into liter D_5W)

OR

DESIRED DOSAGE : AVAILABLE DOSAGE

=

DESIRED VOLUME : AVAILABLE VOLUME

Example: D is desired volume (amount to be administered)
15 mEq potassium: 40 mEq potassium = D:20 ml
Multiply the means by the extremes

$$300 = 40\,D$$

$$\frac{300}{40} = D$$

$$D = 7.5 \text{ ml}$$

Desired dosage is the dosage ordered
Available dosage equals the dosage on hand (eg, the number of milligrams or the number of milliequivalents)
Vehicle is the drug form (number of tablets or amount of solution containing the available dosage)
Desired volume is the volume of the drug to be administered (eg, number of milliliters, minims, tablets)
Available volume is the amount of solution or number of tablets containing the drug (eg, ml minims, tablets) on hand

Action	Rationale
IF YOU ARE UNCERTAIN OF THE ACCURACY OF YOUR CALCULATIONS, CHECK WITH ANOTHER NURSE.	*Provides safety check*
8. Check label on each medication: - Before removing drug from drawer or storage area - Before pouring or drawing up medication (or once medication is in hand, if unit dose)	

Action	Rationale
- Before replacing multiple-dose containers on shelf (or before removing your hands from the drug once it is on the medicine tray, if unit dose)	
9. Recheck medication administration record for appropriate client identification record.	*Ensures that nurse is focusing on right client record*
10. Using aseptic technique, pour or draw up each medication after second label check (Fig. 11.1); use guidelines in Table 11.1 in preparing drugs for various routes of administration.	*Prepares drug using aseptic technique* *Ensures accurate measurement of drug amount*
11. Place each drug on medication tray after checking label a third time and before proceeding to prepare the next drug.	*Provides third label check*
12. Recheck medication record or cards with each drug on tray; if using medication cards, make certain that medicines are placed in front of appropriate cards.	*Provides safety check and identifying information on drug once on medication tray*
13. Place all administration equipment on tray.	*Ensures that proper equipment for administration is present*
14. Lock medication cart or cabinet.	*Adheres to accreditation guidelines*

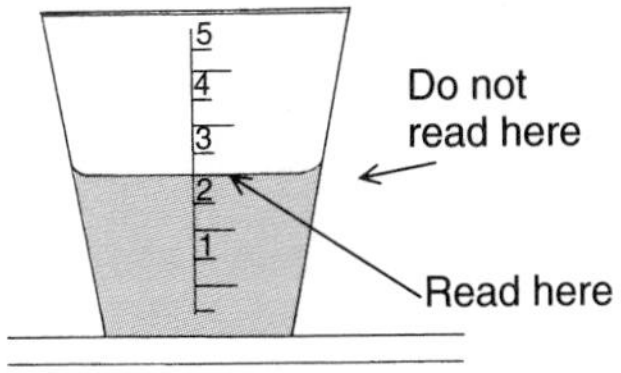

Do not read here

Read here

FIGURE 11.1

TABLE 11.1	Guidelines for Preparing Various Forms of Medication	
Guideline	*Rationale*
1. Most agencies require that certain medications (such as heparin, insulin, IV digoxin) be checked by a second nurse during preparation. Check agency policy and procedure manuals for the full listing of these drugs.	Prevents error in preparation of drugs with potentially lethal effects
2. Do not open unit-dose packages in advance if dosages are exact (ie, pills, oral liquids, and suppositories). Open just before administering.	Provides identifying drug information Prevents waste
3. When preparing topical, nasal, ophthalmic, and other boxed medications, remove medication from box and check labels of actual containers.	Prevents administration of wrong drug
4. If pouring pills from multiple-dose containers, pour pill into cap and then into medicine cup. Pour liquids away from label. Read amount of medication poured in medicine cups at bottom of meniscus (see Fig. 11.1).	Maintains asepsis Prevents destruction of label Measures liquid drug correctly
5. Separate drugs requiring preassessment data, such as vital signs.	Prevents administration before vital sign assessment
6. When preparing any drug, check for expiration date.	Eliminates administering drugs that no longer have full therapeutic effect

See Procedures 11.2 through 11.18 for additional information on the preparation and administration of drugs for various routes.

Evaluation

Were desired outcomes achieved?

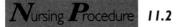

 Eye (Ophthalmic) Instillation

EQUIPMENT

- Two to six cotton balls, one to three per eye (some agencies recommend use of sterile cotton balls)
- Disposable gloves
- Medication record or card
- Pen
- Medication to be administered

Purpose

Instills medications in mucous membranes of eye for various therapeutic effects, such as decreasing inflammatory and infectious processes and preventing drying of cornea, conjunctiva, and other delicate eye structures

Assessment

Assessment should focus on the following:

Presence in structures of eye (sclera, cornea, conjunctival sacs, eyelids) of lesions, redness, or drainage
Status of vision before drug administration
Complaints of pain or eye discomfort

Nursing Diagnoses

The nursing diagnoses may include the following:

Altered comfort: pain related to infectious process

Outcome Identification and Planning

Desired Outcome (sample)
Client shows no redness, edema, or drainage from eye.

Special Consideration

Geriatric and Home Health

For elderly clients at home who have difficulty remembering, use
 a calendar to remind them when to administer eye medication.

 Transcultural

In some cultures (such as the Vietnamese), touching the head may
 be viewed as taking away the spirit. The nurse should consult
 the client, or parents if a child is involved, regarding what is culturally appropriate.

Ask family member to assist in positioning the client's head, if
 necessary or desired.

Delegation

As a basic standard, medication preparation, teaching, and administration are done by a licensed registered or vocational
 nurse. Some drugs may be given by registered nurses only. Policies vary by agency and state. BE SURE TO NOTE SPECIFIC
 AGENCY POLICIES FOR A GIVEN ROUTE AND DRUG BE-
 FORE DELEGATING ADMINISTRATION!

IMPLEMENTATION

Action	Rationale
1. Wash hands.	*Decreases microorganism transfer*
2. Prepare drug to be admini-stered according to the five rights of drug administra-tion (see Procedure 11.1).	*Promotes safe drug administra-tion*
3. Identify client by identifi-cation bracelet and by addressing client by name.	*Verifies identity of client*
4. Explain procedure and purpose of medication to client.	*Reduces anxiety* *Promotes cooperation*
5. Don gloves.	*Prevents exposure to secretions from eye*
6. Position client in supine or sitting position, with fore-head tilted back slightly.	*Facilitates proper placement of medication*
7. If drainage or excess tearing is noted around lower lashes and eyelids, wipe eye with a cotton ball from the inner to outer aspect (if both eyes	*Removes excess secretions and debris to facilitate absorption of medication through mucous membranes* *Prevents cross-contamination*

Action	Rationale
need to be wiped, use a separate cotton ball for each eye).	
8. If using bottle with a dropper, squeeze top of medication dropper to aspirate solution into dropper tube.	*Creates suction to draw up medication in dropper*
9. Holding dropper or ointment to be administered in dominant hand, place heel of dominant hand on client's forehead (Fig. 11.2)	*Provides strategic placement of nurse's hand to prevent accidental eye injury to client*
10. Using cotton ball, gently pull lower eyelid down.	*Exposes lower conjunctival sac for placement of medication*
11. Instruct client to look up toward forehead.	*Eliminates corneal-reflex stimulation*
12. Administer ordered number of drops (or quantity of ointment) into conjunctival sac of appropriate eye without letting dropper touch client; apply ointment from inner to outer canthus, ending administration smoothly with a twisting motion.	*Places medication in conjunctival sac for absorption without contaminating dropper*

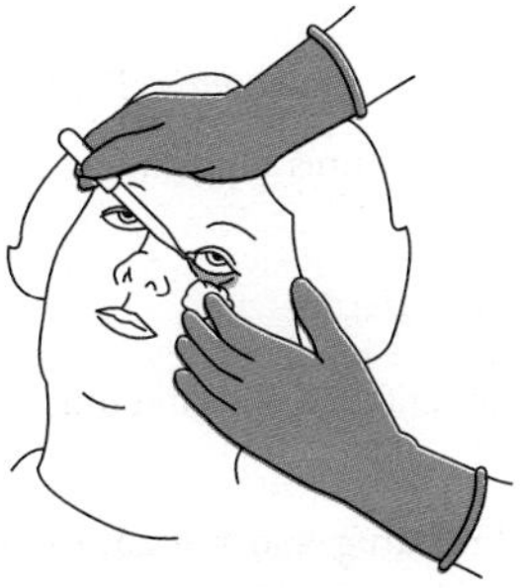

FIGURE 11.2

Action	Rationale
13. Remove hands and instruct client to close and roll eyes around, unless prohibited or unless client is unable to do so.	*Spreads medication evenly over eye*
14. Remove excess medication and secretions from around eye with cotton balls.	*Prevents local irritation and discomfort*
15. Discard gloves.	*Reduces microorganism transfer*
16. If ointments or drops temporarily affect vision, instruct client not to move about until vision is clearer.	*Prevents accidental injury*
17. Lift side rails.	*Prevents falling accidents*
18. Place call light within reach.	*Facilitates communication with nurse*
19. Discard or restore equipment properly.	*Facilitates clean and orderly environment*
20. Document administration on medication record.	*Provides legal record of medication administration and prevents accidental remedication*

Evaluation

Were desired outcomes achieved?

Documentation

The following should be noted on the client's chart:

- Condition of eye structures (appearance of skin, presence of drainage, redness, lesions)
- Status of vision
- Reports of pain or tenderness
- Eye in which drug was instilled
- Name of drug, amount, and date and time administered   .
- Adverse reactions to medication
- Effects of drug
- Teaching regarding drug and self-administration of medications

SAMPLE DOCUMENTATION

DATE	TIME	
7/7/02	1115	One drop of gentamycin solution (3 mg/ml) administered in each eye as initial dose of medication. Client states left eye is slightly painful but no blurred vision. Slight redness in right eye and small amount of creamy, mucous-colored secretions from right eye.

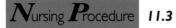

Nursing Procedure 11.3

Ear (Otic) Instillation

EQUIPMENT

- Two or three cotton balls or tissue
- Disposable gloves
- Small basin of warm water
- Soap
- Washcloth
- Small dry towel
- Medication record or card
- Pen
- Medication to be administered

Purpose

Instills liquid medication into external auditory canal for such therapeutic effects as decreasing inflammation and infection and softening ear wax for easy removal

Assessment

Assessment should focus on the following:

Condition of external ear (excess wax production, cleanliness, drainage, and odor)
Hearing ability of client
Client's balance and coordination
Ability of client to follow instructions

Nursing Diagnoses

The nursing diagnoses may include the following:

Altered comfort related to inner ear inflammation
Impaired hearing ability related to excessive wax buildup

Outcome Identification and Planning

Desired Outcomes (sample)

Client states that pain is relieved following treatment.
There is no evidence of redness, edema, or discharge from the affected ear.
Ear canal is clear, with no excess wax buildup.

Special Considerations

Geriatric

For elderly clients who have difficulty remembering, use a calendar to remind them when to administer ear medication.

Pediatric

It may be necessary to have a parent assist by holding the child in position in order to avoid ear damage when administering ear medications.

 Transcultural

In some cultures (such as the Vietnamese), touching the head may be viewed as taking away the spirit. The nurse should consult the client, or parents if a child is involved, regarding what is culturally appropriate.

Ask a family member to assist in positioning the client's head, if necessary or desired.

Delegation

As a basic standard, medication preparation, teaching, and administration are done by a licensed registered or vocational nurse. Some drugs may be given by registered nurses only. Policies vary by agency and state. BE SURE TO NOTE SPECIFIC AGENCY POLICIES FOR A GIVEN ROUTE AND DRUG BEFORE DELEGATING ADMINISTRATION!

IMPLEMENTATION

Action	Rationale
1. Wash hands.	*Reduces spread of micro-organisms*
2. Prepare medication, adhering to the five rights of drug administration (see Procedure 11.1).	*Decreases chance of drug error*
3. Identify client by reading identification bracelet and by addressing client by name.	*Confirms identity of client*
4. Explain procedure and purpose of drug.	*Decreases anxiety*
5. Verify client's allergies.	*Prevents unnecessary allergic reactions and injury*

Action	Rationale
6. Don gloves.	*Decreases nurse's exposure to ear secretions*
7. Wash ear if excess wax is noted.	*Helps clear path for channeling of drug into ear canal*
8. Assist client into side-lying, sitting, or semi-Fowler's position, with ear to receive medication either facing directly upward (in side-lying position) or forehead tilted upward and turned toward opposite side (in sitting or semi-Fowler's position).	*Positions client for channeling of drug into ear canal*
9. Using nondominant hand, gently pull auricle of the ear up and back (for adults and children older than 3 years [Fig. 11.3]) or down and back (for children younger than 3 years).	*Straightens ear canal for correct channeling of drug into ear*
10. While resting heel of dominant hand on side of client's face near temporal area, drop ordered number of ear drops into ear canal without touching ear with medicine dropper.	*Prevents accidental injury of tympanic membrane* *Delivers medication* *Decreases contamination of solution remaining in bottle*

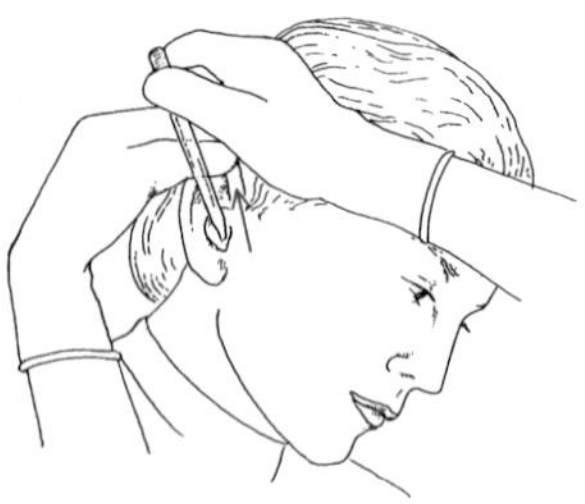

FIGURE 11.3

Action	Rationale
11. Release ear and remove excess medication from around outside of ear with cotton ball or tissue.	*Reduces skin irritation and promotes comfort*
12. Replace cap on medicine container.	*Maintains medication sterility*
13. Instruct client to remain in position for 3 to 5 min.	*Allows time for medication to be absorbed*
14. Remove gloves and discard with soiled materials.	*Reduces transfer of microorganisms*
15. Raise side rails and place call light within reach.	*Prevents falls due to disequilibrium and facilitates communication with nurse*
16. Wash hands.	*Reduces spread of microorganisms*
17. Document administration on medication record.	*Provides legal record of medication administration and prevents accidental remedication*

Evaluation

Were desired outcomes achieved?

Documentation

The following should be noted on the client's chart:
- Condition of ear (appearance of skin, presence of drainage, redness, edema, excess wax buildup)
- Status of hearing
- Reports of pain or tenderness
- Ear in which drug was instilled
- Name and amount of drug
- Adverse reactions to medication
- Effects of drug
- Teaching regarding drug information and techniques for self-administration of medications

SAMPLE DOCUMENTATION

DATE	TIME	
4/7/02	1100	Client received first dose of neomcyin (0.01%) ear drops. Given 2 drops in right ear, without report of pain. Slight redness and a small amount of yellowish discharge from ear. No excess wax buildup noted. Client able to repeat statements without visual cues, indicating unimpaired hearing.

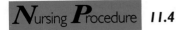

Nursing Procedure 11.4

Nasal Instillation

EQUIPMENT

- Nasal drops to be given
- Medication record or card
- Pen
- Disposable gloves
- Tissue
- Pillow roll (or large towel made into pillow roll)
- Wet washcloth

Purpose

Delivers medication for local or systemic absorption through nasal membranes for such therapeutic effects as resolving infections, treating inflammation, and relieving congestion

Assessment

Assessment should focus on the following:

Condition of nasal mucosa
Patency of nasal airway
Presence of nosebleed or discharge
Respiratory character
Contraindications, if any, to client blowing nose

Nursing Diagnoses

The nursing diagnoses may include the following:

Ineffective breathing pattern related to bronchial congestion and nasal inflammation

Outcome Identification and Planning

Desired Outcomes (sample)

Client's respirations are even and smooth, at rate of 16 breaths per minute.
Nasal passage is clear; septum is pink.

Special Considerations

Geriatric

For elderly clients who have difficulty remembering, use a calendar to remind them when to use nose drops.

Pediatric

It may be necessary to obtain the assistance of a parent to hold the child in position for nasal instillations.

Home Health

Instruct client on administration of nasal medications and provide information about the drugs involved. Caution client against overuse of nasal medications.

 Transcultural

In some cultures (such as the Vietnamese), touching the head may be viewed as taking away the spirit. The nurse should consult the client, or parent if a child is involved, regarding what is culturally appropriate.

Ask a family member to assist in positioning the client's head, if necessary or desired.

Delegation

As a basic standard, medication preparation, teaching, and administration are done by a licensed registered or vocational nurse. Some drugs may be given by registered nurses only. Policies vary by agency and state. BE SURE TO NOTE SPECIFIC AGENCY POLICIES FOR A GIVEN ROUTE AND DRUG BEFORE DELEGATING ADMINISTRATION!

IMPLEMENTATION

Action	Rationale
1. Wash hands.	*Reduces microorganism transfer*
2. Prepare medication, adhering to the five rights of drug administration (see Procedure 11.1).	*Decreases chance of drug error*
3. Identify client by reading identification bracelet and by addressing client by name.	*Confirms identity of client*
4. Explain procedure and purpose of drug.	*Decreases anxiety*

Action	Rationale
5. Verify client's allergies listed on medication record or card.	*Prevents unnecessary allergic reactions and injury*
6. Don gloves.	*Decreases nurse's exposure to nasal secretions*
7. If excess mucus is noted in nares, instruct client to blow nose gently (unless contraindicated).	*Clears nares for proper medication absorption*
8. Wipe excess secretions with tissue.	*Removes secretions and cleans skin*
9. Place client in sitting position with head tilted slightly backward, or supine with head tilted back in a slightly hyper-extended position (it may be necessary to place a pillow roll or rolled towel under client's neck).	*Facilitates proper channeling of drug through nasal passage for optimal absorption*
10. Squeeze top of medication dropper with dominant hand.	*Suctions solution into dropper*
11. Stabilize client's forehead with palm of nondominant hand while gently lifting nose open (Fig. 11.4).	*Prevents accidental damage to nasal mucosa if client suddenly tries to move head when dropper is in place*
12. Without touching client's nose or skin with dropper, hold dropper about ¼ to ½ inch above naris and tilt tip of dropper toward nasal septum (center of nose).	*Maintains asepsis of remaining drug* *Directs dropper to center of nose for proper placement of drug*

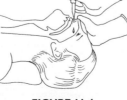

FIGURE 11.4

Action	Rationale
13. Squeeze top of dropper and deliver the appropriate number of drops.	*Delivers correct dose of medication*
14. Instruct client to take one short, deep breath and to remain in position for 3 to 5 min.	*Facilitates full absorption of drug*
15. Replace dropper in bottle.	*Maintains medication sterility*
16. Remove nasal secretions or solution from client's skin (use warm, wet washcloth, if necessary).	*Prevents local skin irritation and client discomfort*
17. Lift side rails and place call light within reach.	*Facilitates client–nurse communication and safety*
18. Discard gloves and restore other equipment properly.	*Promotes cleanliness*
19. Wash hands.	*Prevents spread of infection*
20. Document administration on medication administration record.	*Serves as legal record of medication administration and prevents accidental remediation*

Evaluation

Were desired outcomes achieved?

Documentation

The following should be noted on the client's chart:
- Name, dosage, and route of medication
- Assessment data relevant to purpose of medication
- Effects of medication
- Teaching of information about drug used and techniques of self-administration of medication

SAMPLE DOCUMENTATION

DATE	TIME	
9/6/02	2100	Client received final dose of Neosynephrine nasally, 2 drops in right naris. Client states pain in nose relieved. No redness or swelling of nasal mucosa. No drainage from nares. Respirations smooth and even.

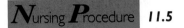

Administration of Oral Medication

EQUIPMENT

- Medication record or cards
- Pen
- Disposable gloves, if possibility of exposure to oral secretions
- Medication to be administered
- Medication cup
- Water, juice, or beverage
- Drinking straw

Purpose

Delivers medication for absorption through alimentary tract

Assessment

Assessment should focus on the following:

Complete medication order
Condition of client's mouth (presence of lesions, tears, bleeding, tenderness)
Ability of client to swallow without difficulty
Client nausea or inability to retain oral medications

Nursing Diagnoses

The nursing diagnoses may include the following:
Altered comfort: pain related to surgical incision
Altered sleep pattern related to unfamiliarity with hospital environment

Outcome Identification and Planning

Desired Outcomes (sample)
Client states that pain is relieved within an hour of administration of pain-killing drug.
Client falls asleep within 1 hour of administration of sleep enhancer.

Special Considerations

When preparing and administering oral drugs, many factors must be taken into account to ensure adequate drug absorption and proper action.

Consult a drug reference manual or pharmacist about drugs with which you are unfamiliar. Some general factors to take into consideration are the following:

- Many solid forms of medication (eg, capsules, enteric-coated tablets) should not be crushed or chewed.
- Many oral medications require administration with milk or food to avoid gastric irritation.
- Frequently, several oral medications are given at the same time. When this occurs, the effects of one or more drugs may be potentiated or decreased.
- When a client receives a medication for the first time, monitor the client closely for an adverse reaction or sensitivity.
- Schedule first doses of new medications at different hours from other medications to obtain a clear picture of the client's response to the new drug.

Geriatric

For elderly clients who have difficulty remembering, use devices that remind the client to take medications, such as daily pill dispensers and calendars.

Pediatric

Holding and cuddling an infant may elicit a positive response when administering oral medications. If drugs are being mixed with food or liquid, use as small an amount of these as possible so the child will take all of the drug.

Medicine can also be given through nipples or droppers.

Toddlers tend to cooperate more when they are given a choice of method of drug delivery—spoon, dropper, syringe—and are allowed to help with drug administration. Most prefer to hold and take pills without assistance.

Home Health

Be alert for self-prescribed medications, usually obtained from previous doctors, friends, or family members. These medications may have adverse reactions when combined with current medications. Ask to see all drugs taken within the past 24 to 72 h.

 Transcultural

If client prefers a substance that is hot or cold for treatment of the condition, and the medication can be warmed or cooled without contraindications, the nurse should acknowledge and accommodate cultural beliefs.

The nurse should inquire if folk medications have been or are currently being ingested before administering ordered medications to prevent potential drug interactions. Consult pharmacy and the physician as indicated.

Delegation

As a basic standard, medication preparation, teaching, and administration are done by a licensed registered or vocational nurse. Some drugs may be given by registered nurses only. Policies vary by agency and state. BE SURE TO NOTE SPECIFIC AGENCY POLICIES FOR A GIVEN ROUTE AND DRUG BEFORE DELEGATING ADMINISTRATION!

IMPLEMENTATION

Action	Rationale
1. Wash hands.	*Reduces microorganism transfer*
2. Prepare medication, adhering to the five rights of drug administration (see Procedure 11.1).	*Prepares drug* *Decreases chance of drug error*
3. Identify client by reading identification bracelet and by addressing client by name.	*Confirms identity of client*
4. Explain procedure and purpose of drug.	*Decreases anxiety* *Promotes cooperation*
5. Verify client's allergies listed on medication record or card.	*Alerts nurse to potential allergic reaction*
6. Separate drugs that might be withheld based on preassessment data.	*Prevents accidental administration of drugs*
7. Obtain preassessment data before administration.	*Determines if medication should be held or given*
8. Assist client into semi-Fowler's or sitting position.	*Prevents aspiration*
9. Don gloves if there is a possibility of nurse's exposure to oral secretions.	*Avoids exposure to client secretions*
10. Open unit-dose packages and place one drug in client's hand or pour in medication cup and give to client; provide assistance if needed.	*Maintains asepsis while administering*

Action	Rationale
11. Instruct client to place tablets or capsules into mouth and to follow with enough liquid to ensure that drug is swallowed.	*Ensures that drug is swallowed and that tablets are not lodged in throat or esophagus*
12. Administer liquid medications after pills, instructing client to drink all of the solution; provide assistance, if needed.	*Facilitates proper absorption of certain liquids that are not to be followed by a beverage*
13. Remain with client until all medications are taken; check client's mouth if there is any question of whether drug has actually been swallowed.	*Ensures that drug is taken*
14. Reposition client and place call light within reach.	*Facilitates comfort and communication*
15. Lift side rails.	*Prevents accidental falls*
16. Discard or restore equipment properly:	*Promotes clean environment*
- If client refuses drug or drug has not been given for any reason, DO NOT leave drug at the bedside.	*Eliminates question of what happened to drug at later time*
- Remove drug from room and restore in medication drawer or cabinet only if in unopened unit-dose package.	*Allows nurse to administer drug at later date*
- If unit-dose package has been opened, discard in sink with witness present if necessary.	*Witness needed when destroying controlled drugs for compliance with federal regulations*
17. Wash hands.	*Prevents spread of infection*
18. Document administration on medication record.	*Serves as legal record of medication administration and prevents accidental remedication*
19. Check client 30 to 60 min later for effects of medication.	*Detects beneficial or toxic effects of drug*

Evaluation

Were desired outcomes achieved?

Documentation

The following should be noted on the client's chart:

- Name, amount, and route of drug given
- Purpose of administration if drug is given on a when-needed (p.r.n.) basis
- Assessment data relevant to purpose of medication
- Effects of medication on client
- Teaching of information about drug used or about self-administration technique

SAMPLE DOCUMENTATION

DATE	TIME	
7/8/02	2200	Dalmane (15 mg PO) given for complaint of inability to sleep at 2100. Client asleep, with even, nonlabored respirations; rate 16.

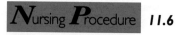
 Administration of Buccal and Sublingual Medication

EQUIPMENT

- Medication record or card
- Pen
- Disposable gloves
- Medication to be administered

Purpose

Delivers medication for absorption through oral mucous membranes

Assessment

Assessment should focus on the following:

Complete medication order
Condition of mouth (presence of lesions, tears, bleeding, tenderness)

Nursing Diagnoses

The nursing diagnoses may include the following:

Altered comfort: chest pain related to oxygen deficit to cardiac muscle
Anxiety related to learning results of diagnostic tests

Desired Outcomes (sample)

Client states pain is relieved within 5 min of administration of one sublingual nitroglycerin tablet.
Client demonstrates signs of decreased anxiety (relaxed facial expression and respiratory rate of 20 breaths per minute).

Special Considerations

Geriatric and Home Health

For elderly clients at home who have difficulty remembering, use devices that remind the client when to take medications, such as calendars and daily pill dispensers.

Delegation

As a basic standard, medication preparation, teaching, and administration are done by a licensed registered or vocational nurse. Some drugs may be given by registered nurses only. Policies vary by agency and state. BE SURE TO NOTE SPECIFIC AGENCY POLICIES FOR A GIVEN ROUTE AND DRUG BEFORE DELEGATING ADMINISTRATION!

IMPLEMENTATION

Action	Rationale
1. Wash hands.	*Reduces microorganism transfer*
2. Prepare medication, adhering to the five rights of drug administration (see Procedure 11.1).	*Prepares drug* *Decreases chance of drug error*
3. Identify client by reading identification bracelet and addressing client by name.	*Confirms identity of client*
4. Explain procedure and purpose of drug.	*Decreases anxiety* *Promotes cooperation*
5. Verify allergies listed on medication record or card.	
6. Don gloves.	*Decreases nurse's exposure to client's body secretions*
7. Place tablet: - Under tongue for sublingual medication - Between cheek and gum on either side of mouth for buccal administration (avoid broken or irritated areas) *Note:* If client's mucous membranes are dry, offer a sip of water before giving medication.	*Facilitates dissolving and absorption through oral mucous membranes* *Reduces additional irritation*
8. Instruct client not to swallow drug but to let drug dissolve.	*Facilitates absorption by proper route*
9. Discard gloves and wash hands.	*Reduces transfer of microorganisms*
10. Document administration on medication record.	*Serves as legal record of medication administration and prevents accidental remedication*

Evaluation

Were desired outcomes achieved?

Documentation

The following should be noted on the client's chart:
- Name, amount, and route of drug given
- Purpose of administration if drug is given on a when-needed (p.r.n.) basis
- Assessment data relevant to purpose of medication
- Effects of medication on client
- Teaching of information about drug used or about self-administration of medication

SAMPLE DOCUMENTATION

DATE	TIME	
1/9/02	1100	Nitroglycerin gr. 1/150 SL for c/o sharp, nonradiating, midsternal chest pain, with relief in 2 minutes. No dysrhythmias noted. Blood pressure 110/70 after 1 tablet.

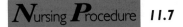

 *Medication Preparation
From a Vial*

EQUIPMENT

- Medication administration record or medication card
- Vial with prescribed medication
- Appropriate-size syringe and needle for type of injection and viscosity of solution
- Extra needle
- Alcohol swabs
- Medication label or small piece of tape
- Medication tray
- Access pin and sterile cap (for needleless procedure) and multidose vials

Purpose

Obtains medication from vial, using aseptic technique, for administration by a parenteral route

Assessment

Assessment should focus on the following:

Appearance of solution (clarity, absence of sediment, color indicated on instruction label)
Vial label for expiration date of drug

Outcome Identification and Planning

Desired Outcome (sample)
Correct amount and type of drug is drawn into syringe using aseptic technique.

Special Considerations
If medication requires reconstitution, follow the guidelines on the vial.
Sterility of the syringe, needle, and medication must be maintained while preparing the drug. Figure 11.5 identifies those parts of a syringe and needle assembly that must be kept sterile.

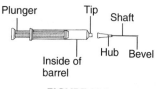

FIGURE 11.5

In a needleless system, the needle is replaced by an access pin with a sterile cap to allow frequent withdrawal of medication. Although exposure to a contaminated needle by the nurse is unlikely at this point in the medication administration procedure, use of a needleless system minimizes the nurse's risk of broken skin integrity.

Geriatric

For elderly clients who have difficulty remembering, use devices that remind them when to take medications, such as calendars and daily medication dispensers.

For elderly clients with special visual deficits, carefully note if client is able to withdraw an accurate amount of solution from the vial.

Home Health

Assess area in which client or family member will be preparing drug for adequacy of lighting.

Delegation

As a basic standard, medication preparation, teaching, and administration are done by a licensed registered or vocational nurse. Some drugs may be given by registered nurses only. Policies vary by agency and state. BE SURE TO NOTE SPECIFIC AGENCY POLICIES FOR A GIVEN ROUTE AND DRUG BEFORE DELEGATING ADMINISTRATION!

IMPLEMENTATION

Action	Rationale
1. Wash hands	*Reduces microorganism transfer*
2. Organize equipment	*Promotes efficiency*
3. Check label of medication vial with medication record or card, using principles of the five rights of drug administration (see Procedure 11.1).	*Avoids client injury from wrong drug or dosage*

Action	Rationale
4. Perform dosage calculations if vial contains more medication than client requires.	*Determines correct amount of solution to be prepared*
5. Remove thin seal cap from top of vial without touching rubber stopper.	*Exposes rubber top for insertion of needle while maintaining asepsis*
6. Firmly wipe rubber stopper on top of vial with alcohol swab. If needleless system is used, insert the spike of the access pin into the vial until the "wing" of the pin touches the vial's rubber stopper. Remove the sterile cap without touching the top of the access pin (Fig. 11.6).	*Ensures asepsis* *Permits access to the fluid in the vial using a syringe only*
7. Pull end of plunger back to fill syringe with a volume of air equal to the amount of solution to be drawn up (Fig. 11.7); do not touch inside of plunger.	*Draws air into syringe to create positive pressure in vial* *Maintains plunger sterility*

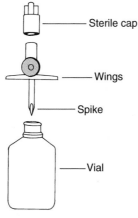

Sterile cap

Wings

Spike

Vial

FIGURE 11.6

Action	Rationale

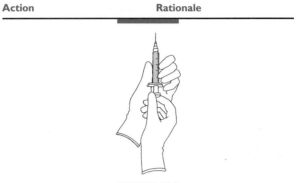

FIGURE 11.7

8. Remove needle cap. (For needleless systems, use syringe only. Remove cap and needle, if necessary. Screw syringe onto access pin and skip steps 9 and 10.)

Prepares for insertion

9. Using a slightly slanted angle, firmly insert needle into center of rubber top of vial, with the sharpest point of the needle (tip of bevel) entering first.

Prevents solution contamination with sediment from rubber top

10. Continue insertion until needle is securely in vial.

Prevents accidental slip of needle from vial

11. Press end of plunger down.

Infuses air to create positive pressure in vial

12. Hold vial with non-dominant hand and turn it up, keeping needle/spike inserted; control syringe with dominant hand and keep plunger down with thumb.

Moves solution to area of vial closest to rubber stopper for easy removal

13. Pull needle/spike back to point at which bevel is beneath fluid level; keep needle/spike beneath fluid level as long as fluid is being withdrawn.

Places needle in position in which fluid can be obtained (below level of fluid)

Action	Rationale
14. Slowly pull end of plunger back until appropriate amount of solution is aspirated into syringe.	*Ensures delivery of prescribed amount of medication*
15. If air bubbles enter syringe, gently flick syringe barrel with fingers of dominant hand while keeping a finger on end of plunger;	*Congregates bubbles in one area for removal*
continue holding vial with nondominant hand.	*Prevents plunger from popping out of barrel*
16. Push plunger in until air is out of syringe.	*Displaces bubble of air into vial*
17. Withdraw additional solution, if needed.	*Replaces solution lost when clearing bubbles*
18. Pull needle out of bottle while keeping a finger on end of plunger. (For needleless systems, screw syringe off and detach from access pin; cover pin with a sterile cap. Apply sterile needle to syringe if IM/SQ injection will be given.)	*Prevents plunger from popping out of barrel*
19. If bubbles remain in syringe: - Hold syringe vertically (with needle pointing up, if attached). - Pull back slightly on plunger and flick syringe with fingers. - Slowly push plunger up to release air but not to the point of expelling the solution.	*Removes remaining air bubbles from syringe using principle that air rises*
20. Recheck amount of solution in syringe, comparing with drug volume required.	*Ensures that correct amount of drug has been prepared*
21. Compare drug label with medication record or card.	*Provides additional identification check of drug*

Action	Rationale
22. Change needle if drug is known to be irritating to tissue; replace cap.	*Prevents tissue irritation from drug clinging to outer surfaces of needle when solution is injected into skin; cap replacement is unnecessary if the needleless system is used*
23. Label syringe with drug label; include name and amount of drug.	*Provides identification information at client's bedside*
24. Place syringe, medication cards, and additional alcohol swabs on medication tray.	*Organizes equipment for administration of drug*
25. Discard or restore all equipment appropriately.	*Promotes clean and organized environment*
26. Wash hands.	*Prevents spread of microorganisms*

Evaluation

Were desired outcomes achieved?

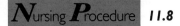

 Medication Preparation From an Ampule

 EQUIPMENT

- Medication administration record or medication card
- Ampule with prescribed medication
- Appropriate-size syringe and needle for type of injection and viscosity of solution (use filtered needle, if available)
- Medication label or small piece of tape
- Extra needle
- Medication tray
- Alcohol swabs
- Paper towel

Purpose

Obtains medication from ampule, using aseptic technique, for administration by a parenteral route

Assessment

Assessment should focus on the following:

Appearance of solution (clarity, absence of sediment, color indicated on instruction label)
Ampule label for expiration date of drug

Outcome Identification and Planning

Desired Outcome (sample)
Correct amount and type of drug drawn into syringe using aseptic technique.

Special Considerations
The sterility of syringe, needle, and medication must be maintained while preparing the drug using principles of asepsis (see Fig. 11.5 for identification of the parts of a syringe and needle assembly that must be kept sterile).

Home Health

In the home, instruct client to discard ampules by wrapping in paper towel and dropping into large coffee can with hole cut in lid. Store can in safe place (away from children) until it becomes full, then transfer to garbage. Evidence of "injectable" goods is not readily detected.

Delegation

As a basic standard, medication preparation, teaching, and administration are done by a licensed registered or vocational nurse. Some drugs may be given by registered nurses only. Policies vary by agency and state. BE SURE TO NOTE SPECIFIC AGENCY POLICIES FOR A GIVEN ROUTE AND DRUG BEFORE DELEGATING ADMINISTRATION!

IMPLEMENTATION

Action	Rationale
1. Wash hands.	*Reduces microorganism transfer*
2. Organize equipment.	*Promotes efficiency*
3. Check label of medication vial with medication record or card, using principles of the five rights of drug administration (see Procedure 11.1).	*Avoids client injury from wrong drug or dosage*
4. Perform dosage calculation if dosage in ampule differs from amount required.	*Determines correct amount of solution to be withdrawn*
5. Holding ampule, gently tap neck (top of ampule) with fingers (Fig. 11.8) or make a complete circle with the ampule by rotating wrist.	*Displaces solution from top of ampule to bottom* *Prevents waste of drug*
6. Place alcohol swab or gauze pad around neck of ampule with fingers of dominant hand; firmly place fingers of nondominant hand around lower part of ampule with thumb placed firmly against junction.	*Promotes easy opening of ampule* *Provides protection against finger cuts*
7. With a quick jolting motion of the wrists, break top of ampule by snapping away from you and others who may be near you (Fig. 11.9).	*Opens ampule* *Prevents injury from glass pieces*

Action	Rationale

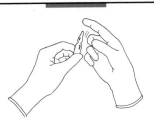

FIGURE 11.8

8. Place top of ampule on paper towel or immediately discard.

Prevents injury from picking up edges of jagged glass

9. Remove needle cap.
10. Press plunger of syringe all the way down; do not aspirate air into syringe.

Prevents accidental displacement and waste of solution

11. Place needle into ampule without letting needle or hub touch cut edges of the ampule (Fig. 11.10).

Maintains needle sterility

12. Withdraw appropriate amount of solution into syringe and remove needle from ampule.
13. Place ampule on paper towel or discard immediately

Prevents injury from picking up edges of jagged glass

14. If bubbles are in syringe:
    - Hold syringe vertically, with needle pointing up.

Removes remaining air bubbles from syringe using principle that air rises

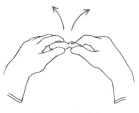

FIGURE 11.9

Action   **Rationale**

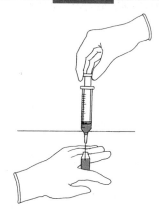

FIGURE 11.10

- Pull back slightly on plunger and flick syringe with fingers.	
- Slowly push plunger up to release air but not to the point of expelling the solution.	
15. Recheck amount of solution in syringe, comparing with drug volume required.	*Ensures that correct amount of drug has been prepared*
16. Compare drug label with medication record or card.	*Provides additional identification check of drug*
17. Change needle if drug is known to cause tissue irritation; replace cap.	*Prevents tissue irritation from drug clinging to outer surfaces of needle when solution is injected into skin*
18. Label syringe with drug label (or tape, if more than one parenteral drug is being given); label should include name and amount of drug.	*Provides identification information once at client bedside*
19. Place syringe, medication cards, and additional alcohol swabs on medication tray.	*Organizes equipment for administration of drug*

Action	Rationale
20. Discard or restore all equipment appropriately.	*Promotes clean and organized environment*
21. Wash hands.	*Prevents spread of micro-organisms*

Evaluation

Were desired outcomes achieved?

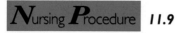
Medication Preparation With a Cartridge System

 EQUIPMENT

- Medication administration record or medication card
- Prefilled medication cartridge with appropriate medication
- Plastic or metal cartridge holder
- Medication tray

Purpose

Secures prefilled medication cartridge in holder
Prepares cartridge medication for administration

Assessment

Assessment should focus on the following:

Sterility of needle on medication cartridge, as indicated by intact needle cover
Adequacy of medication cartridge, as indicated by absence of cracks
Color and clarity of medication solution
Expiration date of medication
Cleanliness of cartridge holder

Outcome Identification and Planning

Desired Outcome (sample)

A prefilled medication cartridge of correct drug and dosage is secured in cartridge holder without contamination.

Special Considerations

Do not use cartridge if there is any indication of previous opening, inappropriate color, or sediment or if expiration date has passed.
Clean reusable cartridge holders with an appropriate disinfectant solution between uses with different clients.

Delegation

As a basic standard, medication preparation, teaching, and administration are done by a licensed registered or vocational nurse. Some drugs may be given by registered nurses only. Policies vary by agency and state. BE SURE TO NOTE SPECIFIC AGENCY POLICIES FOR A GIVEN ROUTE AND DRUG BEFORE DELEGATING ADMINISTRATION!

IMPLEMENTATION

Action	Rationale
1. Wash hands.	*Reduces microorganism transfer*
2. Organize equipment.	*Promotes efficiency*
3. Check label of prefilled medication cartridge with medication record or card, using principles of the five rights of drug administration (see Procedure 11.1).	*Avoids client injury from wrong drug or dosage*
4. Open cartridge holder, slide cartridge (leave needle covered) into barrel, and secure as follows:	*Prevents cartridge movement in holder during usage* *Maintains needle sterility*

Metal Holders
  - Pull plunger straight back (all the way out) and then down at about a 90-degree angle (Fig. 11.11*A*).
  - Insert cartridge, needle end first, into barrel (Fig. 11.11*B*).
  - Pull plunger back up directly in line with barrel of syringe (Fig. 11.11*C*).

Plastic Holders
  - Pull plunger straight back.
  - Insert cartridge through large opening of barrel and guide covered needle through hub of holder (Fig. 11.12*A–C*).

Action	Rationale

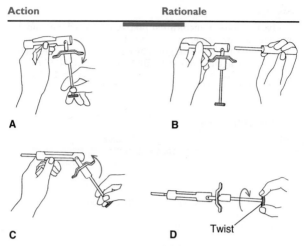

A **B**

C **D** Twist

FIGURE 11.11

Metal and Plastic Holders
- Hold cartridge and barrel stable close to end that has needle.
- Gently twist plunger in a clockwise direction until plunger locks onto cartridge (Fig. 11.11D).

5. Remove needle cover and eject air and excess medication (if discarding a narcotic substance, a witness must

Obtains accurate dosage

Complies with federal narcotic control laws

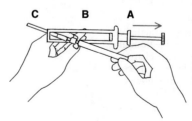

C B A

FIGURE 11.12

Action	Rationale
be present to witness disposal of drug).	
6. Replace needle cover.	*Maintains needle sterility*
7. Place prepared medication on medication tray.	

Evaluation

Were desired outcomes achieved?

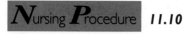
Mixing Medications

EQUIPMENT

- Medication administration record or medication cards
- Prescribed medication
- Appropriate-size syringe and three needles for type of injection and viscosity of solutions
- Medication label or small piece of tape
- Alcohol swabs
- Medication tray

Purpose

Mixes medications (including insulin) from multiple containers into one syringe for parenteral administration

Assessment

Assessment should focus on the following:

Appearance of solutions (clarity, absence of sediment, color indicated on instruction labels)

Drug labels for expiration dates of drugs

Parenteral drug compatibility charts for drug compatibility

Outcome Identification and Planning

Desired Outcome (sample)

Correct amounts of correct drugs are mixed in syringe without incompatibility or contamination.

Special Considerations

If a medication requires reconstitution, follow the guidelines on the vial.

If you are uncomfortable with the mixing process provided in this procedure, draw up medications using two syringes (one with removable needle cap), remove cap from one syringe, and aspirate medication into the other.

Delegation

As a basic standard, medication preparation, teaching, and administration are done by a licensed registered or vocational nurse. Some drugs may be given by registered nurses only. Policies vary by agency and state. BE SURE TO NOTE SPECIFIC AGENCY POLICIES FOR A GIVEN ROUTE AND DRUG BEFORE DELEGATING ADMINISTRATION!

IMPLEMENTATION

Action	Rationale
1. Wash hands.	*Reduces microorganism transfer*
2. Organize equipment.	*Promotes efficiency*
3. Check label of medications to be mixed with medication record or cards, using principles of the five rights of drug administration (see Procedure 11.1).	*Avoids client injury from wrong drug or dosage*
4. Perform dosage calculations, if needed.	*Determines correct amount of solution to be prepared*
5. Remove thin seal caps from tops of both vials without touching rubber stoppers.	*Exposes rubber tops*
	Maintains asepsis
6. Firmly wipe rubber stoppers on top of both vials with alcohol swabs.	*Maintains asepsis*
7. Pull end of plunger of syringe back to fill syringe with air equal to amount of solution to be drawn from first vial (vial A).	*Draws air into syringe needed for creating positive pressure in vial*
(*Note:* If one solution is colored and the other is clear, the colored solution should be vial B and the clear solution should be vial A.	*Allows nurse to determine if clear solution has been contaminated with other solution*
INSULIN IS OFTEN THE EXCEPTION [CHECK AGENCY POLICY]: WITH NPH AND REGULAR INSULIN, REGULAR INSULIN SHOULD BE VIAL B AND NPH INSULIN SHOULD BE VIAL A.	*PREVENTS CONTAMINATION OF SHORT-ACTING REGULAR INSULIN, WHICH IS OFTEN USED IN ACUTE SITUATIONS, WITH NPH INSULIN*

Action	Rationale
- If one vial is multiple dose and one is single dose, the single-dose vial will be vial A and the multiple-dose vial will be vial B (Fig. 11.13A).	*Prevents contamination of solution in multiple-dose container with other solution*
8. Insert air into vial A equal to the volume of solution to be withdrawn (Fig. 11.13B).	*Creates positive pressure in vial* *Prevents excess pressure on plunger that could cause plunger to pop out of barrel when withdrawing solution*
9. Remove needle from vial A and complete additional steps using same syringe.	

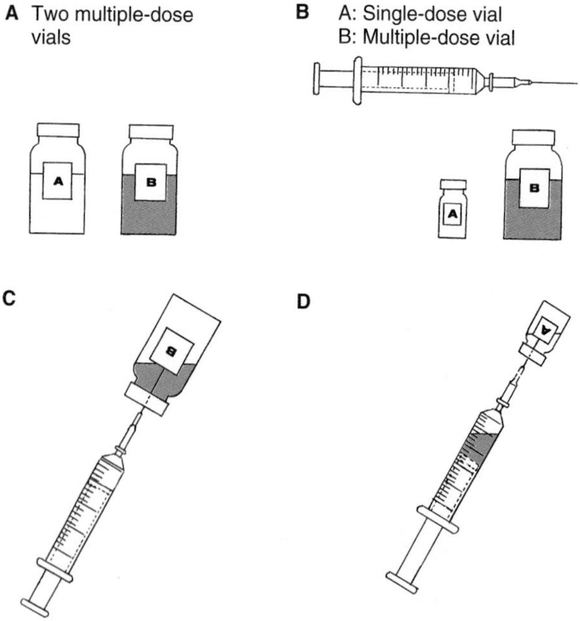

A Two multiple-dose vials

B A: Single-dose vial
   B: Multiple-dose vial

C

D

FIGURE 11.13

Action	Rationale
10. Pull end of plunger back to fill syringe with air equal to amount of solution to be drawn up from vial B.	*Draws air into syringe sufficient to create positive pressure in vial*
11. Insert air into vial B in same manner as first vial; do not, however, remove needle from vial B when air insertion is completed (Fig. 11.13C).	*Creates positive pressure in vial*
12. Invert vial and withdraw exact amount of solution needed from vial B.	*Aspirates solution into syringe*
13. Attach new needle to syringe.	*Prevents dull needle from pushing pieces of rubber top into vial and contaminating solution*
14. Insert needle into vial A, gently holding finger on end of plunger.	*Stabilizes plunger so drug in syringe does not accidentally spill into vial*
15. Invert vial and withdraw exact amount of solution needed from vial A (Fig. 11.13D).	*Withdraws solution from vial A*
16. Leaving needle cap on, attach new needle to same syringe.	*Prevents tissue irritation from dull needle and medication on needle*
17. Recheck amount of solution in syringe.	*Ensures that correct amount of drug has been prepared*
18. Pull plunger back another 0.1 cc.	*Makes air lock*
19. Compare drug labels with medication record or card.	*Provides additional identification check of drug*
20. Label syringe with drug labels.	*Provides identification information*
21. Place syringe, medication cards, and additional alcohol swabs on medication tray.	*Organizes equipment for administration of drug*
22. Discard or restore all equipment appropriately.	*Promotes clean and organized environment*
23. Wash hands.	*Prevents spread of microorganisms*

Evaluation

Were desired outcomes achieved?

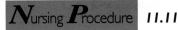

Intradermal Injection

EQUIPMENT

- Medication record or card
- Pen (ink or felt)
- Two alcohol swabs
- Nonsterile gloves
- Medication to be administered
- 1-ml syringe with 26- to 28-gauge needle
- Medication tray

Purpose

Permits exposure of client to small amount of toxin or medication deposited under the skin for absorption

Serves as method of diagnostic testing for allergens or for exposure to specific diseases

Assessment

Assessment should focus on the following:

Complete medication order

Agency protocol regarding specific sites of skin tests

Condition of client's skin (eg, presence of redness, hematomas, scarring, swelling, tears, abrasions, lesions, excoriation, and excessive hair)

Nursing Diagnoses

The nursing diagnoses may include the following:

Potential for biologic injury related to allergen sensitivity

Outcome Identification and Planning

Desired Outcome (sample)

Client shows no signs of local or systemic reaction.

Special Consideration

Allergens used in testing could cause a sensitivity or anaphylactic reaction. Be certain that appropriate antidotal drugs (usually epinephrine hydrochloride, a bronchodilator, and an antihistamine) are available on the unit before beginning. REACTIONS MAY BE FATAL.

Home Health

In the client's home, administer intradermal medication only by order of the attending physician (or with the attending physician's permission, if ordered by another physician).

Delegation

As a basic standard, medication preparation, teaching, and administration are done by a licensed registered or vocational nurse. Some drugs may be given by registered nurses only. Policies vary by agency and state. BE SURE TO NOTE SPECIFIC AGENCY POLICIES FOR A GIVEN ROUTE AND DRUG BEFORE DELEGATING ADMINISTRATION!

IMPLEMENTATION

Action	Rationale
1. Wash hands.	*Reduces microorganism transfer*
2. Prepare medication, adhering to the five rights of drug administration (see Procedures 11.1 and 11.7 through 11.10).	*Decreases chance of drug error* *Prepares drug appropriately from form in which it is supplied*
3. Identify client by reading identification bracelet and addressing client by name.	*Confirms identity of client*
4. Explain procedure and purpose of drug.	*Decreases anxiety* *Promotes cooperation*
5. Verify allergies listed on medication record or card.	*Alerts nurse to possibility of allergic reaction*
6. Don gloves.	*Prevents direct contact with body contaminants*
7. Select injection site on forearm if no other site is required by agency policy or doctor's orders; use alternative sites designated in Fig. 11.14 if forearm cannot be used.	*Forearm is standard beginning point for intradermal injections and the area at which subcutaneous fat is least likely to interfere with administration and absorption*

Action	Rationale

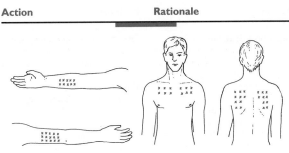

FIGURE 11.14

8. Position client with forearm facing up.

Accesses injection area

9. Cleanse site with alcohol.

Decreases microorganisms

10. Remove needle cap.

11. Place nondominant thumb about 1 inch below insertion site and pull skin down (toward hand).

Pulls skin taut for injection

12. With bevel up and using dominant hand, insert needle just below the skin at a 10- to 15-degree angle (Fig. 11.15).

Places needle just below epidermis

13. Once entry into skin surface is made, advance needle another ⅛ inch.

Prevents back leakage of medication

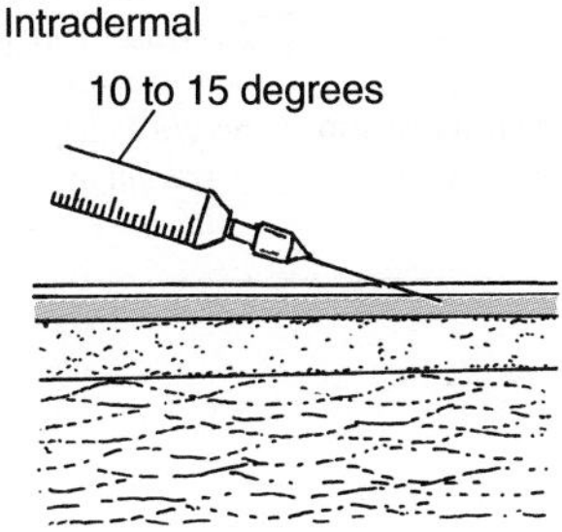

Intradermal

10 to 15 degrees

FIGURE 11.15

Action	Rationale
14. Inject drug slowly and smoothly while observing for bleb (a raised welt) to form. The bleb should be present.	*Delivers medication slowly and allows chance to stop administration if systemic reaction begins*
	Provides visual feedback of proper drug administration
15. Remove needle at same angle inserted.	*Prevents tearing of skin*
16. Gently remove blood, if any, by dabbing with second alcohol swab.	*Cleans area while avoiding pushing medication out*
17. Observe skin for redness or swelling; if this is an allergy test, observe for systemic reaction (eg, respiratory difficulty, sweating, faintness, decreased blood pressure, nausea, vomiting, cyanosis).	*Provides visual assessment of local or systemic reaction*
18. Reassess client and injection site after 5 min, after 15 min, then periodically thereafter during shift.	*Detects occurrence of subsequent reaction*
19. Place uncapped needle on tray.	*Prevents needlesticks*
20. Place a 1-inch circle around bleb and instruct client not to rub the area.	*Serves as guide in locating and reassessing area later*
21. Reposition client.	*Promotes comfort*
22. Discard equipment appropriately.	*Promotes clean and organized environment*
23. Wash hands.	*Decreases transfer of microorganisms*
24. Document administration on medication record.	*Serves as legal record of administration and prevents accidental remedication*

Evaluation

Were desired outcomes achieved?

Documentation

The following should be noted on the client's chart:

- Name of allergen or toxin, dosage, injection site, and route of administration
- Indicators of local or systemic reaction, if any
- Abnormal findings in local skin area
- Results of test 24 to 48 h after administration
- Teaching of information about drug or injection technique

SAMPLE DOCUMENTATION

DATE	TIME	
2/13/02	1440	Tuberculin skin test (0.1 ml) given intradermally in right lower forearm and circled. Noted a 0.5-cm reddened area surrounding injection site after injection, but no other reactions noted.

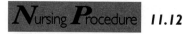

Nursing Procedure 11.12

Intramuscular Injection

 EQUIPMENT

- Medication record or card
- Pen
- Two alcohol swabs
- Disposable gloves
- Medication tray
- Medication to be administered
- 3-ml syringe with 1-, 1.5-, or 2-inch needle (21, 22, or 23 gauge)

Purpose

Delivers ordered medication into muscle tissue

Assessment

Assessment should focus on the following:

Medication order
Site of last injection, allergies, and client's response to previous injections, as noted in client's chart
Intended injection site (presence of bruises, tenderness, skin breaks, nodules, or edema)
Factors that determine appropriate size and gauge of needle (client's size and age, site of injection, viscosity and residual effects of medication)

Nursing Diagnoses

The nursing diagnoses may include the following:
Altered comfort: abdominal pain related to incision
Anxiety related to pain from injections

Outcome Identification and Planning

Desired Outcomes (sample)
There is no redness, edema, or pain at injection site.
Client correctly verbalizes purpose of injection.
Client states that minimum pain was experienced during injection.

Special Considerations

If nausea or pain medication has been ordered in multiple forms (oral, parenteral, or rectal), determine client's preference before preparing the medication.

Pediatric and Geriatric

If client is confused or combative, obtain assistance to stabilize the injection site and avoid tissue damage from the needle.

Delegation

As a basic standard, medication preparation, teaching, and administration are done by a licensed registered or vocational nurse. Some drugs may be given by registered nurses only. Policies vary by agency and state. BE SURE TO NOTE SPECIFIC AGENCY POLICIES FOR A GIVEN ROUTE AND DRUG BEFORE DELEGATING ADMINISTRATION!

IMPLEMENTATION

Action	Rationale
1. Wash hands.	*Reduces microorganism transfer*
2. Prepare medication, adhering to the five rights of drug administration (see Procedures 11.1 and 11.7 through 11.10).	*Decreases chance of drug error* *Prepares drug properly from form in which it is supplied*
3. Identify client by reading identification bracelet and addressing client by name.	*Confirms identity of client*
4. Explain procedure and purpose of drug.	*Decreases anxiety* *Promotes cooperation*
5. Verify allergies listed on medication record or card.	*Alerts nurse to possibility of allergic reaction*
6. Don gloves.	*Prevents contact with body fluids*
7. Select injection site appropriate for client's size and age (see Fig. 11.16 for injection sites located by anatomical landmarks).	
8. Assist client into position for comfort and easy visibility of injection site.	
9. Clean site with alcohol.	*Maintains asepsis*
10. Remove needle cap.	

Action   Rationale

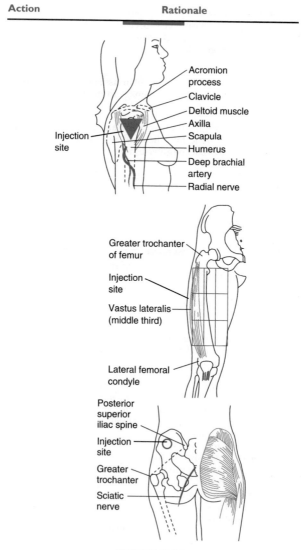

FIGURE 11.16

Action	Rationale

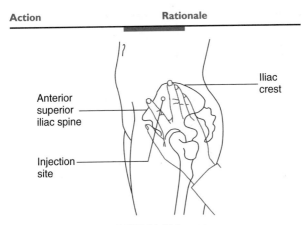

FIGURE 11.16 (cont.)

11. Pull skin taut at insertion area by using the following sequence:
    - Place thumb and index finger of nondominant hand over injection site (taking care not to touch cleaned area) to form a V.
    - Pull thumb and index finger in opposing directions, spreading fingers about 3 inches apart.

    Facilitates smooth and complete insertion of needle into muscle

12. Quickly insert needle at a 90-degree angle with dominant hand (as if throwing a dart).

    Minimizes pain from needle insertion

13. Move thumb and first finger of nondominant hand from skin to support barrel of syringe; fingers should be placed on barrel so that when you aspirate, you can see the barrel clearly (Fig. 11.17).

    Maintains steady position of needle and prevents tearing of tissue

Action	Rationale

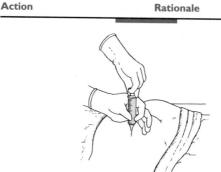

FIGURE 11.17

14. Pull back on plunger and observe for possible blood return in syringe (Fig. 11.18). — *Determines if needle is in a blood vessel rather than in muscle*

15. If blood does return when aspirating, pull the needle out, apply pressure to the insertion site, and repeat steps 7 to 14. — *Prevents inadvertent intra-venous injection*

16. If no blood returns, push plunger down slowly and smoothly; encourage client to talk. — *Delivers medication* *Decreases client anxiety*

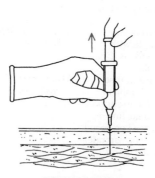

FIGURE 11.18

Action	Rationale
17. Remove needle at same angle as angle of insertion.	*Prevents needless tearing of tissue*
18. Massage and clean insertion area with second alcohol wipe (if contraindicated for drug, apply firm pressure instead).	*Prevents escape of drug into subcutaneous tissue*
19. Place needle on tray; do not recap.	*Prevents accidental needle stick*
20. Remove gloves.	
21. Reposition client; raise side rails and place bed in lowest position with call light within reach.	*Maintains safety, comfort, and communication*
22. Dispose of equipment properly.	*Prevents injury and spread of infection*
23. Wash hands.	*Reduces microorganism transfer*
24. Document administration on medication record.	*Serves as legal record of administration and prevents accidental remedication*

Evaluation

Were desired outcomes achieved?

Documentation

The following should be noted on the client's chart:

- Client's tolerance to injection
- Condition of site following injection (ie, local reactions)
- Effect of medication
- Injection site
- Time of injection
- Status of side rails

SAMPLE DOCUMENTATION

DATE	TIME	
7/8/02	1200	50 mg Demerol given intramuscularly in right deltoid for complaint of nagging pain in left hip. No local redness or swelling after injection. Side rails up and bed in low position.

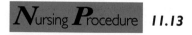

Nursing Procedure 11.13

Z-Track Injection

EQUIPMENT

- Medication record or card
- Pen
- Two alcohol swabs
- Disposable gloves
- Medication tray
- Medication to be administered
- 3-ml syringe with 2- to 3-inch needle (20 to 22 gauge)

Purpose

Delivers irritating or caustic medications deep into muscle tissue to prevent seepage

Assessment

Assessment should focus on the following:

Complete medication order
Intended injection site (presence of bruising, tenderness, skin breaks, nodules, or edema)
Site of last injection, allergies, and client's response to previous injections
Factors that determine size and gauge of needle (client's size and age, site of injection, viscosity and residual effects of medication)

Nursing Diagnoses

The nursing diagnoses may include the following:
Altered nutrition: less iron intake than required to support bodily functions

Outcome Identification and Planning

Desired Outcomes (sample)

Client offers no complaint of extreme pain after medication is administered by Z-track method.
Skin remains intact, without bruise or hematoma formation.

Special Consideration

Skin staining can occur if incorrect technique is used in giving iron injections. Drugs given by this method are generally so irritating to the skin and subcutaneous tissue as to cause sloughing.

Delegation

As a basic standard, medication preparation, teaching, and administration are done by a licensed registered or vocational nurse. Some drugs may be given by registered nurses only. Policies vary by agency and state. BE SURE TO NOTE SPECIFIC AGENCY POLICIES FOR A GIVEN ROUTE AND DRUG BEFORE DELEGATING ADMINISTRATION!

IMPLEMENTATION

Action	Rationale
1. Wash hands.	*Reduces microorganism transfer*
2. Prepare syringe with medication, adhering to the five rights of drug administration (see Procedures 11.1 and 11.7 through 11.10).	*Prepares drug properly* *Decreases chance of drug error* *Prepares drug properly from form in which it is supplied*
3. Change needle after drug has been fully drawn up.	*Prevents staining and irritation of skin and subcutaneous tissue when needle is inserted into skin*
4. Pull plunger back another 0.3 ml.	*Makes air lock in syringe*
5. Identify client by reading identification bracelet and addressing client by name.	*Confirms identity of client*
6. Explain procedure and purpose of drug.	*Decreases anxiety* *Promotes cooperation*
7. Verify allergies listed on medication record or card.	*Alerts nurse to possibility of allergic reaction*
8. Provide privacy.	*Decreases embarrassment*
9. Don gloves.	*Prevents direct contact with body secretions*
10. Assist client into prone position with toes pointed inward.	*Promotes comfort by relaxing gluteal muscles*
11. Outline dorsogluteal site by identifying appropriate landmarks (may also use	*Prevents sciatic nerve damage*

Action	Rationale

ventrogluteal and vastus lateralis areas); see Procedure 11.12 and Fig. 11.16 for information on locating injection sites using anatomical landmarks.

12. Clean site with alcohol. — *Maintains asepsis*

13. Remove needle cap.

14. Hold syringe with needle pointed down and observe for air bubble to rise to top (away from needle). — *Ensures that air clears needle after drug so drug can be "sealed" into muscle tissue*

15. Using fingers of non-dominant hand, pull skin laterally (away from midline) about 1 inch and down (Fig. 11.19). — *Retracts skin and subcutaneous tissue from muscle*

16. While maintaining skin retraction, rest heel of nondominant hand on skin below fingers (Fig. 11.20). — *Allows nurse to maintain retraction and stability of needle while aspirating or if client suddenly moves*

17. Talk to client, pausing to warn of impending needle stick. — *Provides distraction* / *Prevents jerking response*

18. With dominant hand, quickly insert needle at a 90-degree angle (as if throwing a dart). — *Minimizes pain from insertion* / *Ensures that needle enters muscle mass*

19. Pull plunger back and aspirate for blood return. — *Determines if accidental insertion into blood vessel has occurred*

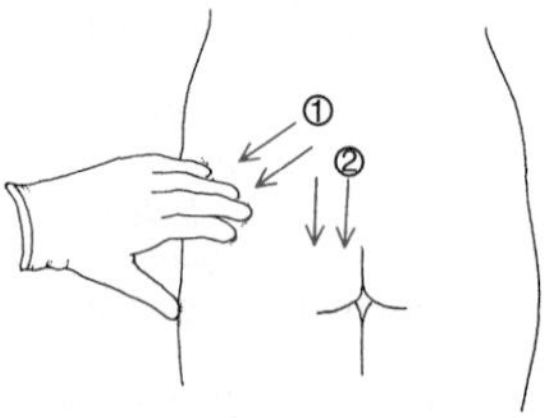

FIGURE 11.19

Action	Rationale

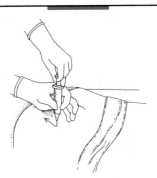

FIGURE 11.20

20. If blood returns, remove needle, clean site with antiseptic swab, assess site, apply adhesive bandage, and begin at step 1.

21. If no blood returns, inject drug slowly and hold needle in place for 10 sec.

Prevents leakage into subcutaneous tissue

Gives adequate absorption time

22. Remove needle at same angle as angle of insertion while releasing skin at the same time.

Prevents needless tearing of tissue

Avoids direct track between muscle and surface of skin

23. Place alcohol swab over insertion area but DO NOT MASSAGE.

Avoids displacing drug into tissues and causing irritation and pain

24. Place needle on tray; do not recap.

Prevents accidental needlestick

25. Reposition client, raise side rails, and lower bed to lowest position; place call light button within reach.

Maintains safety, comfort, and communication

26. Dispose of equipment properly.

Prevents injury and spread of infection

27. Wash hands.

Reduces microorganism transfer

Action	Rationale
28. Document administration on medication record.	*Serves as legal record of administration and prevents accidental remediation*
29. Check site 15 to 30 min later.	*Verifies that no seepage of medication has occurred*

Evaluation

Were desired outcomes achieved?

Documentation

The following should be noted on the client's chart:

- Name of medication, dosage, route, and site of injection
- Assessment and laboratory data relevant to purpose of medication
- Effects of medication
- Condition of site following injection
- Teaching of information about drug or injection technique

SAMPLE DOCUMENTATION

DATE	TIME	
7/8/02	1600	Client received first dose of Imferon 150 mg by Z-track injection in left dorsogluteal area. No local redness, swelling, or skin stain. No complaint of nausea or headache.

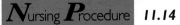

Intermittent Intravenous Medication

EQUIPMENT

- Medication record or card
- Pen
- Disposable gloves
- Four or five alcohol swabs
- Medication to be administered mixed in 50 to 100 ml of appropriate IV fluid (usually 0.9% saline or 5% dextrose) and attached to 22- or 23-gauge needle
- Small roll of 1/2- to 1-inch width tape

If administering medication by piggyback method, include:
- 1 ml of sterile saline

If administering medication through IV lock, include:
- Two syringes of sterile saline (1.5 to 2 ml)
- One syringe with 1 to 2 ml of heparin flush solution (if permitted by agency policy)

Purpose

Intermittently delivers medication through IV route for various therapeutic effects, most frequently treatment of infections

Assessment

Assessment should focus on the following:

Complete medication order
Condition of IV site (patency, discoloration, edema, and pain)
Appearance of IV fluid with added medication (discoloration, sediment)
Expiration dates on medication that has been mixed
Condition of tubing presently hanging, if any

Nursing Diagnoses

The nursing diagnoses may include the following:

Potential for infection related to open abdominal skin wound
Altered comfort: pain related to increased gastric secretion of hydrochloric acid

Outcome Identification and Planning

Desired Outcomes (sample)

IV antibiotics and medications were infused without signs of contamination.
Within 2 days of beginning cimetidine infusions, client states that upper abdominal pain has decreased.

Special Considerations

Pediatric

When infusing intermittent medications to pediatric clients, always regulate by an electronic infusion regulator (IV pump or controller) and a volume-controlled chamber (such as a Buretrol or Volutrol) to prevent infusion errors related to increased rates or volumes (see Procedure 5.6). Check the agency procedure manual.

Delegation

In most agencies, drugs administered by IV route may only be administered by registered nurses. POLICIES VARY BY AGENCY AND STATE, HOWEVER. BE SURE TO CONSULT SPECIFIC AGENCY POLICIES FOR DELEGATION OF DRUG ADMINISTRATION FOR A GIVEN ROUTE AND/OR DRUG. Registered nurses generally administer IV push medications and medications given through central line catheters and PICC lines. IV sedation drugs are given by registered nurses. In many facilities, selected IV piggyback medications and peripheral IV saline flush may be given by licensed vocational nurses.
BE SURE TO CHECK AGENCY POLICY BEFORE DELEGATING *ANY* DRUG ADMINISTRATION TO OTHER PERSONNEL!

IMPLEMENTATION

Action	Rationale
1. Wash hands.	*Reduces microorganism transfer*
2. Prepare medication, adhering to the five rights of drug administration (see Procedure 11.1).	*Prepares drug* *Decreases chance of drug error*

Action	Rationale
3. Calculate infusion flow rate (see Procedure 5.5).	*Determines accurate infusion rate*
4. Identify client by reading identification bracelet and addressing client by name.	*Confirms identity of client*
5. Explain procedure and purpose of drug.	*Decreases anxiety* *Promotes cooperation*
6. Verify allergies listed on medication record or card.	*Alerts nurse to possibility of allergic reaction*
7. Hang medication with attached tubing and needle on IV pole.	
8. Don gloves at any point during procedure when there is a risk of exposure to blood or body secretions (such as when untaping site for in-depth assessment).	*Decreases nurse's exposure to body secretions*
9. Assess patency of catheter or heparin lock:	*Confirms that established IV line is open*

IV lock

Action	Rationale
- Cleanse rubber port of lock with alcohol.	*Reduces microorganisms*
- Stabilize lock with thumb and first finger of nondominant hand.	*Prevents pulling out of catheter*
- Insert needle of sterile saline syringe into lock.	
- Pull back on end of plunger and observe for blood return.	*Aspirates blood* *Ensures catheter is functional*
- If no blood returns, reposition extremity in which catheter is placed and reassess site for redness, edema, or pain.	*Checks for problems related to positioning, local infiltration, or phlebitis*
- Discontinue IV lock and restart if unable to get blood return (see Procedures 5.2 and 5.4).	*Discontinues nonfunctional catheter* *Establishes functional line*
- If blood returns, insert saline and proceed to next step.	*Flushes catheter*

Action	Rationale

Primary line

- Insert needle of syringe containing sterile saline into center of port nearest insertion site.

  Provides access to port near catheter site for easy observation when aspirating

- Pinch IV tubing just above the port (Fig. 11.21).

  Allows for one-way flow during aspiration

- Pull back on plunger and observe for blood return in the tubing; or lower fluid and tubing below level of extremity for 1 to 2 min.

  Aspirates for blood return

- If no blood returns, reposition extremity in which catheter is placed and reassess site for redness edema, or pain.

  Verifies catheter placement
  Checks for problems related to positioning, phlebitis, or infiltration

- Discontinue primary IV and restart if unable to get blood return (see Procedures 5.2 through 5.4)

  Establishes patent IV line

- If blood returns, instill saline and proceed to next step.

  Flushes blood from catheter

10. Cleanse rubber port to be used (see step 11) with alcohol.

    Reduces microorganisms

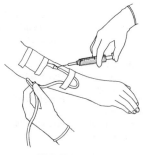

FIGURE 11.21

Action	Rationale
11. Insert needle attached to tubing of mixed medication into IV lock port; for piggyback method, insert needle into port closest to top of primary tubing.	*Connects to main infusion line*
12. Secure needle with tape.	*Prevents needle dislodgment*
13. For piggyback method, lower primary bag to about 6 inches below secondary bag (mixed medication bag; Fig. 11.22).	*Provides more gravitational pull for secondary bag than for primary infusion*
14. Slowly open tubing roller clamp and adjust drip rate (see Procedure 5.6).	*Prevents adverse reactions from too rapid an infusion rate*
15. Periodically assess client during infusion.	*Monitors for adverse reactions and good infusion*
16. When infusion is complete, leave medication and tubing on pole if tubing is not expired; for IV lock (and when administering several different piggyback	*Provides greater mobility for client while maintaining*

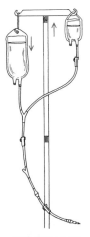

FIGURE 11.22

Action	Rationale
medications), carefully remove needle from primary tubing and recap; for piggy back method, leave connected to port.	*cleanliness of IV tubing for future use* *Decreases destruction of primary tubing port*
17. If tubing has expired, disconnect and discard.	*Reduces contamination of system*
18. Insert needle of second syringe of sterile saline and inject into IV lock; then insert heparin flush or readjust drip rate for primary infusion.	*Clears catheter and tubing*
19. Discard or restore all equipment appropriately.	*Promotes clean environment*
20. Wash hands.	*Reduces microorganism transfer*
21. Document administration on medication record.	*Serves as legal record of administration and prevents accidental remedication*

Evaluation

Were desired outcomes achieved?

Documentation

The following should be noted on the client's chart:

- Name, amount, and route of drug given
- Purpose of administration, if given on a when-needed (p.r.n) basis or one-time order
- Assessment data relevant to purpose of medication
- Effects of medication on client
- Teaching of information about drug

SAMPLE DOCUMENTATION

DATE 7/8/02	TIME 1100	Client received initial dose of IV tobramycin, 80 mg. No redness or drainage from abdominal wound. Client denies having abdominal pain. Temperature, 99.8°F. Other vital signs within normal limits.

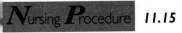

Administration of
Subcutaneous Medication

EQUIPMENT

- Pen
- Medication record or card
- Two alcohol swabs
- Nonsterile gloves
- Adhesive bandage
- Medication to be administered
- 2- to 3-ml syringe with 1/2- to 7/8-inch needle (25, 26, or 27 gauge) or insulin syringe
- Medication tray

Purpose

Delivers medication into subcutaneous tissues for absorption

Assessment

Assessment should focus on the following:

Medication order
Condition of skin at intended injection site (presence of tears, abrasions, lesions, and scars)
Chart or medication administration record for site of last injection

Nursing Diagnoses

The nursing diagnoses may include the following:

Potential altered skin integrity related to repeated insulin injections
Knowledge deficit regarding technique for self-administration of insulin related to newly diagnosed diabetic status

Outcome Identification and Planning

Desired Outcomes (sample)
No scars, craters, or lumps are noted on skin.
Client performs insulin self-injection with 100% accuracy within 1 week of receiving instructions.

Special Considerations

Some agencies recommend that aspiration after needle insertion not be performed with heparin administration. Check agency procedure manual BEFORE heparin administration.

Many agencies require that heparin and insulin be checked with another nurse when preparing. Check agency policy manual before beginning.

Geriatric

Elderly clients often experience a loss of subcutaneous fat tissue.

Choose needle length carefully to avoid painful injections and trauma to the underlying bone.

Pediatric

For clients less than 1 year old, SUBCUTANEOUS INJECTION IN THE DORSAL GLUTEAL AREA CAN BE HAZARDOUS because of possible damage to sciatic nerve.

Enlist assistant to restrain child during procedure to avoid tissue damage from needle during sudden movement.

Home Health

Arrange supplies (eg, insulin, alcohol, needles) in line on a table to assist the client and family in learning the sequence of steps in the procedure.

Delegation

As a basic standard, medication preparation, teaching, and administration are done by a licensed registered or vocational nurse. Some drugs may be given by registered nurses only. Policies vary by agency and state. BE SURE TO NOTE SPECIFIC AGENCY POLICIES FOR A GIVEN ROUTE AND DRUG BEFORE DELEGATING ADMINISTRATION!

IMPLEMENTATION

Action	Rationale
1. Wash hands.	*Reduces microorganism transfer*
2. Prepare medication, adhering to the five rights of drug administration (see Procedures 11.1 and 11.7 through 11.10).	*Prepares drug* *Decreases chance of drug error* *Prepares drug properly from form in which it is supplied*
3. Identify client by reading identification bracelet and addressing client by name.	*Confirms identity of client*
4. Explain procedure and purpose of drug.	*Decreases anxiety* *Promotes cooperation*

Action	Rationale
5. Verify allergies listed on medication record or card.	*Alerts nurse to possible allergic reaction*
6. Provide privacy.	*Decreases embarrassment*
7. Don gloves.	*Prevents direct contact with body fluids*
8. Perform or instruct client to perform the remaining steps.	*Helps client learn procedures*
9. Select injection site on upper arm or abdomen. (*Note:* Heparin should be injected in abdomen.) Use one of the following alternative sites if these two areas are not available because of tissue irritation, scarring, tubes, or dressings: thighs, upper chest, scapular areas (Fig. 11.23); the sites should be rotated.	*Prevents repeated and permanent tissue damage*
10. Position client for site selected.	*Accesses injection area* *Promotes comfort*
11. Cleanse site with alcohol.	*Reduces microorganism transfer*
12. Remove needle cap.	
13. Grasp about 1 inch of skin and fatty tissue between thumb and fingers.	

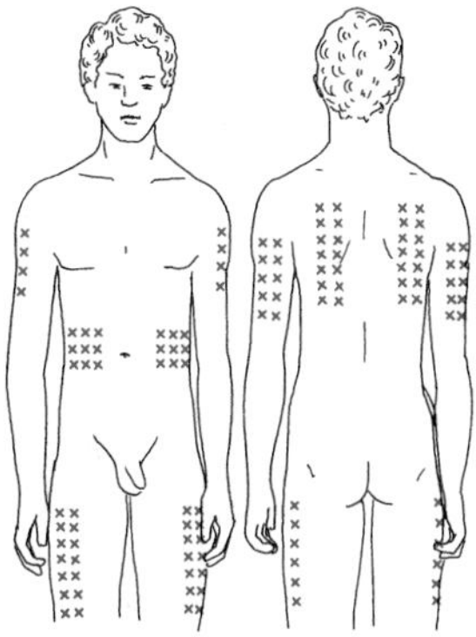

FIGURE 11.23

Action	Rationale
(*Note:* For heparin injection, hold skin gently; do not pinch.)	*Prevents trauma to tissue*
14. With dominant hand, insert needle at a 45-degree angle quickly and smoothly; for a larger person, insert at a 90-degree angle (Fig. 11.24).	*Facilitates injection into subcutaneous tissue (a large person has a thicker layer of subcutaneous tissue)*
15. Quickly release skin fold with nondominant hand.	*Facilitates spread of medication*
16. Aspirate with plunger and observe barrel of syringe for blood return.	*Determines if needle is in a blood vessel*
17. If blood does not return, inject drug slowly and smoothly.	*Delivers the medication*
18. If blood returns: - Withdraw needle from skin. - Apply pressure to site for about 2 min. - Observe for hematoma or bruising. - Apply adhesive bandage, if needed. - Prepare new medication, beginning with step 1, and select new site.	*Prevents injection into blood vessels*
19. Remove needle at same angle at which it was inserted.	*Prevents tissue damage*

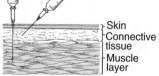

FIGURE 11.24

Action	Rationale
20. Cleanse injection site with second alcohol swab and lightly massage. DO NOT massage after heparin injection.	*Promotes comfort* *Prevents bruising and tissue damage*
21. Apply adhesive bandage, if needed.	*Contains residual bleeding*
22. Place uncapped needle on tray.	*Prevents needlestick*
23. Discard all equipment appropriately.	*Promotes cleanliness*
24. Wash hands.	*Decreases microorganism transfer*
25. Document administration on medication record.	*Serves as legal record of administration and prevents accidental remedication*

Evaluation

Were desired outcomes achieved?

Documentation

The following should be noted on the client's chart:

- Name, dosage, and route of medication; site of injection
- Assessment and laboratory data relevant to purpose of medication
- Effects of medication
- Teaching of information about drug or injection technique

SAMPLE DOCUMENTATION

DATE	TIME	
7/8/02	1400	Client received first dose of regular insulin, 15 units subcutaneously in right upper arm. No scars, abrasions, or lumps noted on skin.

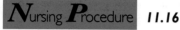

Administration of Rectal Medication

EQUIPMENT

- Medication record card
- Pen
- Disposable gloves
- Suppository to be administered
- Packet of water-soluble lubricant

Purpose

Delivers medication or absorption through mucous membranes of rectum

Assessment

Assessment should focus on the following:

Complete medication order
Condition of anus and skin surrounding buttocks (presence of ulcerations, tears, hemorrhoids, excoriation, abnormal discharge, and foul odor)
Abdominal girth, if distention is present
Client knowledge regarding use of suppositories

Nursing Diagnoses

The nursing diagnoses may include the following:

Altered elimination: constipation related to decreased peristalsis
Altered comfort: pain related to abdominal distention

Outcome Identification and Planning

Desired Outcomes (sample)
Client has normal bowel movement within 24 h.
Abdominal girth decreases to 36 inches in 24 h.
Client verbalizes absence of abdominal pain.

Delegation

As a basic standard medication preparation, teaching, and administration are done by a licensed registered or vocational nurse. Some drugs may be given by registered nurses only. Policies vary by agency and state. BE SURE TO NOTE SPECIFIC AGENCY POLICIES FOR A GIVEN ROUTE AND DRUG BEFORE DELEGATING ADMINISTRATION!

IMPLEMENTATION

Action	Rationale
1. Wash hands.	*Reduces microorganism transfer*
2. Prepare medication, adhering to the five rights of drug administration (see Procedure 11.1).	*Prepares drug* *Decreases chance of drug error*
3. Identify client by reading identification bracelet and addressing client by name.	*Confirms identity of client*
4. Explain procedure and purpose of drug.	*Decreases anxiety* *Promotes cooperation*
5. Verify allergies listed on medication record or card.	*Alerts nurse to possible allergic reaction*
6. Don gloves.	*Decreases nurse's exposure to client's body secretions*
7. Position client in prone or side-lying position.	*Places client for good exposure of anal opening*
8. Place towel or linen saver under buttocks.	*Protects sheets*
9. Remove suppository from wrapper and inspect tip.	*Detects sharp tip*
10. If pointed end of suppository is sharp, gently rub sharp tip until slightly rounded.	*Decreases chance of tearing rectal membranes*
11. Lubricate rounded tip with lubricating jelly.	*Decreases chance of tearing membranes*
12. Gently spread buttocks with nondominant hand.	*Exposes anal opening*
13. Instruct client to take slow, deep breaths through mouth.	*Relaxes sphincter muscles, facilitating insertion*
14. Insert suppository into rectum until closure of anal ring is felt (Fig. 11.25).	

Action	Rationale

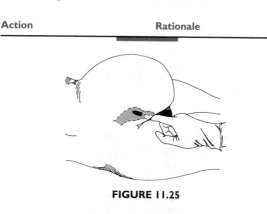

FIGURE 11.25

15. Remove finger, wipe excess lubricant away from skin, and release buttocks.

Promotes client comfort

16. Instruct client to squeeze buttocks together for 3 to 4 min and to remain in position for 15 to 20 minutes. (Note: Suppositories given to expel gas may be released at any time.)

Decreases urge to release suppository

17. Discard gloves and paper wrapper.

Promotes clean environment

18. Raise side rails.

Promotes safety

19. Place call light and bedpan within reach.

Facilitates communication
Anticipates premature expulsion of suppository or feces

20. Wash hands.

Reduces microorganism transfer

21. Document administration on medication record.

Serves as legal record of administration and prevents accidental remedication

Evaluation

Were desired outcomes achieved?

Documentation

The following should be noted on the client's chart:

- Name, dosage, and route of drug
- Condition of anus and surrounding area, if abnormal
- Assessment data relevant to purpose and effects of medication
- Teaching of knowledge about drug and self-administration of medication

SAMPLE DOCUMENTATION

DATE	TIME	
7/8/02	1400	Acetaminophen, gr. XX suppository given for rectal temperature of 103.4°F. Slight protrusion of hemorrhoids noted. Client denies discomfort in anal area.

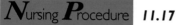

Nursing Procedure 11.17

Topical Application

EQUIPMENT

- Medication to be applied (creams, ointments, gels, medicated disks, sprays)
- Medication record or card
- Pen

For creams, gels, ointments, lotions:
- Two pairs of disposable gloves
- Tongue blade
- Mild soap
- Small towel
- Basin of warm water

For sterile application to open wound or incision
- Two pairs of sterile gloves
- Sterile gauze
- Sterile towel
- Sterile water
- Sterile cleansing solution
- Sterile tongue blade

Purpose

Delivers medication to skin for local or systemic effects, such as skin lubrication and reduction of inflammation

Assessment

Assessment should focus on the following:

Complete medication order
Condition of last treatment area and intended site of this application

Nursing Diagnoses

The nursing diagnoses may include the following:

Altered skin integrity related to local inflammation

Outcome Identification and Planning

Desired Outcome (sample)

Client displays no redness, swelling, drainage, pain, or open skin areas on lower left leg.

Special Considerations

Geriatric

For elderly clients who have problems with memory, use devices that remind them that medication is to be taken (eg, calendars, daily pill dispenser).

Pediatric

Client's cooperation may be improved if the child is allowed to apply the medication under your supervision.

Home Health

Instruct client and family to monitor for side effects and possible reactions to medications.

Delegation

As a basic standard, medication preparation, teaching, and administration are done by a licensed registered or vocational nurse. Some drugs may be given by registered nurses only. Policies vary by agency and state. BE SURE TO NOTE SPECIFIC AGENCY POLICIES FOR A GIVEN ROUTE AND DRUG BEFORE DELEGATING ADMINISTRATION!

IMPLEMENTATION

Action	Rationale
1. Wash hands.	*Reduces microorganism transfer*
2. Prepare medication, adhering to the five rights of drug administration (see Procedure 11.1).	*Prepares drug* *Decreases chance of drug error*
3. Identify client by reading identification bracelet and addressing client by name.	*Confirms identity of client*
4. Explain procedure and purpose of drug.	*Decreases anxiety* *Promotes cooperation*
5. Verify allergies listed on medication record or card.	*Alerts nurse to possibility of an allergic reaction*

Action	Rationale
6. Don disposable gloves if applying gel, cream, ointment, or lotion; apply sterile gloves if applying to open wound or incision, and use sterile technique throughout procedure.	*Decreases nurse's exposure to client's body secretions* *Prevents nurse from receiving effects from the drug*
7. Wash intended application site with warm, soapy water, rinse, and pat dry (unless contraindicated); if applying drug to open skin area, use sterile cleaning solution and gauze to clean area.	*Removes surface skin debris* *Facilitates absorption*
8. Wash hands and change gloves.	*Maintains asepsis*
9. Apply drug to treatment area, using appropriate application method:	*Delivers medication with appropriate technique*

Ointments, creams, lotions, gels

- Pour or squeeze ordered amount onto palmar surface of fingers; or use tongue blade to obtain if removing from multiple-dose container or jar.	*Removes drug from container*
- Lightly spread with fingers of other hand.	*Thins texture of the substance* *Warms cold gels and creams*
- Gently apply to treatment area, lightly massaging until absorbed or as per package directions.	*Spreads drug for intended effect*

Nitroglycerin ointment
(Special preparation and application)

- Remove previous ointment pad and wash area.	*Prevents adverse reactions from dose greater than ordered dose*
- Squeeze ordered number of inches of drug onto paper measuring rule that comes with ointment.	*Obtains ordered amount of drug*

Action	Rationale
- Place on skin surface that is less hairy than other areas (such as upper chest, upper arm); DO NOT apply to areas where there is a heavy skinfold (abdomen) or heavy muscle mass (gluteal muscles) or to the axilla or groin.	*Facilitates optimal absorption for dilation of coronary vessels*
- Secure with adhesive application pad (comes with ointment) or plastic wrap or tape.	*Prevents premature removal of pad*
Medication disks (such as nitroglycerin or clonidine [Catapres])	
- Remove outer package.	
- Carefully remove protective back (usually a plastic shield).	*Obtains disk containing premeasured drug*
- Place patch on skin surface that is less hairy than other areas (such as upper chest, upper arm); DO NOT apply to areas where there is a heavy skinfold (abdomen) or heavy muscle mass (gluteal muscles) or to the axilla or groin.	*Facilitates optimal absorption*
- Gently press around edges with fingers.	*Provides stability during long-term use*
Sprays	
- Instruct client to close eyes or turn head if spray is being applied to upper chest and above.	*Protects against inhaling aerosol particles*
- Apply a light coat of spray onto treatment area (usually 2 to 10 sec, depending on size of treatment area).	
10. Discard or restore all equipment properly.	*Promotes cleanliness*

Action	Rationale
11. Wash hands.	*Prevents spread of infection*
12. Document administration on medication administration record.	*Serves as legal record of administration and prevents accidental remediation*

Evaluation

Were desired outcomes achieved?

Documentation

The following should be noted on the client's chart:

- Name, dosage, and route of medication
- Assessment data relevant to purpose of medication
- Condition of treatment area
- Effects of medication
- Teaching of information about medication and techniques of self-administration

SAMPLE DOCUMENTATION

DATE	TIME	
7/8/02	2100	Tolnaftate 1% cream applied to abdomen for treatment of tinea. Client still has dry, flaky circles (2 cm in diameter) scattered on left lower quadrant of abdomen. States no itching. No other skin abnormalities noted.

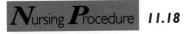

 Administration of Vaginal Medication

EQUIPMENT

- Medication record or card
- Pen
- Basin of warm water
- Disposable gloves
- Washcloth
- Soap
- Towel
- Sanitary pad
- Vaginal applicator
- Vaginal suppository or cream to be administered

Purpose

Delivers medication for absorption through vaginal membranes for such therapeutic effects as resolving infections and treating inflammation

Assessment

Assessment should focus on the following:

Complete medication order
Condition of vaginal area (presence of lesions, tears, bleeding, tenderness, discharge, or odor)

Nursing Diagnoses

The nursing diagnoses may include the following:
Altered vaginal mucous membranes related to inflammatory process

Outcome Identification and Planning

Desired Outcomes (sample)

No redness, heat, swelling, abnormal drainage, or pain is present in vaginal area.

Special Considerations

Delegation

As a basic standard, medication preparation, teaching, and administration are done by a licensed registered or vocational nurse. Some drugs may be given by registered nurses only. Policies vary by agency and state. BE SURE TO NOTE SPECIFIC AGENCY POLICIES FOR A GIVEN ROUTE AND DRUG BEFORE DELEGATING ADMINISTRATION!

IMPLEMENTATION

Action	Rationale
1. Wash hands.	*Reduces microorganism transfer*
2. Prepare medication, adhering to the five rights of drug administration (see Procedure 11.1).	*Prepares drug* *Decreases chance of drug error*
3. Identify client by reading identification bracelet and addressing client by name.	*Confirms identity of client*
4. Explain procedure and purpose of drug.	*Decreases anxiety* *Promotes cooperation*
5. Verify allergies listed on medication record or card.	*Alerts nurse to possibility of allergic reaction*
6. Provide privacy.	*Decreases embarrassment*
7. Don gloves.	*Decreases nurse's exposure to client's body secretions*
8. Assist client into dorsal recumbent or Sims' position.	*Places client in appropriate position for drug placement*
9. Wash and dry perineum, if discharge or odor noted.	*Promotes cleanliness* *Facilitates drug absorption* *Removes excess secretions*
10. Insert medication into vaginal applicator:	*Assists nurse with insertion of drug into vagina at length necessary to facilitate absorption*
- Cream—place applicator over top of open medication tube, invert applicator-tube combination, and squeeze tube.	*Forces medication into applicator*
- Suppository—insert suppository into applicator (or insert suppository	

Action	Rationale
without applicator, if desired).	
11. Spread labia if vagina is not easily visible.	*Exposes vaginal opening*
12. Insert applicator into vagina about 2.5 to 3.0 inches and press applicator top down (Fig. 11.26); if using finger to insert suppository, also insert 2.5 to 3.0 inches.	
13. Remove applicator or finger.	*Completes process*
14. Instruct client to remain in bed in a flat position for 15 to 20 min.	*Allows time for medication to be absorbed*
15. Apply sanitary pad.	*Contains discharge secretions*
16. Discard gloves.	*Decreases transfer of micro-organisms*
17. Raise side rails.	*Facilitates client safety*
18. Place call light within reach.	*Provides client with means to communicate needs*
19. Discard or restore equipment properly (applicators may be washed with soap and water and stored in plastic wrapping, box, or washcloth).	*Promotes cleanliness*
20. Wash hands.	*Reduces microorganism transfer*

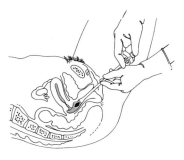

FIGURE 11.26

Action	Rationale
21. Document administration on medication record.	*Provides legal record of administration and prevents accidental remediation*

Evaluation

Were desired outcomes achieved?

Documentation

The following should be noted on the client's chart:

- Name, dosage, and route of medication
- Assessment data relevant to purpose of medication
- Effects of medication
- Teaching of information about medication and techniques of self-administration

SAMPLE DOCUMENTATION

DATE	TIME	
7/8/02	2100	Client received final dose of Monistat vaginally. States pain and itching relieved. No redness, edema, or drainage in vaginal area.

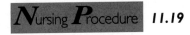

Home Preparation of Solutions

EQUIPMENT

- Glass containers with tight-fitting lids (pint, quart, or larger for acetic acid)
- Large saucepan
- Tongs or oven mitts
- Salt
- White, distilled vinegar
- Bleach

Purpose

Prepares solutions for use in care

Assessment

Assessment should focus on the following:

Economic need to prepare solutions at home instead of purchasing already prepared solutions
Client/caregiver ability to learn and perform procedure

Outcome Identification and Planning

Desired Outcome (sample)

Client/caregiver will demonstrate correct technique in preparation of solution.

Special Considerations
Home Health

If sterile saline, Dakins, or acetic acid solution is ordered for a client, check with the physician to determine if home preparation is acceptable. In some instances, it may be necessary to use purchased solutions and the nurse should access community resources if cost to the client is a factor.

Delegation

As a basic standard, medication preparation, teaching, and administration are done by a licensed registered or vocational nurse. Some drugs may be given by registered nurses only. Policies vary by agency and state. BE SURE TO NOTE SPECIFIC AGENCY POLICIES FOR A GIVEN ROUTE AND DRUG BEFORE DELEGATING ADMINISTRATION!

IMPLEMENTATION

Action	Rationale
1. Wash hands.	*Reduces microorganism transfer*
2. Organize equipment: glass jars with metal lids, clean saucepans large enough to hold jar, tongs, or oven mitts, measuring spoons.	*Promotes efficiency*
3. Clean all equipment with warm soapy water and rinse thoroughly.	*Reduces microorganism transfer*
4. Prepare container:	*Sterilizes container for use*
- Lay jar on its side in the saucepan.	
- Fill with water; be sure jar is filled, as well.	
- Cover pan, bring water to a boil and boil for 20 min.	
- Remove from heat.	
- Using tongs or oven mitt and handling only the outside of the jar and lid, remove the jar, and stand it, empty, in a clean area.	
- Remove the lid, handling only the outside. Place the lid loosely on the jar.	
5. *Sterile water*	
- Prepare jar as in step 4.	
- Boil 6 cups of water for 20 min in a clean saucepan.	*Removes microorganisms*
- Slowly pour water into jar until almost full.	
- Place lid on jar.	
- Allow to cool.	
- Tighten lid and label.	*Indicates date of preparation.*
- Prepare new solution every day.	*Prevents growth of microorganisms*
6. *Sterile saline 0.9%*	
- Prepare jar as in step 4.	

Action	Rationale
- Boil 6 cups of water as above.	
- Pour 4 cups of sterile water into sterile jar.	
- Using a clean teaspoon, add 2 teaspoons of table salt.	*Creates proper percentage solution*
- Put lid on jar and shake well.	
- Label with contents and date.	
- Allow to cool before use.	*Prevents growth of micro-organisms*
- Prepare new solution every day.	

7. *Acetic acid 0.25%*
   - Prepare jar as in step 4.
   - Boil 6 cups of water for 20 min.
   - Pour 5 cups of water into prepared jar.
   - Let cool.
   - Using a clean measuring spoon, add 4 tablespoons of white distilled vinegar.   *Creates proper percentage of solution.*
   - Close lid and shake to mix.
   - Label with contents and date.
   - Prepare new solution every day.   *Prevents growth of micro-organisms*

8. *Dakins' solution*
   - Prepare pint jar as in step 4.
   - Boil water for 20 min.
   - *For ½ strength Dakins,* put 25 ml of bleach in the pint jar and fill to top with prepared, cooled, sterile water.
   - *For full-strength Dakins,* put 50 ml of bleach in the jar and fill to top with prepared, cooled, sterile water.
   - Place lid on jar.
   - Label contents and date.
   - Prepare new solution at least weekly.

Evaluation

Were desired outcomes achieved?

Documentation

The following should be noted on the client's chart (visit note for home health):

Solution prepared
Client/caregiver ability to prepare solution
Order from physician for home preparation

SAMPLE DOCUMENTATION

DATE	TIME	
10/11/02	1200	MD order received for instruction in home-prepared sterile saline. Observed client and caregiver preparing sterile container, sterile water, proper measurement of salt to create 0.9% solution of sterile saline. Instructed in labeling, need to prepare daily. Caregiver demonstrates competence in procedure.

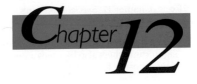

Special Procedures

OVERVIEW

▶ The automatic implantable cardioverter defibrillator (AICD) is a life-saving device. This device also presents a risk of great physical and emotional injury to the client if the device is improperly used or the client is inadequately prepared for the sensation associated with it. Appropriate use of this device requires that the nurse, client, and family members or significant other be fully educated regarding its use and maintenance before an incident requiring intervention by the AICD to reverse a life-threatening dysrhythmia.

▶ Aggressive temperature-control therapy is crucial to regain the delicate balance necessary for vital organ function. If not closely monitored, temperature-control techniques can cause problems greater than those originally being treated. Potential complications of hypothermia/hyperthermia include cardiac, vascular, pulmonary, and metabolic compromise.

▶ A thorough assessment is imperative before beginning any intervention. Improperly performed postmortem techniques could result in serious legal, ethnic/cultural, or ethical/moral dilemmas.

685

▶ When there is a threatened or actual death, the care of significant others also becomes a nursing concern.

▶ Any exposure to body fluids presents a threat to the safety of the caregiver. Self-protective precautions, such as the use of gloves and gown in postmortem care, should be taken.

▶ Some major nursing diagnostic labels related to special procedures are decreased tissue perfusion, altered temperature, risk of ineffective coping, and risk of spread of infection.

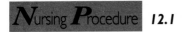

Automatic Implantable Cardioverter Defibrillator (AICD) Management

EQUIPMENT

- No equipment except gloves if contact with body fluids is likely

Purpose

To continuously monitor the heart rate and rhythm and deliver countershocks to the heart to terminate life-threatening recurrent ventricular dysrhythmias

Third-generation AICDs can also pace the heart

Assessment

Assessment should focus on the following:

Level of knowledge of the client and family related to the AICD and follow-up care
Cardiovascular and pulmonary status
Signs of infection
Effects of antiarrhythmia medications
AICD activity diary
Environmental safety
Location of telephone
Client's or significant other's reliability in carrying out home care instructions

Nursing Diagnoses

The nursing diagnoses may include the following:

Decreased tissue perfusion related to decreased cardiac output and dysrhythmia
Anxiety related to life-threatening dysrhythmia

Outcome Identification and Planning

Desired Outcomes (sample)

Client maintains stable vital signs within the client's normal limit parameters.

Surgical incisions and abdominal pocket healing without signs of infection.

Client articulates feelings of acceptance and adaptation to the AICD.

The client and/or significant other will demonstrate consistent ability to follow home care instructions.

Special Considerations

Anxiety and/or residual neurologic impairment as a result of an episode of sudden cardiac death can interfere with integration and processing of information. Repeated teaching sessions may be necessary before the client and significant other can demonstrate an acceptable level of understanding.

Touching the client when the AICD discharges will not cause harm.

Local emergency medical services (EMS) should be informed in advance that the client has an AICD; encourage patient to wear a Medic-Alert bracelet.

IMPLEMENTATION

Action	Rationale
1. Explain procedure to client.	*Reduces anxiety*
2. Wash hands.	*Decreases microorganisms*
3. Clean incisions daily with soap and water (Fig. 12.1).	*Decreases microorganisms*
4. Inspect insertion and generator site daily for redness, swelling, excessive warmth, or pain. The client may use a mirror to examine the lower aspects of the device pocket.	*Fever or signs of infection must be reported to the physician immediately*
5. Instruct the client to avoid wearing tight clothing.	*Prevents chafing the skin over the protruding generator box*
6. Examine the client's written diary of events resulting from each AICD discharge.	*Identifies malfunction of the AICD*
7. Instruct the client to lie down when the AICD discharges.	*Psychological preparation decreases anxiety* *Lying down will prevent falling*

Action	Rationale

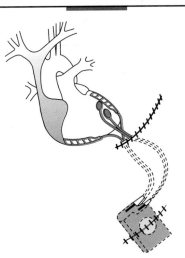

FIGURE 12.1

8. Instruct significant others to activate EMS and initiate cardiopulmonary resuscitation should cardiac arrest occur.

In the event of cardiac arrest, the client will need basic life support until EMS personnel arrive

9. Reinforce and complete teaching begun in the hospital.

Fear and anxiety may interfere with processing of information

10. Assess for the effects of cardiac medications.

Maximizes the chance of arrhythmia control

11. Assess the home for environmental interference. Instruct the client to move away from any device that causes the AICD to emit a beeping tone.

Electromagnetic sources may cause inappropriate firing or deactivation of the AICD; beeping tones from the AICD signal AICD deactivation; household appliances and microwave ovens will not interfere with the device

12. Review any activity restrictions.

Any activity that involves rough contact that could damage the implant site or dislodge the device should be avoided

Action	Rationale
13. Assess adaptation to the AICD.	*Negative thoughts may create unpleasant emotions; ongoing support may be needed*

Evaluation

Were desired outcomes achieved?

Documentation

The following should be noted on the client's chart:

- Teaching done and outcome of teaching
- Condition of the surgical sites and generator pocket
- Responses to AICD shocks and whether or not they are appropriate
- Plans for future visits
- Discharge planning

SAMPLE DOCUMENTATION

DATE	TIME	
9/26/02	0900	Left lateral thoracotomy and abdominal pulse generator pocket incisions without redness, drainage, swelling, or warmth. Temperature 99°F. Denies dizziness or chest pain. Has Medic-Alert necklace on. Reviewed hospital discharge instructions with client and spouse.

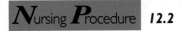

Hyperthermia/ Hypothermia Unit Management

EQUIPMENT

- Hyperthermia/hypothermia unit
- Hyperthermia/hypothermia blanket
- Disposable gloves
- Rectal probe
- Linen blanket (optional)
- Two sheets
- Linen savers (optional)

Purpose

To attain and maintain client's body temperature within acceptable to normal range

Assessment

Assessment should focus on the following:

Baseline data (ie, vital signs, temperature, neurostatus, skin condition, circulation, and ECG)

Signs of shivering

Hyperthermia/hypothermia unit and blanket (properly functioning)

Condition of electrical plugs (properly grounded) and wires (not frayed or exposed)

Nursing Diagnoses

The nursing diagnoses may include the following:

Altered temperature: elevation, related to sepsis

Altered temperature: decreased, related to prolonged exposure to cold

Potential skin impairment related to excess exposure to heating/ cooling unit

Outcome Identification and Planning

Desired Outcomes (sample)

Client's temperature is within acceptable or normal limits.

No skin breakdown or shivering is noted.

Nail beds and mucous membranes are pink; capillary refill time is 3 to 5 sec.

The client demonstrates minimal or no shivering.

Special Considerations

There is a potential for skin damage with any electrical temperature-control device; therefore, treatment and temperature must be monitored closely.

Pediatric and Geriatric

The temperature-control mechanisms of chronically ill elderly and very young pediatric clients are often very sensitive to changes in heat and cold.

Use blanket device to decrease or increase temperature gradually.

IMPLEMENTATION

Action	Rationale
1. Wash hands and organize equipment.	*Reduces microorganism transfer* *Promotes efficiency*
2. Connect the blanket pad (may cover with clear plastic cover) to the operating unit:	*Protects blanket from secretions*
- Insert male tubing connector of blanket into inlet opening on unit (Fig. 12.2).	*Secures blanket tubing–unit connection and prevents solution leakage*
- Repeat same for outlet opening.	
- Connect second pad, if used, in same manner.	
3. Check blanket solution-level gauge and add more recommended solution (usually alcohol–distilled water mixture; see user's manual) into reservoir cap; add solution until it reaches the "fill line."	*Facilitates proper functioning* *Solution is circulated through coils in blanket and warmed/cooled to maintain blanket at the desired temperature*

Action	Rationale

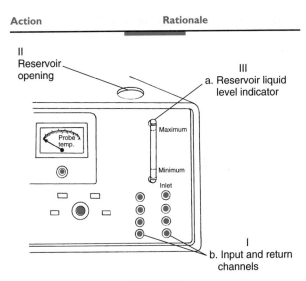

FIGURE 12.2

4. Turn the unit on by moving the temperature control knob to desired temperature (blanket coils will fill with solution automatically).

Activates unit

5. Monitor blanket for adequate filling, watching gauge and adding solution to reservoir as needed to maintain fluid level.

Prevents inadequate filling of blanket and improper functioning of system

6. Turn unit off.

Allows safe transport of unit

7. Set master temperature control knob to either manual or automatic operation.

Adjusts unit to be controlled by temperature probe (automatic) or by nurse (manual)

   If using automatic control:
   - Insert thermistor-probe plug into thermistor-probe jack on unit.

   When using manual control:
   - Set master temperature-control knob to desired temperature.

Action	Rationale
8. Explain procedure to client.	*Reduces anxiety* *Promotes cooperation*
9. Transport equipment into client's room.	
10. Don gloves.	*Prevents microorganism transfer*
11. Bathe client and apply cream, lotion, or oil to skin.	*Increases circulation* *Provides opportunity for skin assessment*
12. Place blanket on bed, place a sheet over the blanket, and apply linen saver, if needed.	*Protects skin from direct contact with blanket and decreases soiling of blanket*
13. Place client on blanket (may use side-to-side rolling, bed scales, or lifting apparatus).	
14. Remove gloves.	
15. Obtain baseline assessment data.	*Allows detection of changes in status*
16. Initiate therapy: don gloves, lubricate rectal probe, and insert probe into rectum.	*Allows machine to warm or cool to desired temperature, with constant automatic monitoring to ensure safe regulation of temperature to desired range*
17. *Automatic control:*	
- Check temperature control for accuracy of setting.	*Ensures that machine is functioning properly*
- Check that automatic mode light is on.	
- Check pad temperature range for safe limits.	
Manual control:	
- Check that manual mode light is on.	*Allows nurse to monitor client's temperature continually and to adjust blanket temperature, as needed, to achieve desired body temperature*
- Check that temperature setting and safety limits are accurate.	
- Monitor client's temperture.	
- Adjust blanket temperature to maintain body temperature.	
18. Monitor client's status:	
- Temperature—every 15 min until desired temperature is reached	*Ensures that no excess change in body temperature occurs*

Action	Rationale
- Vital signs—every 15 to 30 min, or as ordered initially, and every 1 to 2 h until treatment is discontinued	*Initial treatment might cause adverse changes (eg, arrhythmias, hyperventilation)*
- Onset of shivering—verbalized sensations, muscle twitching, ECG artifact; if present, obtain order for medication to prevent	*Shivering increases body metabolism and energy needs* *Medication (tranquilizer) will decrease shivering*
19. Every 4 h, remove rectal probe and clean; use glass thermometer to check temperature.	*Allows monitoring for rectal irritation and maintains probe accuracy*
20. Maintain client in supine position with every-2-hour range of motion, massage to bony prominences, and support stockings as ordered.	*Provides for maximum body surface area exposure* *Decreases venous stasis*
21. Turn client every hour, and have client cough and deep breathe.	*Increases ventilation of airways and secretion removal*
22. Observe for edema.	*Detects edema related to increased cell permeability*
23. Adjust master temperature control gradually until 98.6°F is reached over a period of 6 h.	*Rapid changes in temperature could result in severe vital sign changes and/or arrhythmia*

Evaluation

Were desired outcomes achieved?

Documentation

The following should be noted on the client's chart:

- Time treatment was initiated and initial temperature settings
- Initial and subsequent client response to treatment
- Baseline vital signs and client status

SAMPLE DOCUMENTATION

DATE	TIME	
12/3/02	1400	Client placed on hypothermia blanket with master temperature set at 36°C and patient temperature probe indicating 39°C. Vital signs stable. No shivering noted. Skin intact, with capillary refill less than 5 seconds.

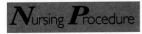

Postmortem Care

EQUIPMENT

- Disposable gloves
- Clean linens
- Clean gown
- Wash basin
- Death certificate
- Isolation bags (optional)
- Cloth or disposable gown
- Two washcloths and towels
- 4 × 4-inch gauze or other dressing (optional)
- Moist cotton balls (optional)
- Identification bracelets or body tags
- Shroud (optional, unless agency policy)
- Dilute bleach mixture (optional)

Purpose

Provides proper preparation of body of deceased client for viewing by family members and for transport to funeral home or morgue, with minimum exposure of staff to body fluids and excrement

Assessment

Assessment should focus on the following:

Hospital policy regarding postmortem care and notification process

Need for autopsy (if death occurs within 24 h of hospitalization or is the result of suicide, homicide, or unknown causes; or if the family requests an autopsy)

Nursing Diagnoses

The nursing diagnoses may include the following:

Risk of ineffective coping by family with the death of loved one

Risk of spread of infection related to contact with contaminated body fluids

697

Outcome Identification and Planning

Desired Outcomes (sample)

Body and environment are clean, with a natural appearance.

Family views body with no signs of extreme distress at its physical appearance.

There is no spead of disease.

Special Considerations

The bodies of deceased clients with known infections requiring blood and body fluid precautions or isolation (eg, tuberculosis, AIDS) should be tagged accordingly, and there should be appropriate disposal of soiled items and cleaning of nondisposable items (see Display 10–1).

In some states, death may be pronounced by a nonphysician (eg, coroner, advance practice nurse, home health nurse), particularly in out-of-hospital settings. Be familiar with agency and state policy and procedure related to pronouncement of death.

Home Health

The client must be pronounced dead before removal of the body from the home (unless being taken to a hospital or health facility). Follow home-health agency policy for recording the pronouncement on the client's chart.

When an autopsy is required or requested, the body must be left basically undisturbed until transported to the morgue.

 Transcultural

Many religious rites and cultural practices may be employed by a variety of cultures. It is important that the nurse demonstrate respect for the deceased, as well as allow the family privacy.

Communicate with the family to determine what is important before preparing the body. It may be important to summon a priest, minister, rabbi, or other religious leader after the client is deceased.

IMPLEMENTATION

Action	Rationale
1. Record time of death (cessation of heart function) and time pronounced dead by physician, or other appropriate authority.	*Required for death certificate and all official records*

Action	Rationale
2. Notify family members that client's status has changed for the worse and assist them to a private room until physician is available.	*Provides privacy for family during initial grief and allows time for physician to notify family of client's death*
3. Close door to client's room.	*Prevents exposure of body to other patients and visitors and prevents accidental viewing of body by family before body is prepared*
4. Don gloves and isolation gown.	*Protects nurse from body secretions*
5. Hold eyelids closed until they remain closed or place moist 4 × 4-inch gauze or cotton balls on lids.	*Fixes eyelids in a natural, closed position before rigor mortis onset*
6. Remove tubes, such as IV line, nasogastric (NG) catheter, or urinary catheter, if allowed and no autopsy is to be done.	*Provides a more natural appearance for viewing by family members*

7. If unable to remove tubes:
  - Clamp IVs and tubes.
  - Coil NG and urinary tubes and tape them down.
  - Cut IV tubings as close to clamp as possible, cover with 4 × 4-inch gauze, tape securely.
	Retains secretions and provides as clean and natural an appearance for family viewing as possible

8. Transfer extra equipment from room to utility room.	*Allows free mobility around bed and improves appearance of environment*
9. Wash secretions from face and body.	*Improves appearance of body and decreases room odor*
10. Replace soiled linens and gown with clean articles.	*Provides clean appearance and decreases odor*
11. Place linen savers under body and extremities, if needed.	*Catches secretions and excrement escaping from open sphincters or oozing wounds*
12. Put soiled linens and pads in bag (isolation bag, if appropriate) and remove from room.	*Decreases exposure to body fluids Removes odor and improves appearance of environment*

Action	Rationale
13. Position body supine with arms at side, palms down.	*Provides a natural appearance*
14. Place dentures (if present) in mouth, put a pillow under head, close mouth, and place rolled towel under chin.	*Gives face a natural appearance and sets mouth closed before onset of rigor mortis*
15. Remove all jewelry (except wedding band, unless band is requested by family members) and give to family with other personal belongings; record the name(s) of receiver(s).	*Prevents loss of property during transfer of body and ensures proper disposal of belongings*
16. Place clean top covering over body, leaving face exposed.	*Allows family to view client, and covers remaining tubes and dressings*
17. Place chair at bedside.	*Provides for family member unable to stand or if momentary weakness occurs*
18. Dim lighting.	*Makes atmosphere more soothing and minimizes abnormal appearance of body*
19. After body has been viewed by family, tag with appropriate identification (some agencies require that body be placed in a covering or shroud and that an outer covering identification tag be applied).	*Ensures proper identification of body before transfer to funeral home or morgue*
20. Send completed death certificate with body to funeral home or complete paperwork as required by hospital and send body to morgue.	*Fulfills legal requirements for documentation of death*
21. Close rooms of clients on hall through which body is transported, if hospital policy.	*Prevents distress of other clients and visitors*

Action	Rationale
22. Restore or dispose of equipment, supplies, and linens properly; remove gown and gloves and wash hands.	*Reduces microorganism transfer* *Maintains clean and orderly environment*
23. Have room cleaned: use special cleaning supplies if client had infection (eg, 1:10 bleach dilution for AIDS clients, special germicides for isolation situations).	*Prevents transfer of micro-organisms*

Evaluation

Were desired outcomes achieved?

Documentation

The following should be noted on the client's chart:

- Time of death and code information, if performed
- Notification of physician and family members
- Response of family members
- Disposal of valuables and belongings
- Time body was removed from room

SAMPLE DOCUMENTATION

DATE	TIME	
12/3/02	1200	Client pronounced dead by Dr. Brown; family members notified by doctor. Body viewed by family with no extreme reactions. Gold-colored wedding band taped to finger on body; gold-colored watch, clothing, and shoes given to Mr. Dale Smith (son). Body removed to James Funeral Home, accompanied by completed death certificate.

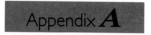

Stress Management Techniques*

The following techniques can be taught to provide an individual with an opportunity to control his or her response to stressors and, in turn, to increase the ability to manage stress constructively. Suggested readings are listed at the end to provide more specific information.

Progressive Relaxation Technique

Progressive relaxation is a self-taught or instructed exercise that involves learning to constrict and relax muscle groups in a systematic way, beginning, with the face and finishing with the feet. This exercise may be combined with breathing exercises that focus on inner body processes. It usually takes 15 to 30 minutes and may be accompanied by a taped instruction that directs the person concerning the sequence of muscles to be relaxed.

1. Wear loose clothing; remove glasses and shoes
2. Sit or recline in a comfortable position with neck and knees supported; avoid lying completely flat.
3. Begin with slow, rhythmic breathing.
   a. Close your eyes or stare at a spot and take in a slow deep breath.
   b. Exhale slowly.
4. Continue rhythmic breathing at a slow steady pace and feel the tension leaving your body with each breath.
5. Begin progressive relaxation of muscle groups.
   a. Breathe in and tense (tighten) your muscles and then relax the muscles as you breath out.
   b. Suggested order for tension–relaxation cycle (with tension technique in parentheses):
   Face, jaw, mouth (squint eyes, wrinkle brow)
   Neck (pull chin to neck)
   Right hand (make a fist)
   Right arm (bend elbow in tightly)
   Left hand (makes a fist)
   Left arm (bend elbow in tightly)
   Back, shoulders, chest (shrug shoulders up tightly)
   Abdomen (pull stomach in and bear down on chair)

*Carpenito, L.J. (2000) *Nursing diagnosis: Application to clinical practice,* 8th ed. Philadelphia: Lippincott-Raven.

     Right upper leg (push leg down)
     Right lower leg and foot (point toes toward body)
     Left upper leg (push leg down)
     Left lower leg and foot (point toes toward body)

6. Practice technique slowly
7. End relaxation session when you are ready by counting to three, inhaling, deeply, and saying, "I am relaxed."

Self-Coaching

Self-coaching is a procedure to decrease anxiety by understanding one's own signs of anxiety (such as increased heart rate or sweaty palms) and then coaching oneself to relax.

For example, "I am upset about this situation but I can control how anxious I get. I will take things one step at a time, and I won't focus on my fear. I'll think about what I must do to finish this task. The situation will not be forever. I can manage until it is over. I'll focus on taking deep breaths."

Thought Stopping

Thought stopping is a self-directed behavioral procedure learned to gain control of self-defeating thoughts. Through repeated systematic practice, a person does the following:

1. Says "stop" when a self-defeating thought crosses the mind (eg, "I'm not smart enough" or "I'm not a good nurse").
2. Allows a brief period—15 to 30 seconds—of conscious relaxation (because of an increased focus on negative thoughts, it may seem at first that self-defeating thoughts increase; however, eventually the self-defeating thoughts will decrease).

Assertive Behavior

Assertive behavior is the open, honest, empathic sharing of your opinions, desires, and feelings. Assertiveness is not a magical acquisition but a learned behavioral skill. Assertive persons do not allow others to take advantage of them and thus are not victims. Assertive behavior is not domineering but remains controlled and nonaggressive. An assertive person

Does not hurt others
Does not wait for things to get better
Does not invite victimization
Listens attentively to the desires and feelings of others

Takes the initiative to make relationships better

Remains in control or uses silences as an alternative

Examines all the risks involved before asserting

Examines personal responsibilities in each situation before asserting

Refer to Suggested Readings for specific techniques or participate in an assertiveness training course led by a competent instructor. Assertive behavior is best learned slowly in several sessions rather than in one lengthy session or workshop.

Guided Imagery

This technique is the purposeful use of one's imagination in a specific way to achieve relaxation and control. The person concentrates on the image and pictures being involved in the scene. The following is an example of the technique:

1. Discuss with the person an image he or she has experienced that is pleasurable and relaxing, such as
   a. Lying on a warm beach
   b. Feeling a cool wave of water
   c. Floating on a raft
   d. Watching the sun set
2. Choose a scene that will involve at least two senses.
3. Begin with rhythmic breathing and progressive relaxation.
4. Have person travel mentally to the scene.
5. Have the person slowly experience the scene; how does it look? sound? smell? feel? taste?
6. Practice the imagery.
   a. Suggest tape recording the imagined experience to assist with the technique.
   b. Practice the technique alone to reduce feelings of embarrassment.
7. End the imagery technique by counting to three and saying, "I am relaxed" (if the person does not use a specific ending, he or she may become drowsy and fall asleep, which defeats the purpose of the technique).

Suggested Readings

Alberti, R. E., & Emmons, L. (1974). Your Perfect Right: A Guide to Assertive Behavior (2nd ed.). San Luis Obispo, CA: Impact.

Bloom, L., Coburn, K., & Pearlman, J. (1976). The new Assertive Woman. New York: Dell.

Chenevert, M. (1978). Special Techniques in Assertiveness Training for Women in the Health Professions. St. Louis: C. V. Mosby.

Chenevert, M. (1985). Pro-Nurse Handbook. St. Louis: C. V. Mosby.

Frisch, N. C., & Kelley, J. (1996). Healing Life's Crisis: A Guide for Nurses. Albany, NY: Delmar.

Gridano., D., & Everly, G. (1979). Controlling Stress and Tension. Englewood Cliffs, NJ: Prentice-Hall.

Herman, S. (1978). Becoming Assertive: A Guide for Nurses. New York: D. Van Nostrand.

Hill, L., & Smith, N. (1985). Self-Care Nursing. Englewood Cliffs, NJ: Prentice-Hall. (Especially Part II, Self Care Primarily Associated with the Mind).

McCaffery, M. (1979). Nursing Management of the Patient with Pain (2nd ed.). Philadelphia: J. B. Lippincott. (especially Ch. 10, Imagery, and Ch. 9, Relaxation).

Rancour, P. (1991). Guided imagery: Healing when curing is out of the question. *Perspectives in Psychiatric Care, 27(4)*:30–33.

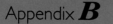

Appendix *B*

Pain Management

Basic Principles

- Pain is subjective and an individual experience; therefore, the client's report of pain characteristics must be considered accurate and valid.
- Pain tolerance is subjective and varies among individuals.
- Acute pain, by definition, generally lasts less than 6 months.
- Chronic pain, by definition, lasts more than 6 months.
- Successful assessment and management of pain depends, in part, on a good nurse–client relationship.
- Anticipatory pain management is best; intervene when pain is anticipated and before pain becomes significant.

Pain Assessment

- Self-report of the client's perceptions regarding pain must be considered valid.
- Assess factors/characteristics of client's pain:
  Location (Where is the pain? Can you point to it?)
  Intensity (On a scale of 1–10, how bad is it? Or use visual pain analog scale)
  Quality (Is it dull, sharp, nagging, burning?)
  Radiation (Does it radiate? Where does it radiate to?)
  Precipitating factors (What were you doing when it occurred?)
  Aggravating factors (What makes it worse?)
  Associating factors (Do you get nauseated or dizzy with the pain?)
  Alleviating factors (Do you know of anything that has made it better at times?)
- The following factors must be considered in assessing and managing the client's pain: Medical diagnosis, age, weight, sociocultural affiliation (religion, race, gender)
- Self-management devices (such as patient-controlled analgesia pumps, PCA pumps) DO NOT exempt the nurse from performing frequent and careful client assessments.
- Assess clients receiving drug therapy for pain management every 1 to 2 hours (more often, if needed) to ensure adequate pain control and avoid complications of uncontrolled pain and complications of drug therapy.

General Pain Management Strategies

- Always assess pain first.
- Client/family teaching should be included as part of nonpharmacologic management to include factors such as what causes the pain, what the client can expect, what needs to be reported, instructions for reducing activity and treatment-related pain, and relaxation techniques.
- Consider general comfort measures such as client repositioning, back rub, pillows at lower back, bladder emptying, and cool or warm washcloth to area.
- Consider management of anxiety along with pain, using strategies of relaxation.
- Escalating and repetitive pain may be difficult to control. Early intervention is best.
- Around-the-clock (ATC) pain-therapy drug protocols are used to treat persistent pain, using the analgesia ladder standard as set forth by the World Health Organization. The use of oral medications, when possible, is recommended. Nonopioid or nonsteroidal anti-inflammatory drugs (NSAIDS) are used in the initial treatment, with progression to an ATC opioid and steroids, antidepressants, or anticonvulsants, as needed to control pain. Treatment proceeds to step 2 and step 3 of the analgesia ladder with increased potency of opioids and use of parenteral routes.
- Unrelieved pain has negative physical and psychological consequences.
- Take into consideration what the client believes will help relieve the pain and the client ability to participate in treatment.
- If pain cannot be realistically relieved completely, educate client as to what would be considered a tolerable level of pain in consideration of the condition.
- Nonsteroidal anti-inflammatory drugs and drugs that inhibit platelet aggregation should be used with caution in clients with bleeding tendencies and conditions such as thrombocytopenia or gastrointestinal ulceration.

Postoperative Pain Management

- Always check the general surgical area for manifestations of postoperative complications when the client complains of pain. Watch for problems such as compromised circulation, excessive edema, bleeding, wound dehiscence and evisceration and infection.
- Goals of postoperative pain management regimens include attaining a positive client outcome and reducing the length of stay.

- Administering nonsedative pain medications before ambulation should be considered to facilitate early and consistent ambulation postoperatively.
- The Agency for Health Care Policy and Research (AHCPR) and American Pain Society (APS) guidelines for management of acute pain indicate that surgical clients should receive nonsteroidal anti-inflammatory drugs or acetaminophen around the clock, unless contraindications prohibit use.
- Opioid analgesics are considered to be the cornerstone for management of moderate to severe acute pain. Effective use of opioid analgesics may facilitate postoperative cooperation in activities such as coughing and deep breathing exercises, physical therapy, and ambulation.
- Intravenous administration is the parenteral route of choice after major surgery.
- Oral drug administration is the primary choice of drug routes in the ambulatory surgical population.
- Oral administration of drugs should begin as soon as the client can tolerate oral intake.
- Acute or significant pain, not explained by surgical trauma, may warrant a surgical evaluation.

Complications of Drug Therapy

Watch for signs of narcotic overdose carefully—decreased respiratory rate and/or depth, decreased mentation, decreased blood pressure.

Administer naloxone as indicated by orders/agency policy immediately if signs of respiratory depression occur in clients receiving narcotics. Naloxone may increase rather than reverse the effects of meperidine.

Major signs of drug dependence are client need for increased dosages of medication (after other methodologic and drug alternatives have been attempted).

Check if narcotic administration produces consistent euphoria rather than just pain relief.

Pain Management in the Elderly

- Elderly clients often have complex pain because of multiple medical problems. Elderly clients are at a greater risk for drug–drug and drug–disease interactions.
- Elderly clients may experience a longer duration and higher peak effect of opioids. It is best to start with more conservative

doses and increase as needed from that point. Meperidine (Demerol) should be given with caution, and monitor particularly for neurologic changes and seizures.
- Some elderly clients may experience more severe postsurgical pain than other age groups. In these cases, consider options such as oral morphine or hydromorphone, if ordered.

Special Considerations

- As a routine, pain medications are not given to clients with acute neurologic conditions, since assessment of the true status of the neurologic status may be skewed with central or peripheral nervous system effects.
- The pain status of clients who have had recent vascular surgery should be monitored carefully. Excessive pain may result in increased blood pressure in response to stress, with subsequent rupture of newly grafted or anastamosed vessels.
- Note procedures on Patient-Controlled Analgesia (PCA) Management, Transelectrical Nerve Stimulation (TENS) Unit Management, Epidural Catheter Management, and Application of Heat/Cold Therapy in this procedure book.

Evaluation of Therapy

- Note verbal statement of pain decrease or increase.
- Note accompanying clinical indicators of pain increase or decrease.
- Note appearance of area of pain.
- Coping skills successfully used by client.
- Anxiety-reducing techniques successfully used

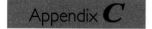

Nursing Diagnoses, North American Nursing Diagnosis Association 2001–2002*

Activity intolerance
Activity intolerance, Risk for
Acute confusion
Acute pain
Adaptive capacity, Decreased intracranial
Adjustment, Impaired
Adult failure to thrive
Airway clearance, Ineffective
Alcoholism, Dysfunctional family processes
Allergy response, Latex
Allergy response, Latex, Risk for
Anticipatory grieving
Anxiety,
 Death
Aspiration, Risk for
Attachment, Risk for impaired parent/infant/child
Autonomic dysreflexia
Autonomic dysreflexia, Risk for
Bathing/hygiene self-care deficit
Bed mobility, Impaired
Body image, Disturbed
Body temperature, Risk for imbalanced
Bowel incontinence
Breastfeeding,
 Effective
 Ineffective
 Interrupted

Breathing pattern, Ineffective
Cardiac output, Decreased
Caregiver role strain
Caregiver role strain, Risk for
Chronic,
 Confusion
 Pain
 Sorrow
Communication, Impaired verbal
Compromised family coping
Conflict,
 Decisional
 Parental role
Confusion
 Acute
 Chronic
Constipation
Constipation, Perceived
Constipation, Risk for
Coping,
 Defensive
 Ineffective
Coping, Community
Coping, Community Ineffective
Coping, Community, Readiness for enhanced
Coping, Family,
 Compromised
 Disabled
 Readiness for enhanced
Death anxiety
Decisional conflict

*Reprinted courtesy of North American Nursing Diagnosis Association, Philadelphia, PA.

Decreased cardiac output
Denial, Ineffective
Dentition, Impaired
Development, Risk for delayed
Diarrhea
Disproportionate growth, Risk for
Disturbed body image
Disuse syndrome, Risk for
Diversional activity, Deficient
Dressing/grooming self-care deficit
Dysreflexia, Autonomic
Elimination, Impaired urinary
Energy field, Disturbed
Environmental interpretation syndrome, Impaired
Excess fluid volume
Failure to thrive, Adult
Falls, Risk for
Family processes,
 Dysfunctional: Alcoholism
 Interrupted
Fear
Feeding self-care deficit
Fluid volume,
 Deficient
 Excess
 Risk for deficient
 Risk for imbalanced
Gas exchange, Impaired
Grieving,
 Anticipatory
 Dysfunctional
Growth and development, Delayed
Growth, Risk for disproportionate
Health maintenance, Ineffective
Health-seeking behaviors
Home maintenance, Impaired
Hopelessness
Hyperthermia
Hypothermia
Identity, Disturbed personal

Imbalanced fluid volume, Risk for
Incontinence,
 Bowel
 Functional urinary
 Reflex urinary
 Stress urinary
 Total urinary
 Urge urinary
 Urge urinary, Risk for
Infant behavior,
 Disorganized
 Readiness for enhanced organized
 Risk for disorganized
Infant feeding pattern, Ineffective
Infection, Risk for
Injury,
 Perioperative-positioning
 Risk for
Intracranial adaptive capacity, Decreased
Interrupted breastfeeding
Knowledge, Deficient
Latex allergy response
Latex allergy response, Risk for
Loneliness, Risk for
Memory, Impaired
Mobility, Impaired,
 Bed
 Physical
 Wheelchair
Mucous membrane, Impaired oral
Nausea
Neglect, Unilateral
Neurovascular dysfunction, Risk for peripheral
Noncompliance
Nutrition,
 Imbalanced: Less than body requirements
 Imbalanced: More than body requirements
 Risk for imbalanced: More than body requirements

Oral mucous membrane, Impaired
Organized infant behavior, Readiness for enhanced
Pain,
Acute
Chronic
Parental role conflict
Parent/infant/child attachment, Risk for impaired
Parenting, Impaired,
Risk for
Perceived constipation
Perioperative-positioning injury, Risk for
Peripheral neurovascular dysfunction, Risk for
Personal identity,
Disturbed,
Physical mobility, Impaired
Poisoning, Risk for
Post-trauma syndrome,
Risk for
Powerlessness,
Risk for
Protection, Ineffective
Rape-trauma syndrome,
Compound reaction
Silent reaction
Recovery, Delayed surgical
Relocation stress syndrome,
Risk for
Retention, Urinary
Role conflict, Parental,
Role performance,
Ineffective
Role strain, Caregiver,
Risk for
Self-care deficit,
Bathing/hygiene
Dressing/grooming
Feeding
Toileting
Self-esteem, Low,
Chronic
Situational,
Risk for situational

Self-mutilation,
Risk for
Sensory perception,
Disturbed
Sexual dysfunction
Sexuality patterns, Ineffective
Skin integrity, Impaired,
Risk for
Sleep deprivation
Sleep pattern, Disturbed
Social interaction, Impaired
Social isolation
Sorrow, Chronic
Spiritual distress,
Risk for
Spiritual well-being, Readiness for enhanced
Suffocation, Risk for
Suicide, Risk for
Surgical recovery, Delayed
Swallowing, Impaired
Syndrome,
Disuse, Risk for
Environmental interpretation, Impaired
Post-trauma
Risk for post-trauma
Rape-trauma
Rape-trauma, Compound reaction
Rape-trauma, Silent reaction
Relocation stress
Therapeutic regimen management,
Effective
Ineffective
Ineffective community
Ineffective family
Thermoregulation, Ineffective
Thought processes, Disturbed
Tissue integrity, Impaired
Tissue perfusion, Ineffective
Toileting self-care deficit
Transfer ability, Impaired
Trauma, Risk for
Unilateral neglect
Urinary elimination, Impaired

Appendix *D*

Common Clinical Abbreviations

*When multiple meanings are possible, consider the context.

abd	abdomen	FBS	fasting/fingerstick blood sugar
ac	before meals		
ADLs	activities of daily living	FHT	fetal heart tones
		fl, fld	fluid
ad. lib.	as desired	ft	feet
adm	admission	fx	fracture/fractional
AKA	above-the-knee amputation	g/gm	gram
		gr	grain
alb	albumin	grav	gravida
amb	ambulate	gt, gtt	drops
ant	anterior	h, hr	hour
AP	anterior-posterior	hg	mercury
ATC	around-the-clock	hct	hematocrit
ax	axillary	hgb	hemoglobin
approx	approximately	HOB	head of bed
b.i.d.	twice a day	hs	hour of sleep
BKA	below-the-knee amputation	hx	history
		I & D	incision and drainage
BM	bowel movement		
BP	blood pressure	I & O	intake and output
BRP	bathroom privileges	ID	intradermal
C	Centigrade, Celsius	IM	intramuscular
c̄	with	irriga	irrigation
Ca	calcium	IV	intravenous
CA	cancer	K	potassium
CC	chief complaint	kg	kilogram
cc	cubic centimeter	L	liter
C & S	culture and sensitivity	L, lt	left
		lat	lateral
c/o	complains of	lb	pound
CVP	central venous pressure	lymph	lymphatic
		MAE	moves all extremities
cysto	cystoscopy		
DC	discontinue	m	minims
diab	diabetic	mcg	microgram
diag, DX	diagnosis	mEq	milliequivalent
DOA	dead on arrival	mg, mgm	milligrams
dr	dram	MI	myocardial infarction
ECG	electrocardiogram	ml	milliliter
EENT	eye, ear, nose, throat	neg	negative
et	and	NKA	no known allergies
exam	examination	noct	nocturnal
F	Fahrenheit	NPO	nothing by mouth

N & V	nausea and vomiting	SOB	short of breath or side of bed
OOB	out of bed	sol	solution
oz	ounce	sp. gr.	specific gravity
OD	right eye	S & S	signs/symptoms
OS	left eye	stat	immediately
OU	each eye	supp	suppository
p.c.	after meals	T, temp	temperature
PO	by mouth, orally	T & A	tonsillectomy and adenoidectomy
pr	per rectum		
PRN	when needed	tab	tablet
q	every	tbsp	tablespoon
qAM	every morning	t.i.d.	three times a day
qd	every day	tinc	tincture
q.i.d.	four times a day	TKO	to keep open
q.o.d.	every other day	trach	tracheostomy
qs	quantity sufficient	tsp	teaspoon
R	rectal	TUR	transurethral resection
RBC	red blood cell		
rt, R	right	tx	treatment
resp	respirations	UA	urinalysis
RLQ	right lower quadrant	UGI	upper gastrointestinal
RO or r/o	rule out	vag	vaginal
ROM	range of motion	vol	volume
Rx	prescription	VS	vital signs
sø	without	WBC	white blood cell
SC/sub q	subcutaneous	WNL	within normal limits
sm	small	wt	weight
SL	sublingual		

Selected Abbreviations Used for Specific Descriptions

ASCVD	arteriosclerotic cardiovascular disease	GYN	gynecology
		H_2O_2	hydrogen peroxide
		HA	hyperalimentation or headache
ASHD	arteriosclerotic heart disease		
		HCVD	hypertensive cardiovascular disease
BE	barium enema		
CMS	circulation movement sensation	HEENT	head, ear, eye, nose, throat
CNS	central nervous system or Clinical Nurse Specialist	HVD	hypertensive vascular disease
		ICU	intensive care unit
DJD	degenerative joint disease	LLE	left lower extremity
		LLQ	left lower quadrant
DOE	dyspnea on exertion	LOC	level of consciousness; laxatives of choice
DTs	delerium tremens		
D_5W	5% dextrose in water		
FUO	fever of unknown origin	LMP	last menstrual period
GB	gallbladder	LUE	left upper extremity
GI	gastrointestinal	LUQ	left upper quadrant

Neuro	neurology; neurosurgery	Psych	psychology; psychiatric
NS	normal saline	PT	physical therapy
NWB	non-weight bearing	RL (or LR)	Ringer's lactate; lactated Ringer's
OPD	outpatient department		
		RLE	right lower extremity
ORIF	open reduction internal fixation	RR	recovery room
		RUE	right upper extremity
Ortho	orthopedics	RUQ	right upper quadrant
OT	occupational therapy	Rx	prescription
		STSG	split-thickness skin graft
PAR	postanesthesia room		
PE	physical examination	Surg	surgery, surgical
		THR; TJR	total hip replacement; total joint replacement
PERRLA	pupils equal, round, and react to light and accommodation		
		URI	upper respiratory infection
PID	pelvic inflammatory disease	UTI	urinary tract infection
PI	present illness	VD	venereal disease
PM & R	physical medicine and rehabilitation	WNWD	well-nourished, well-developed

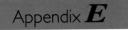

Diagnostic Laboratory Tests: Normal Values

Test	Normal Values	(SI units)
Serum/Plasma Chemistries		
Arterial blood gases:		
pH	7.35–7.45	7.35–7.45 pH units
pCO_2	35–45 mm Hg	4.7–5.3 kPa
HCO_3	21–28 mEq/L	21–28 mmol/L
pO_2	80–100 mm Hg	10.6–13.3 kPa
	60–70 mm Hg (newborn)	8–10.33 kPa
O_2 saturation	95%–100%	Fraction saturated: > 0.95
	40%–90%	Fraction saturated: 0.4–0.9
Base excess	± 2mEq/L	±2 mmol/L
AST (aspartate aminotransferase), formerly SGOT	8–35 U/L 16–72 U/L (newborn)	—same— —same—
Bilirubin:		
Direct (conjugated)	0.0–0.4 mg/dl	<5 umol/L
Indirect (unconjugated)	0.2–0.8 mg/dl	3.4–13.6 umol/L
Total	0.3–1 mg/dl	5–17 umol/L
Newborns	6–10 mg/dl	103–171 umol/L
Blood urea nitrogen (BUN)	5–20 mg/dl 4–16 mg/dl (newborn)	1.8–7.1 mmol/L 1.4–5.7 mmol/L
Calcium (total)	8–10 mg/dl	2.05–2.54 mmol/L
Chloride	98–107 mEq/L	98–107 mmol/L
Cholesterol	120–200 mg/dl	—same—
Creatinine	0.7–1.3 mg/dl	62–115 umol/L
Creatinine phosphokinase (CPK)	25–175 U/ml	—same—
CPK isoenzymes	MM (skeletal) band 5–70 U/MB band (cardiac) < 5%	—same— —same—
Erythrocyte sedimentation rate (ESR)	Up to 20 mm/hr	—same—
Erythrocyte indices:		
Mean corpuscular volume 80–96 cu micron/micrometer (MCV)	80–96 fL	

Test	Normal Values	(SI units)
Mean corpuscular hemoglobin (MCH)	27–31 picograms/cell	27–31 pg
Mean corpuscular hemoglobin concentration (MCHC)	32%–36%	0.32–0.36 (mean concentration fraction)
Reticulocytes	0.5%–1.5% of red cells	0.005–0.15 fraction
Glucose	70–120 mg/dl	3.9–6.7 mmol/L
Hematocrit:		
Newborns	44%–64%	0.44–0.64 (volume fraction)
Infants	30%–40%	0.30–0.40 (volume fraction)
Children	31%–43%	0.31–0.43 (volume fraction)
Men	40%–54%	0.4–0.59 (volume fraction)
Women	38%–47%	0.38–0.47 (volume fraction)
Hemoglobin concentration:		
Newborns	14–24 g/dl	135–240 g/L
Infants	10–15 g/dl	100–150 g/L
Children	11–16 g/dl	110–160 g/L
Men	14–18 g/dl	135–180 g/L
Women	12–16 g/dl	120–160 g/L
Lactic dehydrogenase (LDH)	70–200 IU/L	—same—
Platelet count	150,000–450,000 cell/ul	$150–450 \times 10^9$/L
Potassium	3.5–5.1 mEq/L	3.5–5.1 mmol/L
Partial thromboplastin time (PTT); (activated APTT)	20–45 seconds	—same—
Prothrombin time	10–13 seconds	—same—
Red blood cells (RBCs):		
Newborns	4.8–7.1 million/cu mm	4.8–7.1 10^{12}/L
Infants/children	3.8–5.5 million/cu mm	3.8–5.5 10^{12}/L
Men	4.6–6.2 million/cu mm	4.6–6.2 10^{12}/L
Women	4.2–5.4 million/cu mm	4.2–5.4 10^{12}/L
Serum glutamic oxaloacetic transaminase (SGOT)	5–40 U/ml	
Sodium	136–145 mEq/L	136–145 mmol/L

Test	Normal Values	(SI units)
White blood cells (leukocyte 5000–10,000 cu mm count)		
Neutrophils	60%–70%	0.60–0.70 (mean number fraction)
Eosinophils	1%–4%	0.01–0.04 (mean number fraction)
Basophils	0%–0.5%	0.0–0.005 (mean number fraction)
Lymphocytes	20%–30%	0.20–0.30 (mean number fraction)
Monocytes	2%–6%	0.02–0.06 (mean number fraction)
Urine Chemistry		
Calcium	100–300 mg/24 h	2.5–7.5 mmol/24h
Creatine	0–200 mg/24 h	< 5.0 mmol/24h
Creatinine	0.8–2.0 g/24 h	7.1–17.7 mol/24h
Creatinine clearance	100–150 ml of blood cleared of creatine per minute	
Osmolality	Males: 390–1090 mM/kg Females: 300–1090 mM/kg	
Potassium	25–125 mEq/24 h	25–125 mmol/24 h
Protein	40–150 mg/24 h	—same—
Sodium	40–220 mEq/24 h	40–220 mmol/24 h
Urea nitrogen	9–16 g/24 h	90–160 g/L
Uric acid	250–750 mg/24 h	1.48–4.43 mmol/24 h

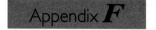

Types of Isolation*

There are two tiers of isolation precautions recommended by the Hospital Infection Control Practices Advisory Committee (HIC-PAC). The tiers include Standard Precautions and Transmission-based Precautions for clients with known or suspected infections with epidemiologically important pathogens. The major category of isolation involves the use of standard precautions, which combine the major features of universal precautions and body substance isolation. HAND WASHING IS REQUIRED WITH ALL CLIENT CONTACT AND WITH ALL FORMS OF ISOLATION.

Standard precautions (blood and body fluid) involve the use of protective coverings whenever contact with blood and certain other body fluids is a possibility. These precautions are intended to prevent contact of the skin and mucous membranes of health care workers with blood and body fluids of the client.

Standard precautions are applied to blood; all body fluids, secretions, and excretions except sweat, regardless of the presence of visible blood; nonintact skin; and mucous membranes. If a client is known to have an infection involving highly transmissible pathogens, additional precautions are employed to interrupt transmission. Three types of precautions—airborne, droplet, and contact—are used. The appropriate disease-specific or transmission-specific isolation system is initiated (see table for protective barriers required).

Standard precautions involve the use of protective barrier coverings whenever contact with any body fluid is expected. These precautions are based on the principle that not all clients infected with blood-borne pathogens can be reliably identified before the possible exposure of health-care team members. Health-team members are instructed to use precautions with all clients and to add transmission precautions when indicated.

Precautions are posted in all clients' rooms. Gloves are used when handling any body part with broken skin, body secretion or secretion-soiled item. A gown is added when soiling of clothing is likely. A mask and goggles are worn whenever secretions are projectile or when an infection with a microorganism that is transmitted through air droplet transmission is suspected (an additional mask-precautions notice may be posted). All linens are handled with care to prevent contamination of the nurse's clothing. Reusable items used on clients known to be infected are tagged accordingly when sent for disinfecting.

*CDC Isolation Guidelines, AJIC, February 1996, pp. 32–52.

Disease-specific transmission precautions involve the use of isolation precautions identifying required barrier coverings when caring for clients with diseases caused by specific microorganisms that are identified by the mode of disease transmission. Many facilities design isolation precautions that identify the necessary precautions (eg, the use of gloves, gown, masks, goggles, or special disposal of contaminated materials) in a yes/no format. The table includes information found on most cards.

Precautions Used by Health-Care Team Members

Isolation/Precaution Systems	Gloves	Gown	Mask	Goggles	Special Handling of Reusable Equipment
Standard precautions	Y	With possible soiling	If splashing likely	Y with projectile secretions	Y if contaminated with body substances
Transmission-based precautions	D	D	D	D	D
Contact	Y	Y	Y	Y with secretions	Y
Droplet	Y	Y	Y	Y if splashing	Y if soiled
Airborne	N	Y/D	Y	Y with secretions	Y if soiled

D = depends on disease; N = no, item is not generally required; Y = yes, item is needed in most circumstances (some listed). Some agencies require double-bagging of soiled materials before removal from the room; isolation card should identify these requirements.

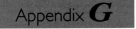

Medication Interactions: Drug–Drug*

Some drugs (P 450 metabolism) may interact with other similarly metabolized drugs. Administer these medications with caution and explore possible need to avoid administering together. Choose times for drug administration that will place 2 to 4 hours between administering each drug (6 hours after taking extended-release dosage forms). Drugs with P450 metabolism include: amitriptyline, caffeine, haloperidol, theophylline, tacrine, cyclophosphamide, carbamazepine, cyclophosphamide, diazepam, ibuprofen, naproxen, omeprezole, phenytoin, propranolol, tolbutamide, chlorpromazine, codeine, dextromethorphan, encainide, nortriptyline, timolol, verapamil, acetaminophen, ethanol, halothane, amiodarone, cisapride, cocaine, cortisol, cyclosporine, dapsone, dexamethasone, diltiazem, erythromycin, imipramine, lidocaine, lovastatin, nifedipine, progesterone, tacrolimus, tamoxifen, testosterone, valproate, vincristine, warfarin.

Type of Drug (examples)	Interacting Drug Type (examples)	Common Interaction
1. Analgesics		
Acetaminophen	Alcohol	Increased risk of liver damage
Ketoprofen (Orudis) Aspirin	Methotrexate (for cancer chemotherapy)	Increased risk of methotrexate toxicity: fever, mouth sores, low white blood cell production
Aspirin	Anticoagulants (oral) such as warfarin (Coumadin, Panwarfin)	Increases bleeding
Barbituates amobarbital (Amytal) phenobarbital (Luminal) pentobarbital (Nembutal) and others . . .		Decrease in anti-coagulation effect (Note: if dosage maintained and barbituates are discontinued bleeding may occur.)

Type of Drug (examples)	Interacting Drug Type (examples)	Common Interaction
Ibuprofen Indocin	Lithium	Elevated levels of Lithium and risk of toxicity Sx: nausea, slurred speech, muscle twitching . . .
Meperidine (Demerol)	Chlorpromazine (Thorazine)	Increased sedation
2. *Antihypertensives* ACE inhibitors enalapril (Vasotec) lisinopril (Zestril) Atenolol (Tenorim) Thiazide drugs Bumex Lasix Hydralazine	Indomethacin (Indocin)	Inhibition of the antihypertensive drugs results in lack of control of hypertension
3. *Anticoagulants* Oral: dicumarol and warfarin (Coumadin, Panwarfin)	Amiodarone (Cordarone) Aspirin Ibuprofen Diflunisal (Dolobid) Naproxen and other NSAIDs	Increased risk of bleeding; enhanced anticoagulant effect Sx: hematemesis, blood in urine, stool, sputum . . .
4. *Anticonvulsives* Phenytoin (Dilantin)	Amiodarone (Cordarone) Disopyramide (Norpace)	Increased phenytoin levels and toxicity Sx: confusion, rapid eye movement, lack of muscle coordination Dysrhythmia and anti-cholinergic Sx: dry mouth, tachycardia . . .
5. *Antidepressants* Monoamine oxidase (MAO) Inhibitors such as: isocarboxazid (Marplan) phenelzine (Nardil) tranylcypromine (Parnate) and others	Meperidine (Demerol)	Severe hypotension or hypertension, impaired breathing, convulsions, coma, and death

Type of Drug (examples)	Interacting Drug Type (examples)	Common Interaction
MAO Inhibitors	Pseudoephedrine Phenylpropanolamine Phenylephrine	(SEE RESP. DRUGS)
MAO Inhibitors Tricyclic drugs amitriptyline (Elavil) doxepin (Sinequan) and others . . .	Metaraminol (Aramine) Guanethidine (Ismelin)	Severe hypertension Hypertension due to the decreased anti-hypertensive effect of Ismelin
6. Heart medications Procainamide (Procan SR)	Pyridostigmine (Mestinon) for myasthenia gravis	Decreased effect Pyridostigmine with increased myasthenia gravis symptoms
Quinidine (Quinaglute)	Digoxin (Lanoxin) Digitoxin (Crystodigin)	Increased digoxin/digitoxin effect Risk for toxicity Sx: poor appetite, visual abnormality, weakness, irregular heart beat
7. Gastrointestinal meds Antacids	Anti-infection drugs: Ketoconazole (Nizoral), Tetracyclines. Ex: (Sumycin) (Doxycycline) (Vibramycin)	Reduced absorption with diminished effects of anti-infective drug
Acid Inhibitors Cimetidine (Tagamet)	Theophylline (Theo-Dur, Primatene)	Increased levels of theophylline with risk for toxicity: nausea, tremor, diarrhea, tachycardia, seizures
Cimetidine (Tagamet)	Warfarin (Coumadin)	Increased risk of bleeding Sx: blood in emesis, urine, stool
Famotidine (Pepcid) Omeprazole (Prilosec) Rantidine (Zantac) Sulcrafate (Carafate)	Varied oral anti-infection drugs: ciprofloxacin (Cipro) norfloxacin (Noroxin)	Decreased effectiveness of anti-infection drugs due to reduced absorption

Type of Drug (examples)	Interacting Drug Type (examples)	Common Interaction
8. Antidiabetic drugs Oral agents: chlorpropamide (Diabinese) glipizide (Glucotrol) glyburide (Micronase)	Sulfonamides Ex: sulfamethoxazole (Bactrim)	Increased effect of antidiabetic drugs, hypoglycemia Sx: tachycardia, tremors, diaphoresis, nausea, convulsions, coma and death
	Phenylbutazone (Butazolidin)	Risk for hypoglycemia
	Alcohol	Increased hypoglycemic effect from antidiabetic agents with moderate to large intake of alcohol
	Nonselective beta blockers Ex: propranolol (Inderal), pindolol (Viskin), timolol (Blocadren), carteolol (Cartrol), nadolol (Corgard)	May decrease secretion of Insulin, thus reducing effectiveness of antidiabetic drugs resulting in continued or increased hyperglycemia
9. Respiratory drugs Theophylline (Primatene, Theo-Dur . . .)	Propranolol (Inderal)	Increased theophylline risk for toxicity Sx: nervousness, tachycardia
Asthma drugs: Epinephrine (Primatene, Epifrin) Isoproterenol (Isuprel)	Nonspecific beta blockers Ex: propranolol (Inderal), pindolol (Viskin), timolol (Blocardren), carteolol (Cartrol), nadolol (Corgard)	Decreased effectiveness of epinephrine and isoproterenol Sx: continued respiratory distress or anaphylaxis Hypertension with systemic epinephrine treatment unrelated to allergy
Allergy or cold/ Cough Phenylephrine (Neo-Synephrine, Dristan, Night Relief . . . others)	Several Tricyclic Antidepressants Ex: amitriptyline (Elavil) doxepin (Sinequan)	Acute increase in blood pressure and cardiac contractility Sx: confusion, chest pain, palpitations, headache

Type of Drug (examples)	Interacting Drug Type (examples)	Common Interaction
Phenylpropanol amine (Allerest, Comtrex, Contac, Triaminic, Dimetapp, Sinarest and others); also diet aids Acutrim and Dexatrim	Antidepressants Monoamine oxidase (MAO) Inhibitors such as: isocarboxazid (Marplan), phenelzine (Nardil), tranylcypromine (Parnate) and others	Severe hypertensive reactions Sx: chest pain, flushing face, lightheadedness
Ephedrine (Primatene, broncholate and others)	MAO Inhibitors	Severe hypertension (as above)
OR		
Pseudoephedrine (Actifed, Benadryl, Tylenol cold med)	(See above)	(as above)
10. Antimicrobials		
Aminoglycosides Ex: gentamicin (Garamycin), amikacin (Amikin) tobramycin (Nebcin)	Ethacrynic acid (Edecrin)	Increased risk for hearing loss
Chloramphenicol	Oral antidiabetic drugs (Ex: Tobutamide)	Increased effect of antidiabetic drug and hypoglycemia
Ciprofloxacin (Cipro)	Theophylline (Theo-Dur, Primatene)	Increased levels of theophylline = toxicity: nausea, tremor, diarrhea, tachycardia . . .
Erythromycin (E-Mycin)	Cyclosporine (Sandimmune) Amioderone	Increased levels of each drug, and high risk of kidney or liver damage
Ketoconazole (Nizoral) or Troleandomycin (TAO) Antituberculosis Drugs:	Terfenadine (Seldane)	Increased levels of Terfenadine toxicity: dysrhythmia, dizziness . . .
Rifampin (Rifadin)	Immune suppressant cyclosporine (Sandimmune)	Decreased effect of cyclosporine

Type of Drug (examples)	Interacting Drug Type (examples)	Common Interaction
Rifampin (Rifadin) Tetracyclines	Estrogen-containing oral contraceptives (Ex: Ortho Novum)	Decreased effect of contraceptive, high risk of pregnancy
Tetracyclines (Achromycin, Sumycin)	Calcium supplements or medications containing calcium	Reduced absorption and effect of tetracycline

*(Most interactions included were those known to be severe, with some moderate interactions being noted. The degree of interaction for specific individuals may vary, however, thus this list is not all inclusive.) Attempts were made to eliminate duplicate listings.

Drug and Nutrient Interaction Chart*

Drug	Interaction With Food	Action
Acetaminophen	Ethanol increases hepatotoxicity	Avoid alcohol
Adenosine	Avoid food or drugs with caffeine Increase adenosine's effects	Avoid food or drugs with caffeine (Goody's®, Anacin®, Excedrin®)
Antibiotics		
Amoxicillin	No interaction with food	Take without regard to food
Ampicillin	Food decreases absorption	Take on empty stomach
Azithromycin	Better absorbed on empty stomach, do not give with antacids	Take on empty stomach
Cephalosporins	No interaction with food	Take without regard to food
Dicloxacillin	Food decreases absorption	Take on empty stomach
Erythromycin (take PCE dispertab without food**)	Possible gastric distress	Best if taken on empty stomach but may be taken with food
Fluoroquinolones	Complexes formed when given with iron or dairy products	Avoid iron and dairy products within 2 hours of dose
Nitrofurantoin	Possible gastric distress; improved absorption with food	Should be taken with food
Penicillin	Food decreases absorption (50%–80%)	Take on empty stomach
Sulfonamides		Take with plenty of fluid and on an empty stomach if possible

*Original version from: *Drug Information Newsletter* (Sept.–Oct., 1996), published by the Drug Information Center Pharmacy Department, Medical College of Georgia Hospital and Clinics. Updated 2001: see Bibliography.

Drug	Interaction With Food	Action
Tetracycline	Decreased absorption due to chelation by milk, dairy, iron, antacids	Take with plenty of fluid and avoid interacting products
Antihypertensives Propranolol, metoprolol, HCTZ, and hydralazine	Food enhances bioavailability	Take consistently with food
Atovaquone	Absorption of tablets increased 3–4 times when given with fatty foods	Can take with food
Bisacodyl	Milk breaks down protective coating, which may lead to GI irritation	Avoid milk or antacids 1–2 hours before or after dose
Calcium acetate	Food increases absorption	Best if taken on an empty stomach, avoid antacids
Captopril	Food decreases absorption	Take at a constant time in relation to meals
Carbamazepine	Food-induced bile secretions improve drug dissolution	Take with food
Didanosine	Food decreases absorption due to acid secretion	Take on an empty stomach
Estrogens	Administration with food decreases nausea	Take with food
Etidronate	Forms complexes with polyvalent cations in food, decreasing absorption	Avoid food within 2 hours of dose
Griseofulvin	High-fat foods increase absorption	Take with high fat meal or nonskim milk
Hypoglycemics Chlorpropamide Glipizide Glyburide Tolbutamide	Drug takes 30 minutes to be absorbed and become effective	Take 30 minutes before meals
Iron	Decreased absorption with antacids and certain foods (cheese, milk, ice cream)	Best if taken on empty stomach, but if taken with food, avoid interacting products
Isoniazid	Food decreases and delays absorption	Take on an empty stomach

Drug	Interaction With Food	Action
Ketoconazole	Antacids decrease absorption	May be taken without regard to meals, but not with antacids
Levadopa	Decreased absorption with high protein diet	Take on an empty stomach
Lithium	Sodium is exchanged with lithium, which may lead to elevated lithium levels	Avoid abrupt changes in sodium intake or excretion
Lovastatin -excludes other HMGCoA drugs	Food maximizes absorption and increases bioavailability	Take with meals
Methoxsalen	Food impairs absorption	May take with food if nausea occurs, but better absorption on an empty stomach
Metroprolol	Food enhances absorption	Should be taken in a consistent manner with relationship to meals to avoid fluctuations in drugs levels
Mexiletine		Take with food for stomach irritation associated with administration
Monoamine Oxidase Inhibitors Isocarboxazid Tranylcypromine Phenelzine	Potentially life-threatening hypertensive episode due to tyramine interaction	Avoid cheeses, fermented meats, pickled herring, yeast, meat extracts, chianti wine
Moricizine	Food delays absorption	Best if taken on an empty stomach
Morphine	Food increases bioavailability	Take with food
Nifedipine	Food alters release properties of drug	Take on an empty stomach
NSAIDs diflunisal, fenoprofen, ibuprofen, indomethacin, ketoprofen, meclofenamate, naproxen, piroxicam, salsalate, sulindac, tolmetin	Stomach irritation may occur	Take with food

Drug	Interaction With Food	Action
Olsalazine	Increases residence of drug in body	Take with food
Omeprazole	Food delays absorption	Take on an empty stomach
Ondansetron	Food increases absorption by 17%	Take with food
Phenytoin	May decrease absorption with food	May be taken with or without food, but take consistently with or without food
Potassium (oral)	Stomach irritation and discomfort	Take with plenty of fluid and/or food
Pravastatin		May be taken with or without meals; avoid taking with high-fiber meals
Propafenone	Food increases absorption	Take with food
Quinidine	Possible stomach upset; increased absorption	May take with food if stomach upset occurs; avoid citrus fruit juices
Sotalol	Food decreases absorption	Take on an empty stomach
Sucralfate	Food inhibits therapeutic effects of drug (coats stomach)	Take on an empty stomach 1 hour before meals with plenty of water; avoid antacids 1–2 hours before or after dose
Theophylline	Charcoaled meats cause decreased levels; high-fat foods increase absorption, raising levels	Avoid consumption of barbecued meats during therapy, avoid co-administration with high-fat food
Ticlopidine	High-fat meals increase absorption; antacids decrease absorption	Take with food to decrease GI upset
Warfarin	Vitamin K-containing foods (green leafy vegetables, lettuce, broccoli, brussels sprouts) decrease the PT	Avoid large amounts of, or changes in, consumption of vitamin K-containing foods; avoid alcohol
Zalcitibine	Food decreases bioavailability by 14%	Avoid administration with food

Drug	Interaction With Food	Action
Zidovudine	Food decreases concentration of drug	Take on an empty stomach

Some drugs (P 450 metabolism) may interact with grapefruit juice and cruciferous vegetables. Administer medications with water only and caution patient to avoid drinking grapefruit juice 2 hours before and 4 hours after taking these drugs (6 hours after taking extended-release dosage forms). Drugs with P450 metabolism include: amitriptyline, caffeine, haloperidol, theophylline, tacrine, cyclophosphamide, carbamazepine, cyclophosphamide, diazepam, ibuprofen, naproxen, omeprezole, phenytoin, propranolol, tolbutamide, chlopromazine, codeine, dextromethorphan, encainide, nortriptyline, timolol, verapamil, acetaminophen, ethanol, halothane, amiodarone, cisapride, cocaine, cortisol, cyclosporine, dapsone, dexamethasone, diltiazem, erythromycin, imipramine, lidocaine, lovastatin, nifedipine, progesterone, tacrolimus, tamoxifen, testosterone, valproate, vincristine, warfarin.

Equipment Substitution in the Home

Equipment	Substitution
Bed cradle, footboard	• Folding tray table, cardboard box
Bedrail	• Folding card table with legs under mattress
Male urinal	• Liter plastic soda bottle, cut to enlarge opening, cut edge taped
Electric adjustable bed	• Concrete block under corners of bed to elevate entire bed • Tightly rolled blankets under mattress to elevate head or foot of bed
Heel and elbow protectors	• Heavy-duty socks with padded heels, with the toe cut out
Hand mitts to prevent scratching	• Heavy-duty socks
Ice collar, bag	• Plastic bag of water frozen in desired shape
Linen protector	• Large plastic bag with towel taped on surface touching client
Device to prevent foot drop	• Well-fitted high-top sneakers
IV pole	• Cup hook • Wire hanger • Picture hanger
Trochanter roll	• Large towels rolled and taped
Weights	• Unopened food cans or bags of sugar/flour
Call bell	• Soda can filled with small stones
Medicine organizer and dispenser	• Egg carton, muffin tray

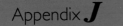

Nursing Management for Selected Diagnostic Procedures

Procedure	Pretest	Posttest
Arteriography (Angiography) -Determines status of blood flow to major arterial areas	-Explain procedure -Obtain Informed Consent form -Check hypersensitivity to iodine, shellfish/ seafood, contrast dyes (such as IV pyelogram). -Laxative or cleansing enema, as ordered -Sedative or narcotic, as ordered -Obtain vital signs -Obtain IV access -NPO 2–8 hours, depending upon site (check radiology manual) -Check if receiving anticoagulants (contact physician) -Remove dental prostheses	Monitor for indication of bleeding: Check dressing or catheter insertion site for bleeding or hematoma along with vital signs Apply pressure to area as ordered or needed. If cardiac catheterization or femoral area used, may require sandbag application. Vital signs every 15 min for 1 hr, then every 30 min for 2 hrs, and every hr for next 4 hrs, every 4 hrs or as ordered there- after Changes in mental status Urine output at least 30 cc/hr Peripheral pulses normal or not further diminished Monitor for infection: Temperature every 4 hrs for 48 hrs If applicable, maintain straight position of extremity for 6 or more hrs or as ordered Maintain 6 to 8 hrs bed rest, as ordered

Procedure	Pretest	Posttest
Biopsy (Breast, bone marrow, endometrial, uterine, liver, kidney)		Monitor IV fluids Note respiratory character, visual changes, slurred speech, changes in mental status, dysphagia (cerebral angiogram) Monitor for delayed dye reaction (tachycardia, dyspnea, rash, hives, headache, vomiting) for up to 6 hrs Resume medications according to agency protocol/doctor's orders when patient is fully alert
-Obtains tissue sample to determine status of tissue in terms of malignancy	Explain procedure Informed Consent form for all biopsies Obtain ordered laboratory tests Vital signs Obtain IV access, if indicated Empty bladder Laxative, as ordered Liver—NPO for 6 hrs NPO for 6–8 hrs for all biopsies performed under general anesthesia	Monitor for bleeding or hematoma at local site and internally (vital signs, changes in mental status, urinary output, peripheral pulses, respiratory character, dressings) Vital signs every 15 min for 1 hr, then every 30 min for 2 hrs, and every hr for next 4 hrs, every 4 hrs or as ordered thereafter Monitor temperature every 4 hrs for 48 hrs Monitor for diminished or absent bowel sounds (kidney, liver, or after general anesthesia) Monitor urine output and increase fluids (kidney) Rest for 24 hrs Avoid lifting heavy objects (liver, kidney, uterine, endometrial)

Procedure	Pretest	Posttest
		Resume medications according to agency protocol/doctor's orders when patient is fully alert Administer pain medications as ordered
Barium swallow (Upper GI series) Detects masses, polyps, ulcerations, or structural abnormalities of upper GI structures	Explain procedure NPO 8 hrs before procedure No smoking morning of test Abdominal assessment	Monitor stools after procedure, watch for constipation Expect chalky appearance of stools until barium evacuated Laxative, if ordered, following procedure Allow to eat as soon as possible Resume medications according to agency protocol/doctor's orders
Barium enema (Lower GI series) Detects masses, polyps, ulcerations, or structural abnormalities of the colon	Explain procedure NPO 6–8 hrs before test or after evening meal, if ordered Diet as ordered 2–3 days before test (clear liquids, 18–24 hrs pretest, low-residue diet up to 3 days before test) Laxative and/or suppository as ordered per bowel evacuation protocol the day before Cleansing enema, if ordered, the evening before the test Saline enemas until clear (solution returns clear) between 4–6 AM	Allow to use toilet/bedpan to evacuate barium as soon as patient returns from procedure Monitor stools after procedure, watch for constipation, expect chalky appearance of stools until barium evacuated. Laxative or enema as ordered following procedure Increase fluids Resume medications according to agency protocol/doctor's orders when patient is fully alert

Procedure	Pretest	Posttest
Bronchoscopy To examine respiratory tree (larynx, trachea, bronchus); remove excess secretions and debris; enhances breathing and drainage of upper respiratory secretions	Explain procedure Informed Consent form NPO 4–8 hrs Cardiorespiratory assessment Vital signs Obtain IV access Remove prostheses	Cardiorespiratory assessment Vital signs every 15 min for 1 hr, then every 30 min for 2 hrs, and every hour for next 4 hrs, every 4 hrs or as ordered thereafter Temperature routinely up to 48 hrs Monitor for bloody sputum. Expect small amount of blood in sputum, but moderate to copious amounts should be reported to doctor. NPO until gag reflex returns and client is fully alert Resume medications according to agency protocol/doctor's orders when patient is fully alert
Colonoscopy and Endoscopy Examines upper (endoscopy) or lower (colonoscopy) GI structures for structural abnormalities, polyps, masses or other lesions, and ulcerations	Explain procedure Informed Consent form Bowel evacuation protocol for agency and as indicated for area of examination (laxatives and enemas until clear, *or* oral electrolyte solution, not both) NPO 6–8 hrs Sedatives or narcotics	Abdominal assessment (flatulence expected, tenderness, increased pain, or distention should be reported) Monitor for indicators of bleeding from perforation (vital signs— pulse increase, respiratory rate increase, blood pressure decrease; changes in mental status, urinary output, peripheral pulses, respiratory character) Vital signs every 15 min for 1 hr, then every 30 min for 2 hrs, and every hr for next 4 hrs every 4 hrs or as ordered thereafter

Procedure	Pretest	Posttest
		Monitor stools for blood Colonoscopy: Oral intake when fully alert, increase fluids unless contraindicated Endoscopy (Upper GI): NPO until gag reflex returns and fully alert Resume medications according to agency protocol/doctor's orders when patient is fully alert
Computed tomography (CT Scan) Detects lesions, injury, vascular problems, edema, or tumors of various organs and structures	Explain procedure Informed Consent form if agency policy Check allergy to iodine, contrast medium (seafood, shellfish) Obtain IV access, if dye used NPO 4–8 hrs Remove clips, pins, dental prostheses, wigs, (if brain CT)	Increase fluids Monitor for delayed dye reaction (tachycardia, dyspnea, rash, hives, headache, vomiting) for up to 6 hrs Resume medications according to agency protocol/doctor's orders when patient is fully alert.
Electroencephalogram (EEG) To examine brain wave activity	Explain procedure Informed Consent form, if required by agency Wash or instruct to wash hair night before to remove sprays, oils, etc. No caffeinated or stimulant products morning of test, but do not hold NPO Hold sedatives and hypnotics and alcohol Check with doctor regarding other medication administration Client receives only 4–5 (adult) or 5–7 (pediatric) hrs of sleep the night before test	Remove paste from skin (acetone may be helpful) Wash hair Side rails up Resume medications as per agency policy or doctor's orders when client is fully alert

Procedure	Pretest	Posttest
Endoscopic retrograde cholangiopancreatography (ERCP)		
Detects biliary disorders (stones, cysts, tumors, strictures) and some pancreatic disorders)	Explain procedure Obtain informed consent form NPO after midnight Vital signs Premedicate with sedative or narcotic, and usually, atropine, if ordered	Vital signs NPO until gag reflex returns Skin color for jaundice Assess abdomen, notify doctor if nausea and vomiting or abdominal pain Resume medications according to agency protocol/doctor's orders when patient is fully alert Instruct patient to use throat lozenges or cool fluid if hoarse for a couple of days
Intravenous pyelogram [IVP or excretory urography (EUG)]		
Examines structure and function of kidneys, renal pelvis, ureters, bladder	Explain procedure Obtain Informed Consent form Check hypersensitivity to iodine, shellfish/seafood, contrast dyes (such as IV pyelogram)	Vital signs Monitor for delayed dye reaction (tachycardia, dyspnea, rash, hives, headache, vomiting) for up to 6 hrs Monitor urinary output Increase fluids Resume medications according to agency protocol/doctor's orders when patient is fully alert
Magnetic Resonance Imaging (MRI)		
Detects lesions, injury, vascular problems, edema, or tumors of various organs and structures	Explain procedure Obtain Informed Consent form Remove all metal objects (pins, dental prostheses, jewelry, credit cards, belts)	Return all personal items

Procedure	Pretest	Posttest
Paracentesis Assesses and removes peritoneal fluid	Explain procedure Obtain Informed Consent form Have client empty bladder Vital signs Weight Abdominal assessment, including girth	Secure specimens, label, and send to lab immediately Abdominal assessment, noting girth Monitor for bleeding or fluid volume deficit (vital signs or continued drainage, report decreased blood pressure, increased pulse, increased respirations, changes in mental status) Monitor electrolytes and serum protein level

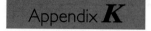
Guide to Nursing Organizations

Keep a copy of this chart in case you need to contact these nursing organizations.

**Academy of Medical-
Surgical Nurses**
E. Holly Ave., Box 56 Pitman,
NJ 08071-0006
(609) 256-2323;
fax: *(609) 589-7463*
E-mail: amsn@mail.ajj.com
Web site:
http://amsn.inurse.com

**American Academy of
Ambulatory Care Nursing**
E. Holly Ave., Box 56 Pitman,
NJ 08071-0056
1-800-262-6877;
fax: *(609) 589-7463*
E-mail: aaacn@mail.ajj.com
Web site: http://aaacn.org

**American Academy of Nurse
Practitioners**
Capitol Station, LBJ Building
P.O. Box 12846
Austin, TX 78711
(512) 442-4262;
fax: *(512) 442-5221*
E-mail: admin@aanp.org
Web site:
http://www.aanp.org

**American Academy of
Nursing**
600 Maryland Ave., SW, Suite
100 West
Washington, DC 20024-2571
(202) 651-7238;
fax: *(202) 544-2641*
E-mail: lzeck@ana.org
Web site: http://www.
nursingworld.org/aan

**American Assembly for Men
in Nursing**
c/o NYSNA, 11 Cornell Rd.
Latham, NY 12110-1499
(518) 782-9400, ext. 346;
fax: *(518) 782-9530*
E-mail: aamn@aamn.org
Web site:
http://www.aamn.org

**American Association for the
History of Nursing**
P.O. Box 175
Lanoka Harbor, NJ 08734
(609) 693-7250;
fax: *(609) 693-1037*
E-mail: nsghistory@aol.com
Web site:
http://www.aahn.org

American Association of Colleges of Nursing
1 Dupont Circle, NW, Suite 530 Washington, DC 20036
(202) 463-6930;
  fax: (202) 785-8320
E-mail:
  webmaster@aacn.nche.edu
Web site:
  http://www.aacn.nche.edu

American Association of Critical-Care Nurses
101 Columbia
Alisa Viejo, CA 92656-1491
1-800-899-2226;
  fax: (714) 362-2020
E-mail: info@aacn.org
Web site:
  http://www.aacn.org

American Association of Diabetes Educators
100 W. Monroe St., 4th floor
Chicago, IL 60603
(312) 424-2426;
  fax: (312) 424-2427
E-mail: styler@aadenet.org
Web site:
  http://www.aadenet.org

American Association of Legal Nurse Consultants
Glenview, IL 60025-1485
(847) 375-4713;
  fax: (847) 375-4777
E-mail: info@aalnc.org
Web site:
  http://www.aalnc.org

American Association of Neuroscience Nurses
224 N. Des Plaines Ave., Suite 601 Chicago, IL 60661
(312) 993-0043;
  fax: (312) 993-0362
E-mail: assnneuro@aol.com
Web site:
  http://www.aann.org

American Association of Nurse Anesthetists
222 S. Prospect Ave.
Park Ridge, IL 60068-4001
(847) 692-7050;
  fax: (847) 692-6968
E-mail: info@aana.com
Web site:
  http://www.aana.com

The American Association of Nurse Attorneys
3525 Ellicott Mills Dr., Suite N
Ellicott City, MD 21043-4547
(410) 418-4800;
  fax: (410) 418-4805
E-mail: taana.assochq.com
Web site:
  http://www.taana.org

American Association of Occupational Health Nurses, Inc.
2920 Brandywine Rd., Suite 100
Atlanta, GA 30341
(770) 455-7757;
  fax: (770) 455-7271
E-mail: aaohn@aaohn.org
Web site:
  http://www.aaohn.org

American Association of Office Nurses
109 Kinderkamack Rd.
Montvale, NJ 07645
(201) 391-2600;
  fax: (201) 573-8543
E-mail: aaonmail@aaon.org
Web site:
  http://www.aaon.org

American Association of Spinal Cord Injury Nurses
75-20 Astoria Blvd.
Jackson Heights, NY 11370-1177
(718) 803-3782 ext 321;
fax: (718) 803-0414
E-mail: scihotline@aol.com
Web site:
http://www.aascin.org

American College of Nurse Practitioners
1111 19th Street, NW, Suite 404
Washington, DC 20036
(202) 659-2190;
fax: (202) 659-2191
E-mail: acnp@acnpweb.org
Web site: http://
www.nurse.org/acnp

American Holistic Nurses Association
P.O. Box 2130
Flagstaff, AZ 86003-2130
1-800-278-2462;
fax: (520) 526-2752
E-mail: ahna-flag@flaglink.com
Web site:
http://www.ahna.org

American Nephrology Nurses Association
E. Holly Ave., Box 56
Pitman, NJ 08071-0056
1-800-203-5561;
fax: (609) 589-7463
E-mail: anna@mail.ajj.com
Web site:
http://anna.inurse.com

American Nurses Association
600 Maryland Ave., SW, Suite 100 West
Washington, DC 20024
1-800-274-4262;
fax: (202) 554-2262
Web site: http://
www.nursingworld.org

American Organization of Nurse Executives
1 N. Franklin St., 34th floor
Chicago, IL 60606
(312) 422-2800;
fax: (312) 422-4503
E-mail: mschonel@aha.org
Web site:
http://www.aone.org

American Psychiatric Nurses Association
1200 19th St., NW, Suite 300
Washington, DC 20036-2422
(202) 857-1133;
fax: (202) 223-4579
E-mail: apna@dc.sba.com
Web site:
http://www.apna.org

American Society for Long-Term Care Nurses
660 Lonely Cottage Dr.
Upper Black Eddy, PA 18972-9313
(610) 847-5396;
fax: (610) 847-5063
E-mail: padona@epix.net

American Society of Ophthalmic Registered Nurses, Inc.
P.O. Box 193030
San Francisco, CA 94119
(415) 561-8513;
fax: (415) 561-8575
Web site:
http://www.asorn.org

American Society of Pain Management Nurses
7794 Grow Dr.
Pensacola, FL 32514
888-342-7766;
fax: (850) 484-8762
E-mail:
aspmn@puetzamc.com
Web site:
http://www.aspmn.org

American Society of Peri-Anesthesia Nurses
10 Melrose Avenue, Suite 11
Cherry Hill, NJ 08003-3696
(877) 737-9696;
fax: (856) 616-9601
E-mail: aspan@slackinc.com
Web site:
http://www.aspan.org

American Society of Plastic Surgical Nurses, Inc.
E. Holly Ave., Box 56 Pitman, NJ 08071-0056
(609) 256-2340;
fax: (609) 589-7463
E-mail: asprsn@mail.ajj.com
Web site:
http://asprsn.inurse.com

Association for Professionals in Infection Control and Epidemiology, Inc.
1275 K St., NW, Suite 1000
Washington, DC 20005-4006
(202) 789-1890;
fax: (202) 789-1899
E-mail: apicinfo@apic.org
Web site:
http://www.apic.org

Association of Nurses in AIDS Care
80 South Summitt Street, Suite 500
Akron, OH 44308
1-800-260-6780;
fax: (330) 762-5813
E-mail: anac@aanacnet.org
Web site:
http://www.anacnet.org

Association of Perioperative Registered Nurses, Inc.
2170 S. Parker Rd., Suite 300
Denver, CO 80231-5711
1-800-755-2676;
fax: (303) 750-3212
Web site:
http://www.aom.org

Association of Pediatric Oncology Nurses
4700 W. Lake Ave. Glenview, IL 60025
(847) 375-4724;
fax: (847) 375-4777
E-mail: apon@amtec.com
Web site:
http://www.apon.org

Association of Rehabilitation Nurses
4700 W. Lake Ave.
Glenview, IL 60025-1485
1-800-229-7530;
fax: (847) 375-4777
E-mail: info@rehabnurse.org
Web site:
http://www.rehabnurse.org

Association of Women's Health, Obstetric and Neonatal Nurses
2000 L St., NW, Suite 740
Washington, DC 20036
1-800-673-8499;
fax: (202) 728-0575
Web site:
http://www.awhonn.org

Case Management Society of America
8201 Cantrell, Suite 230
Little Rock, AR 72227
(501) 225-2229;
fax: (501) 221-9068
E-mail: cmsa@cmsa.com
Web site:
http://www.cmsa.org

Dermatology Nurses Association
E. Holly Ave., Box 56
Pitman, NJ 08071-0056
1-800-454-4362;
fax: (609) 589-7463
E-mail: dna@mail.ajj.com
Web site:
http://dna.inurse.com

Development Disabilities Nurses Association
1733 H Street, Suite 330 PMB 1214
Blaine, WA 98230
1-800-888-6733;
fax: (360) 332-2280
E-mail: ddnahq@aol.com
Web site:
http://www.ddna.org

Emergency Nurses Association
915 Lee Street
Des Plaines, IL 60016-6569
(800) 900-9659;
fax: (847) 460-4001
E-mail: enainfo@ena.org
Web site: http://www.ena.org

Endocrine Nurses Society
4350 East West Highway, Suite 500
Bethesda, MD 20814-4410
Web site:
http://www.endo-nurses.org

Home Healthcare Nurses Association
228 7th Street, SE
Washington, DC 20003
1-800-558-4462;
fax: (202) 547-3540
E-mail: hhnainfo@nahc.org
Web site:
http://www.hhna.org

Infusion Nurses Society
220 Norwood Park South
Norwood, MA 02062
(781) 440-9408;
fax: (781) 440-9409
E-mail: ins@ins1.org
Web site: http://www.ins1.org

International Nurses Society on Addictions
1500 Sunday Drive, Suite 102
Raleigh, NC 27607
(919) 783-5871;
fax: (919) 787-4916
E-mail:
knorris@olsonmgmt.com
Web site:
http://www.intnsa.org

National Association of Hispanic Nurses
1501 16th St., NW
Washington, DC 20036
(202) 387-2477;
fax: (202) 483-7183
E-mail: info@jnahnhq.org
Web site: http://
www.thehispanicnurse.org

National Association of Neonatal Nurses
4700 W. Lake Ave
Glenview, IL 60025-1485
1-800-451-3795; (847) 375-3660;
fax (888) 477-6266
E-mail: info@nann.org
Web site:
http://www.nann.org

National Association of Nurse Practitioners in Women's Health
503 Capitol Court, NE, Suite 300
Washington, DC 20002
(202) 543-9693;
  fax: (202) 543-9858
E-mail: info@npwh.org, or npwhdc@aol.com
Web site:
  http://www.npwh.org

National Association of Orthopaedic Nurses, Inc.
E. Holly Ave., Box 56
Pitman, NJ 08071-0056
(856) 256-2310;
  fax: (856) 589-7463
E-mail: naon@mail.ajj.com
Web site:
  http://naon.inurse.com

National Association of Pediatric Nurse Associates and Practitioners
1101 Kings Hwy. North, Suite 206
Cherry Hill, NJ 08034-1912
(877) 662-7627; (856) 667-1773;
  fax: (856) 667-7187
E-mail: info@napnap.org
Web site:
  http://www.napnap.org

National Association of School Nurses, Inc.
P.O. Box 1300 Scarborough, ME 04070-1300
(877) 627-6476; (207) 883-2117;
  fax: (207) 883-2683
E-mail: nasn@nasn.org
Web site:
  http://www.nasn.org

National Black Nurses Association, Inc.
8630 Fenton Street, Suite 330
Silver Spring, MD 20910-3803
(301) 589-3200;
  fax: (301) 589-3223
E-mail: nbnac@erols.com
Web site:
  http://www.nbna.org

National Council of State Boards of Nursing, Inc.
676 N. St. Clair St., Suite 550
Chicago, IL 60611-2921
(312) 787-6555;
  fax: (312) 787-6898
Web site:
  http://www.ncsbn.org

National Federation of Licensed Practical Nurses, Inc.
893 US Hwy 70 W, Suite 202
Garner, NC 27529-4547
1-800-948-2511;
  fax: (919) 779-5642
E-mail:
  cbarbour@dockpoint.net
Web site:
  http://www.nflpn.org

National Federation of Specialty Nursing Organizations
c/o Anthony J. Jannetti, Inc.
E. Holly Ave., Box 56
Pitman, NJ 08071
(856) 256-2333;
  fax: (856) 589-7463
E-mail: nfsno@ajj.com
Web site:
  http://www.nfsno.org

National Gerontological Nursing Association
7794 Grow Drive
Pensacola, FL 32514
1-800-723-0560;
  fax: (850) 484-8762
E-mail: ngna@puetzamc.com
Web site: www.ngna.org

National League for Nursing
61 Broadway
New York, NY 10006
1-800-669-1656;
fax: (613) 591-4240
E-mail: nlnweb c@nln.org
Web site: http://www.nln.org

National Nursing Staff Development Organization
7794 Grow Dr.
Pensacola, FL 32514
1-800-489-1995;
fax: (850) 484-8762
E-mail: nnsdo@aol.com
Web site:
http://www.nnsdo.org

National Organization of Nurse Practitioner Faculties
1522 K Street, NW #702
Washington, DC 20005
(202) 289-8044;
fax: (202) 289-8046
E-mail: nonpf @nonpf.org
Web site:
http://www.nonpf.com

National Student Nurses Association
555 W. 57th St.
New York, NY 10019
(212) 581-2211;
fax: (212) 581-2368
E-mail: nsna@nsna.org
Web site:
http://www.nsna.org

Oncology Nursing Society
501 Holiday Dr.
Pittsburgh, PA 15220-2749
(412) 921-7373;
fax: (412) 921-6565
E-mail: memberr@ons.org
Web site: http://www.ons.org

Society of Gastroenterology Nurses and Associates
401 N. Michigan Ave.
Chicago, IL 60611-4267
1-800-245-7462;
fax: (312) 527-6658
E-mail: sgna@sba.com
Web site:
http://www.sgna.org

Society of Otorhinolaryngology and Head-Neck Nurses
116 Canal St., Suite A
New Smyrna Beach, FL 32168
(386) 428-1695;
fax: (386) 423-7566
E-mail: sohnnet@ aol.com
Web site:
http://sohnnurse.com

Society of Urological Nurses and Associates
E. Holly Ave., Box 56
Pitman, NJ 08071
(888) TAP-SUNA;
(856) 256-2335;
fax: (856) 589-7463
E-mail: suns@mail.ajj.com
Web site:
http://www.suna.org

Society for Vascular Nursing
7794 Grow Dr.
Pensacola, FL 32514
1-888-536-4786;
fax: (850) 484-8762
E-mail: svna@puetzamc.com;
Web site:
http://www.svnnet.org

Wound, Ostomy and Continence Nurses Society
1550 S. Coast Hwy., #201
Laguna Beach, CA 92651
1-888-224-9626;
fax: (949) 376-3456
E-mail:
coleen@adlerdrozinc.com
Web site:
http://www.wocn.org

Bibliography

Agency for Health Care Policy and Research (US). (1996). *Urinary incontinence in adults: Acute and chronic management.* Rockville, MD: Department of Health and Human Services, AHCPR, Pub. No. 86–0682.

Ahmed, D. (2000). "It's not my job." *American Journal of Nursing,* 100(6), 25.

Alan, J., et al. (2000) Patient-Centered Documentation: an effective and efficient use of clinical information systems. *The Journal of Nursing Administration.* 30(2), 90–96.

Boucher, M. (1998). Delegation alert. *American Journal of Nursing,* 98(2), 26–33.

Brown, S. (2000). The legal pitfalls of home care. *RN,* 63 (11), 75–76, 78, 80.

Campbell, D. B. & Anderson, J. A. (1999). Setting behavioral limits. *American Journal of Nursing,* 99(12), 40–42.

Carroll, P. (2000). Exploring chest drain options. *RN,* 63(10), 50–54.

Derby, S. (1999). Managing adult cancer pain. *American Journal of Nursing,* 99(10), 62–65.

Diagnostic Ultrasound Corporation (2000). BVI Product Brochure. Redmond, WA.

GE Medical Systems Information Technology (2001). Dinamap Pro-400. Tampa, FL.

Gooden, M.B., Porter, C.P., Gonzalez, R.I, & Mims, B.L. (2000). Rethinking the relationship between nursing and diversity. *American Journal of Nursing,* 101(1), 63–65.

Gray, M. (2000). Urinary retention: Management in the acute care setting (Part 2). *American Journal of Nursing,* 100(8), 36–44.

JACE Systems, Inc. (1990). *JACE Universal CPM-K100 Operating Manual,* Moorestown, NJ.

Joint Commission on Accreditation of Healthcare Organizations (JCAHO). (2000). Comprehensive Accreditation Manual for Hospitals. Oakwood, IL: Author.

Keeling, B., Adair, J., Seider, D., & Kirksey, G. (2000). Appropriate delegation: Uncovering opportunities for improvement. *American Journal of Nursing,* 100(12), 24A–24D.

Klenner, S. (2000). Mapping out a clinical pathway. *RN, 63*(6), 33–36.

Macklin, D. (2000). Removing a PICC. *American Journal of Nursing, 100*(1), 52–54.

Metheny, N., Wehrie, M., Wiersema, L. & Clark, J. (1998). Nasally inserted feeding tube placement. *American Journal of Nursing, 98*(5).

Nield-Anderson, L., & Minarik, P. (1999). Responding to difficult patients. *American Journal of Nursing, 99*(12), 26–35.

Peterson, K.J. (2000). Checking feeding tube placement. *AACN News, 17*(12), 4.

Phillips, L. (1999). Pressure ulcers: Prevention and treatment guidelines. *Nursing Standard, 14*(12), 56, 58, 60, 62.

Ray, A., & Mould, C. (2000). Risk assessment in suprapubic catheterization. *Nursing Standard, 14*(36), 43–46.

Rhiner, M. & Kedziera, P. (1999). Managing breakthrough pain: A new approach. *American Journal of Nursing,* Supplement to March, 1999, 1–15.

Rogers, P. D., & Bocchino, N. (1999). Restraint-free care: Is it possible? *American Journal of Nursing, 99*(10), 26–34.

Scale-Tronix, Inc. (2002). 2002 Portable SlingScale—Operating and Service Manual. White Plains, NY.

Seeman, S., & Reinhardt, A. (2000). Blood sample collection from a peripheral catheter system compared with phlebotomy. *Journal of Intravenous Nursing, 23*(5), 290

Seley, J., & Quigley, L. (2000). Blood glucose testing. *American Journal of Nursing, 100*(8), 24A–24F.

Serra, A. (2000). Tracheostomy care. *Nursing Standard, 14*(42), 45–55.

Sienty, M. K., & Dawson, N. (1999). Preventing urosepsis from indwelling urinary catheters. *American Journal of Nursing, 99*(1), 24C–24H.

Sullivan, G. H. (2000). Keep your charting on course. *RN, 63*(5), 75–76.

Thompson, J. (2000). A practical ostomy guide (Part one). *RN, 63*(11), 61–73.

Wooldridge, L. (2000). Ultrasound technology and bladder dysfunction. *American Journal of Nursing,* Supplement to June, 2000, 100(6).

Xavier, G. (2000). The importance of mouth care in preventing infection. *Nursing Standard, 14*(18), 47–52.

Index

Note: Page numbers followed by *f*, *t*, and *d* indicate figures, tables, and displays, respectively.